Mobile Devices and Smart Gadgets in Medical Sciences

Sajid Umair
The University of Agriculture, Peshawar, Pakistan

A volume in the Advances in Medical
Technologies and Clinical Practice (AMTCP) Book
Series

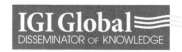

Published in the United States of America by
    IGI Global
    Medical Information Science Reference (an imprint of IGI Global)
    701 E. Chocolate Avenue
    Hershey PA, USA 17033
    Tel: 717-533-8845
    Fax: 717-533-8661
    E-mail: cust@igi-global.com
    Web site: http://www.igi-global.com

Library of Congress Cataloging-in-Publication Data

Names: Umair, Sajid, 1992- editor.
Title: Mobile devices and smart gadgets in medical sciences / Sajid Umair,
  editor.
Description: Hershey, PA : Medical Information Science Reference, [2020] |
  Includes bibliographical references and index. | Summary: "This book
  explores advancements and practices in the use of mobile devices, smart
  gadgets, and other technologies in the medical sciences"--Provided by
  publisher.
Identifiers: LCCN 2019040969 (print) | LCCN 2019040970 (ebook) | ISBN
  9781799825210 (hardcover) | ISBN 9781799825227 (ebook)
Subjects: MESH: Telemedicine | Mobile Applications | Computers, Handheld
Classification: LCC R855.3 (print) | LCC R855.3 (ebook) | NLM W 83.1 |
  DDC 610.285--dc23
LC record available at https://lccn.loc.gov/2019040969
LC ebook record available at https://lccn.loc.gov/2019040970

This book is published in the IGI Global book series Advances in Medical Technologies and Clinical Practice (AMTCP) (ISSN: 2327-9354; eISSN: 2327-9370)

British Cataloguing in Publication Data
A Cataloguing in Publication record for this book is available from the British Library.

All work contributed to this book is new, previously-unpublished material. The views expressed in this book are those of the authors, but not necessarily of the publisher.

For electronic access to this publication, please contact: eresources@igi-global.com.

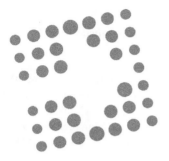

Advances in Medical Technologies and Clinical Practice (AMTCP) Book Series

Srikanta Patnaik
SOA University, India
Priti Das
S.C.B. Medical College, India

ISSN:2327-9354
EISSN:2327-9370

MISSION

Medical technological innovation continues to provide avenues of research for faster and safer diagnosis and treatments for patients. Practitioners must stay up to date with these latest advancements to provide the best care for nursing and clinical practices.

The **Advances in Medical Technologies and Clinical Practice (AMTCP) Book Series** brings together the most recent research on the latest technology used in areas of nursing informatics, clinical technology, biomedicine, diagnostic technologies, and more. Researchers, students, and practitioners in this field will benefit from this fundamental coverage on the use of technology in clinical practices.

COVERAGE

- Nutrition
- Diagnostic Technologies
- Patient-Centered Care
- Clinical Studies
- Medical Informatics
- Neural Engineering
- Medical Imaging
- Biomedical Applications
- Clinical Data Mining
- Nursing Informatics

IGI Global is currently accepting manuscripts for publication within this series. To submit a proposal for a volume in this series, please contact our Acquisition Editors at Acquisitions@igi-global.com or visit: http://www.igi-global.com/publish/.

Titles in this Series

For a list of additional titles in this series, please visit:
https://www.igi-global.com/book-series/advances-medical-technologies-clinical-practice/73682

Applications of Deep Learning and Big IoT on Personalized Healthcae Services
Ritika Wason (Bharati Vidyapeeth's Institute of Computer Applications and Management (BVICAM), India) Dinesh Goyal (Poornima Institute of Engineering and Technology, India) Vishal Jain (Bharati Vidyapeeth's Institute of Computer Applications and Management (BVICAM)) S. Balamurugan (QUANTS IS and Consultancy Services, India) and Anupam Baliyan (Bharati Vidyapeeth's Institute of Computer Applications and Management (BVICAM))
Medical Information Science Reference • ©2020 • 300pp • H/C (ISBN: 9781799821014) • US $275.00

Communicating Rare Diseases and Disorders in the Digital Age
Liliana Vale Costa (University of Aveiro, Portugal) and Sónia Oliveira (University of Aveiro, Portugal)
Medical Information Science Reference • ©2020 • 412pp • H/C (ISBN: 9781799820888) • US $295.00

Exploring the Role of ICTs in Healthy Aging
David Mendes (Universidade de Évora, Portugal) César Fonseca (Universidade de Évora, Portugal) Manuel José Lopes (Universidade de Évora, Portugal) José García-Alonso (University of Coimbra, Spain) and Juan Manuel Murillo (University of Coimbra, Spain)
Medical Information Science Reference • ©2020 • 300pp • H/C (ISBN: 9781799819370) • US $285.00

Artificial Intelligence Paradigms in Smart Health Informatics Systems
Abdel-Badeeh M. Salem (Ain Shams University, Egypt) and Senthil Kumar A V (Hindusthan College of Arts and Science, India)
Medical Information Science Reference • ©2020 • 300pp • H/C (ISBN: 9781799811015) • US $265.00

Incorporating the Internet of Things in Healthcare Applications and Wearable Devices
P. B. Pankajavalli (Bharathiar University, India) and G. S. Karthick (Bharathiar University, India)
Medical Information Science Reference • ©2020 • 288pp • H/C (ISBN: 9781799810902) • US $285.00

Impacts of Information Technology on Patient Care and Empowerment
Roger W. McHaney (Kansas State University, USA) Iris Reychev (Ariel University, Israel) Joseph Azuri (Maccabi Healthcare Services, Israel) Mark E. McHaney (U.S. Air Force, USA) and Rami Moshonov (Assuta Medical Centers, Israel)
Medical Information Science Reference • ©2020 • 452pp • H/C (ISBN: 9781799800477) • US $295.00

Handbook of Research on Clinical Applications of Computerized Occlusal Analysis in Dental Medicine
Robert B. Kerstein, DMD (Tufts University School of Dental Medicine, USA & Private Dental Practice Limited to Prosthodontics and Computerized Occlusal Analysis, USA)
Medical Information Science Reference • ©2020 • 1356pp • H/C (ISBN: 9781522592549) • US $765.00

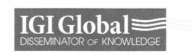

701 East Chocolate Avenue, Hershey, PA 17033, USA
Tel: 717-533-8845 x100 • Fax: 717-533-8661
E-Mail: cust@igi-global.com • www.igi-global.com

This book is dedicated to my father, mother, and sisters.

Table of Contents

Detailed Table of Contents

  Ines Carvalho, Polytechnic Institute of Gaya, Portugal
  Fernando Almeida, Polytechnic Institute of Gaya, Portugal

MHealth involves the provision of health products, services, and information through mobile and wireless technologies. Companies and institutions in the healthcare sector are progressively proposing innovative mhealth solutions that simultaneously reduce costs and improve the quality of life of citizens. In this chapter, a mobile app is proposed to promote healthy food habits through better management of the food each person has at home. This app intends to reduce food waste and promotes the development of good food practices based on the nutritional value of each recipe and the indication of potential allergies to ingredients. The development of the app was based on the best practices of Mobile UX, which is fundamental to offer intuitive interaction and rapid learning for the user. Furthermore, other factors also relevant in the context of mobile apps were considered in the development, namely usability, data backup, performance, security, scalability, and interoperability.

  Rafiullah Khan, The University of Agriculture, Peshawar, Pakistan
  Mohib Ullah, The University of Agriculture, Peshawar, Pakistan
  Bushra Shafi, The University of Agriculture, Peshawar, Pakistan
  Urooj Beenish Orakzai, Government Girls Degree College, Peshawar, Pakistan
  Seema Shafi, Charssada Homeopathic Medical College, Pakistan

Despite the extraordinary progression in modern medicines, alternative medicine has always been practiced. Alternative medicine or complementary medicine is a term referring to any practice that aims to achieve healing effects using pseudoscience or without biological explanation. The major drawback of alternative medicine is that these medicines are not scientifically tested as claimed by different studies. Nevertheless, according to the World Health Organization, more than 70% of the population of developing countries prefer alternative medicine systems. In this work, a review of ten most popular Android based smartphone applications that belongs to two most popular alternative medicines systems i.e. Homeopathy and Ayurveda are presented. The apps are selected based on the number of reviews, user rating, and the number of downloads provided by Google's play store. From the reviews of users, it was noted that most of the users are satisfied with the selected smartphone app. Based on this fact, it can be implicitly concluded that these medical systems can effectively solve user health-related issues.

There is the emerging use of smart and digital (modern) technologies, such as smart TVs, Internet of Things-connected devices, mobile devices, Big Data software and analytics in healthcare practice and administration. The deployment of such technologies is meant to provide quality, prompt, accurate, tangible information and other critical resources for patients. At a national level, drone technology is being used in African countries like Ghana and Rwanda to deliver critical medications and blood supplies to hospitals difficult to reach because of poor road infrastructure. This chapter of the book explores what technologies are being deployed at institutional levels to provide efficient medical care to patients. Fifteen maternal and neonatal health care practitioners in Accra, Ghana, were interviewed on their use of modern technologies in healthcare administration and delivery and what their challenges are. The study also explored what technologies they currently do not have that they think will be of benefit to their practice.

The aim of this research is to examine student acceptance and use of virtual reality technologies in medical education. Within the scope of the research, a questionnaire consisting of 4 sub-dimensions and 21 items was developed by the researchers. This questionnaire consists of sub-dimensions of performance expectancy, effort expectancy, facilitating conditions, and social influence. The study was conducted on 421 university students who participated in courses and activities related to the use of virtual reality applications in medical education. The findings of the research demonstrated that the students' acceptance and use of virtual reality applications were high in medical education. Various suggestions were made for researchers and educators in accordance with the findings.

To reduce healthcare costs and improve human well-being, a promising technology known as wireless body area networks (WBANs) has recently emerged. It is comprised of various on-body as well as implanted sensors which seamlessly monitor the physiological characteristics of the human body. The information is heterogeneous in nature, requires different QoS factors. The information may be classified as delay-sensitive, reliability-sensitive, critical, and routine. On-time delivery and minimum losses are the main QoS-factors required to transmit the captured information. Various researchers have work to provide the required QoS, and some have also considered the other constraints due to the characteristics and texture of the human body. In this research work, we have discussed the communication architecture of WBANS along with the various challenges of WBANS. Furthermore, we have classified and discussed the existing QoS-aware data dissemination mechanisms. In the end, a comparative study of existing QoS-aware data dissemination mechanisms highlights the pros and cons of each mechanism.

Chapter 6

Junaid Ahmad Malik, Government Degree College, Bijbehara, India

With the expanding use of wireless cellular networks, concerns have been communicated about the possible interaction of electromagnetic radiation with the human life, explicitly, the mind and brain. Mobile phones emanate radio frequency waves, a type of non-ionizing radiation, which can be absorbed by tissues nearest to where the telephone is kept. The effects on neuronal electrical activity, energy metabolism, genomic responses, neurotransmitter balance, blood–brain barrier permeability, mental psychological aptitude, sleep, and diverse cerebrum conditions including brain tumors are assessed. Health dangers may likewise develop from use of cellular communication, for instance, car accidents while utilizing the device while driving. These indirect well-being impacts surpass the immediate common troubles and should be looked into in more detail later on. In this chapter, we outline the possible biological impacts of EMF introduction on human brain.

Chapter 7

Muzamil Ahmad, The University of Agriculture, Peshawar, Pakistan
Muhammad Abbas Khan, The University of Agriculture, Peshawar, Pakistan
Mairaj Bibi, Bolan University of Medical and Health Sciences, Pakistan
Zia Ullah, The University of Agriculture, Peshawar, Pakistan
Syed Tanveer Shah, The University of Agriculture, Peshawar, Pakistan

Lack of proper diet causes many diseases like night blindness, gum death, rickets, osteomalacia, etc. Similarly, undernutrition will cause a low intelligence quotient (IQ), osteoporosis, anemia, scurvy, pellagra, etc. Over-nutrition will result in obesity, Type II diabetes mellitus, and ischemic heart diseases. Also, the unhygienic intake of food, intake of food on no fixed time, intake of fast food intake of other unhealthy stuff can lead to irregularities in the human body. Adopting healthy habits, physical activity, exercise, sports, and walking can lead to a healthy lifestyle of an individual. In addition, today's busy schedule and less time availability restricts individuals to visit the doctors or nutritionists. Many mobile applications were developed for monitoring and calculating an energy level as well as healthy nutrition. This review chapter has assessed the use and features of various mobile phone health applications, which helps individuals to overcome and monitor the above-mentioned health-related issues.

Bukhtawar Elahi, National University of Sciences and Technology, Pakistan
Maria Kanwal, National University of Sciences and Technology, Pakistan
Sana Elahi, Dr. A. Q. Khan Institute of Computer Sciences and Information Technology,
   Pakistan

This chapter gives an analysis of various methodologies for detecting cancer cells through image processing techniques. The challenges during such detections are over-segmentation and computational complexities. Therefore, the algorithms dealing with such problems are analyzed in this chapter. In these algorithms, a watershed and setting up threshold are helpful to overcome segmentation issues. A support vector machine is discussed to detect subtypes of pneumoconiosis for disjointing segments of lungs. For finding lung cancer cells, a segmentation weighted fuzzy probabilistic-based clustering has been used. Multiple variants of thresholding along with classifiers are proposed to detect lungs and liver cancer. Other than that, noise-removal, feature extraction and watershed are used to detect breast cancer. For leukemia, a bimodal thresholding over enhanced images of cytoplasm and nuclei regions has been discussed. kNN classifier, k-mean clustering, and feed-forward neural networks have also been discussed. Results from these techniques vary from 60%-100% depending on the proposed methodology.

Rehan Ullah, The University of Agriculture, Peshawar, Pakistan
Abdullah Khan, The University of Agriculture, Peshawar, Pakistan
Syed Bakhtawar Shah Abid, The University of Agriculture, Peshawar, Pakistan
Siyab Khan, The University of Agriculture, Peshawar, Pakistan
Said Khalid Shah, Department of Computer Science, University of Science and Technology,
   Bannu, Pakistan
Maria Ali, The University of Agriculture, Peshawar, Pakistan

DNA sequence classification is one of the main research activities in bioinformatics on which, many researchers have worked and are working on it. In bioinformatics, machine learning can be applied for the analysis of genomic sequences like the classification of DNA sequences, comparison of DNA sequences. This article proposes a new hybrid meta-heuristic model called Crow-ENN for leukemia DNA sequences classification. The proposed algorithm is the combination of the Crow Search Algorithm (CSA) and the Elman Neural Network (ENN). DNA sequences of Leukemia are used to train and test the proposed hybrid model. Five other comparable models i.e. Crow-ANN, Crow-BPNN, ANN, BPNN and ENN are also trained and tested on these DNA sequences. The performance of models is evaluated in terms of accuracy and MSE. The overall simulation results show that the proposed model has outperformed all the other five comparable models by attaining the highest accuracy of over 99%. This model may also be used for other classification problems in different fields because it can achieve promising results.

    Abu Baker, Khyber Coded, Pakistan
    Furqan Iqbal, Stuttgart Technology University of Applied Sciences, Germany
    Mahnoor Laila, University of Peshawar, Pakistan
    Annas Waheed, University of Peshawar, Pakistan

One in four people in the world will be affected by mental or neurological disorders at some point in their lives. Around 450 million people currently suffer from such conditions, placing mental disorders among the leading causes of ill-health and disability worldwide, according to the World Health Organization. Keeping in mind the above facts, Self Assessment Psychology Dictionary and Notes app has been designed and developed to educate psychology students and psychological patients. With the help of this application the user can do different physiological tests like Hads Mood, Internet Addiction Test, The Robertson Emotional Distress Scale, Beck Anxiety Inventory and Zung Self-Rating Anxiety Scale. The application has a smart algorithm that calculates the result on the basis of the user inputs. The application also generates the certificate for the user to share and use it for further treatment. The application provides detail information about psychology and psychologist. Apart from that, the application has a psychology dictionary of psychology-related topics.

    Siyab Khan, The University of Agriculture, Peshawar, Pakistan
    Abdullah Khan, The University of Agriculture, Peshawar, Pakistan
    Rehan Ullah, The University of Agriculture, Peshawar, Pakistan
    Maria Ali, The University of Agriculture, Peshawar, Pakistan
    Rahat Ullah, University of Malakand, Pakistan

Various nature-inspired algorithms are used for optimization problems. Recently, one of the nature-inspired algorithms became famous because of its optimality. In order to solve the problem of low accuracy, famous computational methods like machine learning used levy flight Bat algorithm for the problematic classification of an insulin DNA sequence of a healthy human, one variant of the insulin DNA sequence is used. The DNA sequence is collected from NCBI. Preprocessing alignment is performed in order to obtain the finest optimal DNA sequence with a greater number of matches between base pairs of DNA sequences. Further, binaries of the DNA sequence are made for the aim of machine readability. Six hybrid algorithms are used for the classification to check the performance of these proposed hybrid models. The performance of the proposed models is compared with the other algorithms like BatANN, BatBP, BatGDANN, and BatGDBP in term of MSE and accuracy. From the simulations results it is shown that the proposed LFBatANN and LFBatBP algorithms perform better compared to other hybrid models.

    Abu Baker, Khyber Coded, Pakistan
    Furqan Iqbal, Stuttgart Technology University of Applied Sciences, Germany
    Lala Rukh, The University of Agriculture, Peshawar, Pakistan

For successful life human being needs good health but illness is a part of life. The crowd in the hospitals, long waiting of doctor appointments makes the patients more disturb. Sometimes the patient sees the other serious patients in hospitals which makes him mental sick. Also due to busy life schedules, the peoples have not enough time to visit the doctor's clinics for small health problems which may lead to a serious disease. In this regard, the application UberGP is developed to assist the patients to connect with the doctor on phone to phone consultancy or book appointment to come doctor at home. This application has numerous benefits in case of time saving and quick appointment system at home or office. This study provides the detail documentation and usage of the UberGP Application.

Chapter 13

    Muhammad Roman, The University of Agriculture, Peshawar, Pakistan
    Siyab Khan, The University of Agriculture, Peshawar, Pakistan
    Abdullah Khan, The University of Agriculture, Peshawar, Pakistan
    Maria Ali, The University of Agriculture, Peshawar, Pakistan

A number of ANN methods are used, but BP is the most commonly used algorithms to train ANNs by using the gradient descent method. Two main problems which exist in BP are slow convergence and local minima. To overcome these existing problems, global search techniques are used. This research work proposed new hybrid flower pollination based back propagation HFPBP with a modified activation function and FPBP algorithm with log-sigmoid activation function. The proposed HFPBP and FPBP algorithm search within the search space first and finds the best sub-search space. The exploration method followed in the proposed HFPBP and FPBP allows it to converge to a global optimum solution with more efficiency than the standard BPNN. The results obtained from proposed algorithms are evaluated and compared on three benchmark classification datasets, Thyroid, diabetes, and glass with standard BPNN, ABCNN, and ABC-BP algorithms. The simulation results obtained from the algorithms show that the proposed algorithm performance is better in terms of lowest MSE (0.0005) and high accuracy (99.97%).

Chapter 14

    Numan Ali, University of Malakand, Pakistan
    Sehat Ullah, University of Malakand, Pakistan
    Zuhra Musa, University of Malakand, Pakistan

Various interaction techniques (such as direct, menu-based, etc.) are provided to allow users to interact with virtual learning environments. These interaction techniques improve their performance and learning but in a complex way. In this chapter, we investigated a simple list-liner based interface for gaining access to different modules within a 3D interactive Virtual Learning Environment (VLE). We have implemented a 3D interactive biological VLE for secondary school level students by using virtual mustard plant (VMP), where students interact by using 3D interactive device with the help of list-liner based interface. The aim of this work is to provide an easy interaction interface to use list-liner interaction technique by using 3D interactive device in an information-rich and complex 3D virtual environment. We compared list-liner interface with direct interface and evaluations reveal that the list-liner interface is very suitable and efficient for student learning enhancement and that the students can easily understand and use the system.

xvii

Foreword

The emergence of mobile device technologies has made digital medicine and health enter a new era. Mobile devices and smart gadgets can be used as tools for collecting and analyzing data related to health and help improving patient care. They also are applicable for educational purposes and designing preventive medicine platforms in which patients can participate in monitoring their health status.

Mobile Health (mHealth), which is the use of mobile technologies in medical and healthcare activities, can provide an integrative environment for systems medicine (Tavassoly et al., 2018; Kay et al., 2011).

This book, "Mobile Devices and Smart Gadgets in Medical Sciences", has collected several chapters on applications and implications of mHealth in medicine and healthcare.

These chapters cover a wide range of topics including mHealth in medical education and providing guidelines for patients, mHealth in preventive medicine, mHealth in alternative medicine, digital health, and mHealth in maternal and neonatal healthcare, mHealth and monitoring healthy habits. Some of the chapters provide insights on methods and modalities applied in data analysis in digital health and medicine.

The final goal of using mHealth is to contribute to P4 medicine (Hood, 2013). P4 medicine or Predictive, Personalized, Preventive, and Participatory medicine can benefit from mHealth and mobile devices to a large extent. For P4 medicine, data collection, data analysis, and the participation of the patients in a preventive approach are essential elements that mHealth has all of them.

This book is a perfect introduction for mHealth and mobile devices in medicine, which is useful for biomedical professionals and scientists at different levels.

Iman Tavassoly
Icahn School of Medicine at Mount Sinai, USA

REFERENCES

Hood, L. (2013). Systems biology and p4 medicine: Past, present, and future. *Rambam Maimonides Medical Journal, 4*(2), e0012. doi:10.5041/RMMJ.10112 PMID:23908862

Kay, M., Santos, J., & Takane, M. (2011). mHealth: New horizons for health through mobile technologies. *World Health Organization, 64*(7), 66-71.

Tavassoly, I., Goldfarb, J., & Iyengar, R. (2018). Systems biology primer: The basic methods and approaches. *Essays in Biochemistry, 62*(4), 487–500. doi:10.1042/EBC20180003 PMID:30287586

Preface

Technology, as we all know, has numerous benefits however these benefits are reaped but only by those fortunate who are aware about its use. Technology is transforming each facet of life, whether it be communication, traveling, banking or even in sports the role of technology is significant. The technology has also an enormous role in the field of medical sciences. Like there are a lot of mobile applications, software's, tools, smart gadgets used for medical sciences. With the advent of personal gadgets such as smartphones, laptops and tablet PCs' the role of technology in the field of medical sciences further strengthens. Each day new applications and methods are developed for the appropriate use of technology in the field of medical sciences. However, there are many unraveled areas in this field. This book aims to gather ideas for reaping the maximum potential of innovative mobile technologies used in the medical area for the benefits of the academia and the industry. This book will also investigate the innovative mobile technologies, mobile apps, tools, software's, and algorithms used in medical sciences. The academia will learn new ways of maximizing the efforts to improve the medical sciences using technology while the industry will get a look at the demand of new software's, hardware's, gadgets related to the medical sciences.

AN OVERVIEW OF BOOK CONTENT

Through this book, *Mobile Devices and Smart Gadgets in Medical Sciences*, we mean to explore the various ways in which smart technology is being used for medical sciences in multifarious ways. Being a hot topic of the day, our main objective has been to give a platform to the scholars, researchers and practitioners for sharing issues on hand, ideas, trends, and advancements in relation to the role of technology in medical sciences. The book provides detailed information about different mobile applications, tools, softwares, smart gadgets and algorithms which are being used in medical sciences domain. In addition, through this book we intend to create awareness in the academia, researchers, medical sciences activists and most importantly general public about the role of mobile and smart technologies in medical sciences.

TARGET AUDIENCE

The target audience of the book is university scholars, professionals and researchers, postgraduates and undergraduate students, doctors, medical researchers, mobile apps developers and experts, tools and software experts, ICT innovators, medical practitioners, technology experts and researchers, medical industry experts and professionals, teachers, subject experts, government and non-governmental organizations. The potential users of the book are people associated with medical sciences, health care, computer science and information technology, mobile apps developers and experts, tools and software experts.

SIGNIFICANCE OF THE BOOK

The book contents appeal to anyone with interest in information technology and/or medical sciences. Keeping in view the general readers' interest, we have included and organized the contents so as to disseminate comprehensive knowledge of the smart gadgets applications that have developed and used for medical sciences. This way the book also serves to save researchers' time and money by providing all the necessary information within one handbook. It provides complete information about the applications, their installation modes, their individual usages, benefits of their features, facilities they offer, and competitive advantages they carry against rival software tools in the market, etc.

CHAPTER ORGANIZATION

The book comprises 14 chapters that aim to highlight mobile applications, software's, tools, smart gadgets, algorithms and other technological sources being used for medical sciences.

Chapter 1, "Promoting Healthy Food Habits Through an mHealth Application," by Ines Carvalho and Fernando Almeida, explores that mHealth involves the provision of health products, services, and information through mobile and wireless technologies. Companies and institutions in the healthcare sector are progressively proposing innovative mhealth solutions that simultaneously reduce costs and improve the quality of life of citizens. In this chapter, a mobile app is proposed to promote healthy food habits through better management of the food each person has at home. This app intends to reduce food waste and promotes the development of good food practices based on the nutritional value of each recipe and the indication of potential allergies to ingredients. The development of the app was based on the best practices of Mobile UX, which is fundamental to offer intuitive interaction and rapid learning for the user. Furthermore, other factors also relevant in the context of mobile apps were considered in the development, namely usability, data backup, performance, security, scalability, and interoperability.

Chapter 2, "Knocking at Alternate Doors: Survey of Android-Based Smartphone Applications for Alternate Medicines," by Rafiullah Khan, Mohib Ullah, Bushra Shafi, Urooj Beenish Orakzai, and Seema Shafi, reveals that despite of all the extraordinary progression in modern medicines, alternative medicine has always been practiced. Alternative Medicine or Complementary Medicine is a term referring to any practice that aims to achieve the healing effect using pseudoscience or without biological explanation. The major drawback of alternative medicine is that these medicines are not scientifically tested as claimed by different studies. Nevertheless, according to the World Health Organization, more than 70% population of developing countries prefer alternative medicines systems (WHO). In this work, a review of ten most popular smartphone applications that belongs to two most popular alternative medicines systems i.e. Homeopathy and Ayurveda are presented. The apps are selected based on the number of reviews, user rating and the number of downloads provided by Google's play store. From the reviews of users, it was noted that most of the users are satisfied with the smartphone app. Based on this fact it can be implicitly concluded that these medical systems can effectively solve users' health-related issues.

Chapter 3, "Healthcare Gets Smarter: Smart and Digital Technologies Usage by Maternal and Neo-Natal Healthcare Providers," by Theodora Dame Adjin-Tettey, discusses that there is the emerging use of smart and digital (modern) technologies, such as smart TVs, Internet of Things-connected-devices, mobile devices, big data software and analytics in healthcare practice and administration. The deployment of such technologies are meant to provide quality, prompt, accurate, tangible information and other critical resources for patients. At a national level, drone technology are being used in African countries like Ghana and Rwanda to deliver critical medications and blood supplies to hospitals difficult to reach because of poor road infrastructure. This chapter of the book explores what technologies are being deployed at institutional levels to provide efficient medical care to patients. Fifteen maternal and neonatal health care practitioners in Accra, Ghana were interviewed on their use of modern technologies in healthcare administration and delivery and what their challenges are. The study also explored what technologies they currently do not have that they think will be of benefit to their practice.

Chapter 4, "Virtual Reality in Medical Education," by Ahmet B. Ustun, Ramazan Yilmaz, and Fatma Gizem Karaoglan Yilmaz, examines the use of virtual reality technologies in medical education. Within the scope of the research, a questionnaire consisting of 4 sub-dimensions and 21 items was developed by the researchers. This questionnaire consists of sub-dimensions of 'Performance Expectancy', 'Effort Expectancy', 'Facilitating Conditions' and 'Social Influence'. The study was conducted on 421 university students who participated in courses and activities related to the use of virtual reality applications in medical education. The findings of the research demonstrated that the students' acceptance and use of virtual reality applications were high in medical education. Various suggestions were made for researchers and educators in accordance with the findings.

Chapter 5, "QoS-Aware Data Dissemination Mechanisms for Wireless Body Area Networks," by Javed Iqbal Bangash, Abdul Waheed Khan, Adil Sheraz, Asfandyar Khan, and Sajid Umair, discusses that how to reduce healthcare costs and improve human well-being, a promising technology known as Wireless Body Area Networks (WBANs) is being recently emerged. It comprises of various on-body as well as implanted sensors seamlessly monitor the physiological characteristics of the human body. The information is heterogeneous in nature, requires different QoS factors. The information may be classified as Delay-Sensitive, Reliability-Sensitive, Critical and Routine. On-time delivery and minimum losses are the main QoS-factors required to transmit the captured information. Various researchers have work to provide the required QoS, and some have also considered the other constraints due to the characteristics and texture of the human body. In this research work, we have discussed the communication architecture of WBANS along with the various challenges of WBANS. Furthermore, we have classified and discussed the existing QoS-aware data dissemination mechanisms. In the end a comparative study of existing QoS-aware data dissemination mechanisms highlighting the pros and cons of each mechanism.

Chapter 6, "Effects of Electromagnetic Radiation of Mobile Phones on Human Brain," by Junaid Ahmad Malik, explains that with the expanding use of wireless cellular network, concerns have been communicated about the possible cooperation of electromagnetic radiation with the human life and, explicitly, the mind and brain. Mobile phones emanate radio frequency waves, a type of non-ionizing radiation, which can be absorbed by tissues nearest to where the telephone is kept. The effects on neuronal electrical activity, energy metabolism, genomic responses, neurotransmitter balance, blood–brain barrier permeability, mental psychological aptitude, sleep, and diverse cerebrum conditions including brain tumors are assessed. 4G and 5G cause various diseases in people, and can kill everything that lives however a few types of microorganisms. Health dangers may likewise develop from underhanded results of cellular communication, for instance, car accidents while utilizing telephone during driving.

These indirect well-being impacts surpass the immediate common troubles and should be looked into in more detail later on. In this chapter, we outline the possible biological impacts of EMF introduction on human brain.

Chapter 7, "Mobile Apps for Human Nutrition: A Review," by Muzamil Ahmad, Muhammad Abbas Khan, Mairaj Bibi, Zia Ullah, and Syed Tanveer Shah, explores that lack of proper diet causes many diseases like night blinders, gum dying, rickets, and osteomalacia, etc. Similarly, malnutrition causes diseases like undernutrition will cause low Intelligence Quotient (IQ), osteoporosis, anemia, scurvy, pellagra etc. and over nutrition will result in obesity, Type II diabetes mellitus and ischemic heart diseases. Also, unhygienic intake of food, intake of food on no fixed time, intake of fast food intake of other unhealthy stuff can lead to irregularities in the human body. Adopting healthy habits, physical activity, exercise, sports, gym and walking an entire day can lead to a healthy lifestyle of an individual. In addition, today's busy schedule and less time availability restrict individuals to visit the doctors or nutritionists, etc. So many mobile applications are developed for monitoring and calculating the energy level as well as healthy nutrition. This review paper has assessed the use and features of various mobile phone health applications, which helps individuals to overcome and monitor the above-mentioned health-related issues.

Chapter 8, "Analysis of Different Image Processing Techniques for Classification and Detection of Cancer Cells," by Bukhtawar Elahi, Maria Kanwal, and Sana Elahi, investigates that an analysis of various methodologies for detection of cancer cells through image processing techniques. The challenges during such detections are over-segmentation and computational complexities. Therefore, the algorithms dealing with such problems are analyzed in this chapter. In these algorithms, watershed and setting up threshold are helpful to overcome segmentation issues. A support vector machine is discussed to detect subtypes of pneumoconiosis for disjoint segments of lungs. For finding lung cancer cells, segmentation weighted fuzzy probabilistic based clustering has been used. Multiple variants of thresholding along with classifiers are pro-posed to detect lungs and liver cancer. Other than that, noise-removal, feature extraction and watershed are used to detect breast cancer. For leukemia, a bimodal thresholding over enhanced images of cytoplasm and nuclei regions has been discussed. kNN classifier k-mean clustering and feed-forward neural networks have also been discussed. Results from these techniques are varying from 60%-100% depending on the proposed methodology.

Chapter 9, "CROW-ENN: An Optimized Elman Neural Network With Crow Search Algorithm for Leukemia DNA Sequences Classification," by Rehan Ullah, Abdullah Khan, Syed Bakhtawar Shah Abid, Siyab Khan, Said Khalid Shah, and Maria Ali, explains that DNA sequence classification is one of the main research activities in bioinformatics on which, many researchers have worked and are working on it. In bioinformatics, machine learning can be applied for the analysis of genomic sequences like the classification of DNA sequences, comparison of DNA sequences. This paper proposed a new hybrid meta-heuristic model called Crow-ENN for Leukemia DNA sequences classification. The proposed algorithm is the combination of the Crow Search Algorithm (CSA) and the Elman Neural Network (ENN). DNA sequences of Leukemia are used to train and test the proposed hybrid model. Five other comparable models i.e. Crow-ANN, Crow-BPNN, ANN, BPNN and ENN are also trained and tested on these DNA sequences. The performance of models is evaluated in terms of accuracy and MSE. The overall simulation results show that the proposed model has outperformed all the other five comparable models by attaining the highest accuracy of over 99%. This model may also be used for other classification problems in different fields because it can achieve promising results.

Chapter 10, "Psychology With Mahnoor App: Android-Based Application for Self-Assessment, Psychology Dictionary, and Notes," by Abu Baker, Furqan Iqbal, Mahnoor Laila, and Annas Waheed, explores that one in four people in the world will be affected by mental or neurological disorders at some point in their lives. Around 450 million people currently suffer from such conditions, placing mental disorders among the leading causes of ill-health and disability worldwide. Keeping in mind the above facts, Self-Assessment Psychology Dictionary and Notes App has been designed and developed to educate psychology students and psychological patients. With the help of this application the user can do different physiological tests like Hads Mood, Internet Addiction Test, The Robertson Emotional Distress Scale, Beck Anxiety Inventory and Zung Self-Rating Anxiety Scale. The application has a smart algorithm that calculates the result on the basis of the user inputs. The application also generates the certificate for the user to share and use it for further treatment. The application provides detail information about psychology and psychologist. Apart from that, the application has a psychology dictionary having rich stuff of psychology-related topics.

Chapter 11, "Insulin DNA Sequences Classification Using Levy Flight BAT With Back Propagation Algorithm," by Siyab Khan, Abdullah Khan, Rehan Ullah, Maria Ali, and Rahat Ullah, discusses the various nature inspired algorithms are used for optimization problems. Recently, one of the nature inspired algorithms became famous because of its optimality. In order to prevail problem of low accuracy, famous computational methods like machine learning used by a Levy Flight Bat algorithm for the problematic classification of an insulin DNA sequence of healthy Human, one variant of insulin DNA sequence is used. The DNA sequence is collected from NCBI. In preprocessing alignment is performed in order to obtain the finest optimal DNA sequence with greater number of matches between base pairs of DNA sequence. Further, binaries the DNA sequence for the aim of machine readability. Six hybrid algorithms are used for the classification to check the performance of these proposed hybrid models. The performance of the proposed models is compared with the other algorithms like BatANN, BatBP, BatGDANN and BatGDBP in term of MSE and accuracy. From the simulations results it is shown that the proposed LFBatANN and LFBatBP algorithms perform better as compared to other hybrid models.

Chapter 12, "UBERGP: Doctor Home Consultancy App," by Abu Baker, Furqan Iqbal, and Lala Rukh, explains that for a successful life human being needs good health but illness is a part of life. The crowd in the hospitals, long waiting of doctor appointments makes the patients more disturb. Sometimes the patient sees the other serious patients in hospitals which makes him mental sick. Also due to busy life schedules, the peoples have not enough time to visit the doctor's clinics for small health problems which may lead to a serious disease. In this regard, the application UberGP is developed to assist the patients to connect with the doctor on phone to phone consultancy or book appointment to come doctor at home. This application has numerous benefits in case of time saving and quick appointment system at home or office. This study provides the detail documentation and usage of the UberGP Application.

Chapter 13, "Optimizing Learning Weights of Back Propagation Using Flower Pollination Algorithm for Diabetes and Thyroid Data Classification," by Siyab Khan, Abdullah Khan, Maria Ali, and Muhammad Roman, explains that number of ANN methods are used, but BP is the most commonly used algorithms to train the ANN by using the gradient descent method. Two main problems which exist in BP are slow Convergence and Local Minima. To overcome these existing problems, global search techniques are used. This research work proposed new Hybrid Flower Pollination based Back Propagation HFPBP with Modified Activation Function and FPBP algorithm with Log-Sigmoid Activation Function. The proposed HFPBP and FPBP algorithm search within the search space first and finds the best sub-search space. The exploration method followed in the proposed HFPBP and FPBP allows it to converge to a global optimum solution with more efficiency than the standard BPNN. The results obtained from proposed algorithms are evaluated and compared on three Benchmark classification datasets, Thyroid, Diabetes and Glass with standard BPNN, ABCNN, and ABC-BP algorithms. The simulation results obtained from the algorithms show that the proposed algorithm performance is better in terms of lowest MSE (0.0005) and High Accuracy (99.97%).

Chapter 14, "The Effect of List-Liner-Based Interaction Technique in a 3D Interactive Virtual Biological Learning Environment," by Numan Ali, Sehat Ullah, and Zuhra Musa, investigates that various interaction techniques (such as direct, menu-based etc.) are provided to allow users to interact with virtual learning environments. These interaction techniques improve their performance and learning but in a complex way. In this paper, we investigated a simple list-liner based interface for gaining access to different modules within a 3D interactive Virtual Learning Environment (VLE). We have implemented a 3D interactive biological VLE for secondary school level students by using Virtual Mustard Plant (VMP), where students interact by using 3D interactive device with the help of list-liner based interface. The aim of this work is to provide an easy interaction interface to use list-liner interaction technique by using 3D interactive device in an information-rich and complex 3D virtual environment. We compared list-liner interface with direct interface and evaluations reveal that the list-liner interface is very suitable and efficient for students' learning enhancement and the students can easily understand and use the system.

Sajid Umair
The University of Agriculture, Peshawar, Pakistan

Acknowledgment

All praise is due to Almighty Lord, the Beneficent, the Merciful.

It takes extensive research skills, great writing acumen, deep technological insight, and up-dated knowledge of day to day progresses, being made in the sciences to serve humanity in better ways, to compile an updated handbook of research on *Mobile Devices and Smart Gadgets in Medical Sciences*. A lot of effort and variegated contributions go into the publication of a research handbook such as this one. Therefore, the Editor-in-Chief is specifically thankful to all the authors for their highly informative research papers, reviewers for their insightful reviews, editorial advisory board for their valuable suggestions, and the team of IGI Global for their persistent support.

Without the assistance of any of you, the compilation and publication of this Handbook won't have been possible. Your unfailing support certainly helped with the completion of all necessary processes before the final print.

Thanks a great deal to everyone who has been a part of this project in some way or the other.

Sajid Umair
The University of Agriculture, Peshawar, Pakistan

Chapter 1
Promoting Healthy Food Habits Through an mHealth Application

Ines Carvalho
Polytechnic Institute of Gaya, Portugal

Fernando Almeida
🆔 https://orcid.org/0000-0002-6758-4843
Polytechnic Institute of Gaya, Portugal

ABSTRACT

MHealth involves the provision of health products, services, and information through mobile and wireless technologies. Companies and institutions in the healthcare sector are progressively proposing innovative mhealth solutions that simultaneously reduce costs and improve the quality of life of citizens. In this chapter, a mobile app is proposed to promote healthy food habits through better management of the food each person has at home. This app intends to reduce food waste and promotes the development of good food practices based on the nutritional value of each recipe and the indication of potential allergies to ingredients. The development of the app was based on the best practices of Mobile UX, which is fundamental to offer intuitive interaction and rapid learning for the user. Furthermore, other factors also relevant in the context of mobile apps were considered in the development, namely usability, data backup, performance, security, scalability, and interoperability.

INTRODUCTION

The health sector is being profoundly changed by globalization, from which new challenges arise that impact on the way citizens access health services. With the increasingly intense development of information technologies, new technological innovations are emerging, which is turning the world progressively more interoperable, mobile, connected and dynamic. In fact, characteristics such as mobility, ubiquity, instant connectivity, convenience, and personalization are constantly sought by users as a way to over-

DOI: 10.4018/978-1-7998-2521-0.ch001

come geographical, temporal and organizational barriers (Dunaway et al., 2018; Sarwar & Soomro, 2013; Taniar, 2008).

Mobile technologies offer enormous potential for the healthcare sector. Mobile Health or mhealth aims to improve people's lifestyles by contributing to the remote treatment of health problems, equipping healthcare providers to make better clinical decisions and also enabling the healthcare system to become more sustainable (Machado et al., 2017; Mayes & White, 2016). More broadly, mhealth involves the use of wireless technologies that allow the transmission of various data contents and services, which are easily accessible to healthcare workers, through mobile devices such as laptops, smartphones or PDAs. Therefore, it is possible to have a personalized and interactive health service with the aim of providing ubiquitous and universal access to information and medical advice by any user (Akter et al., 2013).

Nutrition is one of the areas that has gained growing relevance in health services. Campbell and Jacobson (2014) and Gropper et al. (2017) highlight the role of nutrition and nutrition in health promotion, disease prevention and progression, and therapeutic effectiveness is increasingly evident. The World Health Organization (2016) establishes that the main cause of mortality and morbidity throughout the European Region of the World Health Organization is poor nutrition, which contributes to diseases such as obesity, type 2 diabetes, cardiovascular diseases, and some types of cancer. Therefore, it can be considered that adequate nutrition is a key factor for the health of the world population.

The scientific and technological advances that have occurred in recent decades have made food more available and facilitated its consumption, as well as allowing stressful and time-consuming tasks to be carried out in a short period of time and with minimal energy expenditure, thus saving time and money. Apparently, these changes should improve the nutritional status of the world population, contributing to its longevity and quality of life. However, what is observed is an increase in the consumption of fats, sugar, and sodium, to the detriment of the consumption of fruits and vegetables, in addition to the increase in physical inactivity (Marotz, 2014).

People's lifestyles and the increase in new services and food venues have led people to simplify mealtimes. Examples of these practices are industrialized products and self-service restaurants. Feeding outside the home is also another factor contributing to the increased prevalence of chronic non-communicable diseases. According to Seguin et al. (2016), this type of food is fundamentally less healthy, with a higher calorie density, sugar, salt and fat content, low in fibers and high in sodium, when compared to foods prepared at home.

New technological tools have been progressively used by health professionals to help individuals expand their awareness of appropriate choices and prevent the development of chronic non-communicable diseases. Among the new tools are mobile devices that bring together countless resources whose focus is no longer just the traditional process of making and receiving calls. The features of today's mobile devices are agile and easy to use, providing easy access to information and better support for multimedia applications. In fact, Free et al. (2013) and Ventola (2014) point out that mobile apps for the health sector have been very popular with citizens.

One of the difficulties that citizens experience due to the completion of numerous daily tasks and the scarcity of time is to have enough time and adequate ability to prepare a meal quickly and efficiently. It is therefore important to develop a mobile application that allows the person responsible for preparing the meal not to spend too much time thinking about possible recipes or purchasing ingredients that they do not have in their homes for the respective meal.

In this sense, the authors of this study developed a mobile application for Android devices, where the user easily introduces the ingredients they have, as well as the respective quantities, and a wide variety of recipes are automatically generated. It is particularly important to note the creation of this application intends to encourage the avoidance of food waste and pays special attention to the health of the user, allowing them to mention their dietary restrictions. Additionally, the application suggests the substitution of ingredients where the user is potentially allergic and presents nutritional information regarding each recipe. With this, it is intended to promote healthy food habits through the adoption of a mhealth application.

BACKGROUND

Mobile Development Paradigm

The new era of mobile devices (e.g., smartphones, tablets, iPods) offers currently countless possibilities. All these options offer customization options with virtual stores such as Apple's App Store, Microsoft's Cloud Marketplace and Google's Android Market. These stores have free and paid applications for the most varied categories, such as games, web browsers, video, and image editing programs, etc.

The main feature of the mobile device is mobility. Johansson and Andersson (2015) define mobility as the ability of technology to perform multiple and different tasks, in addition to connecting and exchanging information with other people, applications and systems. Loeb, Falchuk and Panagos (2009) argue that for a device to be considered mobile it must have four characteristics:

- **Portability**: The ability of the device to move or to be moved easily. This factor covers the size and weight, including also its accessories (Collins & Ellis, 2015).
- **Usability**: The ability of the device to be used by different people and environments. This feature includes device dimensions, initialization time, data integrity, user interface, robustness, and resilience considering normal and extreme conditions of use (Harrison, Flood & Duce, 2013)
- **Functionality**: Tasks that the device can perform through mobile apps. It is possible to differentiate between two categories of applications: those that require user interaction and those that are fed with automatic information that results from interaction with the operating system and other applications (Iversen & Eierman, 2013).
- **Connectivity**: A fundamental objective of a mobile device is to connect people and exchange information between different systems. Connectivity can be divided into three ways: always connected, intermittent connections and operations that do not require a connection (Iversen & Eierman, 2013).

The development of software for mobile devices is more complex than traditional software for desktop and web environment due to several factors, such as: need to be in real-time, limited device memory, limited input and output channels, need for specific development tools, strong reliance on hardware, existence of different types of technology, and different sizes of devices (Iversen & Eierman, 2013). Despite the small size of many mobile applications, the technical complexity and associated costs can be much greater than in a Web application. Stremetska (2016) highlights that many of these applications need backend access, an object-oriented database and an Application Programming Interface (API). Furthermore, it is essential to design the User Interface (UI) and determine the User Experience

(UX) that encompasses all aspects of user interaction with the application (Abhay, 2018; Almeida & Monteiro, 2017).

Several factors must be taken into account when choosing the architecture for the development of a mobile application. Sommerville (2018) emphasizes the importance of taking into account the functional and non-functional requirements of the business and the user. Another perspective, Pankomera and Greunen emphasize the importance of high availability and scalability. It is necessary to create an application that keeps the performance stable according to the fluctuations of user demand and predict the ability of the application and the server to support the increase in the number of users and requests made. Finally, Gonzalez, Stakhanova and Ghorbani (2016) argue that the ideal solution for developing an application that allows the reuse of code for development between different devices.

In addition to choosing the architecture for the development of a mobile application, it is necessary to analyze the hardware of each technology that the application will be made available. In this sense, Iversen and Eierman (2013) highlight the following items that will be relevant in the development of the application: (i) CPU and memory, defines the speed that the device has to process the instructions of the application and that restricts the execution speed; (ii) operating system, defines the language and tools that will be used in the development of the application; (iii) disk space, limits the amount of data that can be stored locally on the device; (iv) batteries and power supplies, limits the autonomy of the device; (v) connection devices, establishes how information exchange and data synchronization are performed; (vi) screen, defines the dimensions of the device; and (vii) accessories, defines the peripherals that can be used by the application.

Comparison Between Mobile Web Applications and Native Applications

Historically, it has been observed that in the development for mobile devices, and especially to offer a complete user experience, it is necessary to develop applications in a native way, following the language and development process specific to each technology (Fling, 2009). However, the development of mobile web applications has also its advantages. According to Kumar (2018), the evolution of mobile web browsers turned possible to support more complex applications and services. Functionalities like the detection of the user's location and the use of the device's hardware are gradually being added. This situation reduces the need to develop specific applications that request to use the full capacity of the device. Furthermore, native applications are not the exclusive authorship of the developer, as they require the intermediation of the application store provided by the technology manufacturer (Iversen & Eierman, 2013). With this, the financial return of the project is divided and it is not possible to have complete control of the way the application is made available. In short, the mobile web platform is the only one that works independently of the device, being also the easiest to learn and develop, the cheapest to produce, the most standardized, the most available for use and easy to distribute (Ater, 2017; Halvorsen, 2018). However, and despite these benefits, web apps are less interactive and intuitive, typically offer worse performance and are less responsive than native apps (Dossey, 2019; Tandel & Jamadar, 2018).

From another perspective, development using the native structure of the technologies may become a better option, especially if some required device functionality is not allowed or possible through web browsers. Access to location data in the application typically requires access to the device's own resources. In this sense, the native form allows the application access to its location (Verma, Kansal, & Malvi, 2018). The cameras of the device are another resource that through native development becomes possible to have access. This functionality allows applications to take real-time photos, share multimedia content, or process QR codes (Kasinathan, Rahman & Rani, 2014). Access to files (e.g., photos, calendar, calendar, emails) is another very useful feature in the development of native applications. Additionally, in native applications, it is possible for the user to continue using it without being connected to the network. In this sense, Meier and Lake (2018) consider that native applications should have an offline mode and support situations in which there is a need to stay online, but in which the network signal may be lost.

The app development process is one of the factors that best distinguishes these two development paradigms (Viswanathan, 2019). Each manufacturer stipulates its own unique development process. One of the main challenges of developing mobile web applications is to make the code adapt to the specifics of each device because each device has unique characteristics. Each mobile device uses a different native programming language defined by its operating system. For example, iOS uses Objective-C, Android uses Java, Windows Mobile uses C++. On the other hand, web applications use languages such as JavaScript, HTML5, CSS3, and other web frameworks. Furthermore, each mobile platform offers to programmers their own standardized Software Development Kit (SDK), development tools, and other elements that assist in the process of designing the user interface. For the development of mobile hybrid applications, there is much wider panoply of options (e.g., Xamarin, PhoneGap, Ionic, Mobile Angular UI, Kendo UI, among others).

MHealth Solutions

With the increasingly intense development of technologies and technological innovations, and the simultaneous rise in the number of users adopting these technologies, an increasingly dynamic, mobile and interoperable society has been created. In fact, characteristics such as mobility, ubiquity, and personalization are constantly sought by users as a way to overcome geographical, temporal and organizational barriers (Silva et al., 2015). In this sense, the health sector has also undergone several transformations in recent years, with the emergence of health services based on mobility called mobile health or mhealth. According to Nisha et al. (2015), the mhealth involves the use of wireless technologies that allow the transmission of various data contents and services in the health field through mobile devices like smartphones, PDAs, laptops and tablets. Therefore, mhealth may be considered a personalized and interactive health service whose main objective is to provide ubiquitous and universal access to medical information and advice by any user (Akter et al., 2013).

Mobile computing has been one of the main areas of attraction of the research and business communities with the emergence of smart mobile devices that support 3G and 4G mobile networks. Mhealth emerges as a relevant health innovation that aims to overcome geographical, temporal and organizational barriers (Van Velthoven & Cordon, 2019). Furthermore, mhealth systems and associated mobility functionalities have a strong impact on typical systems for monitoring and alerting health care, administrative data collection, record keeping, health care, medical information, and prevention systems (Silva et al., 2015).

The use of smartphones as a platform to facilitate the individual's health care presents a wide range of benefits. Smartphones are agile and portable devices that can be used at anytime and anywhere (Batista & Gaglani, 2013). The continuous connection of smartphones to the Internet also allows the sharing of behavioral and health data with health professionals. Additionally, the growing ability of smartphones to use sensors allows inferring from the individual's context (e.g., location, movement, emotion, etc.), which facilitates the continuous and automated monitoring of health-related behaviors (Hussain et al., 2015).

Despite the unequivocal benefits of using medical apps in smartphones, there are some concerns and issues raised by both end-users and healthcare professionals. Hussain et al. (2015) summarize these challenges into three major groups: (i) poor quality of applications; (ii) concerns about users' privacy and security in the storage, transfer and processing of their personal data; and (iii) unreliability of the self-monitoring process. Regarding this last point, Hussain et al. (2015) point out that applications that provide medical advice based on their own data collection and algorithms may raise unnecessary concerns or lead to false diagnoses. This view is confirmed by Larson (2018) that, in a study conducted in early 2017 based on a sample of 52 mhealth apps in iTunes App Store and Google Play, found that 63.5% do not offer information about the intervention, around 67.3% do not present information about the professional credentials, and only 4% offered information about the efficacy data supporting the apps. Finally, the cultural barrier emerges as another obstacle to greater dissemination of mobile health. Muoio (2017) advocates many mhealth apps ignore the traditions and complexity of the healthcare system and, consequently, the resistance to change on the part of citizens and health professionals is high.

In order to take advantage of the positive effects of using apps in the field of health and nutrition, it is necessary to properly develop mobile applications that have a concrete effect on users' lives. The nutrition field registers a very significant and certain number of mhealth apps. A search conducted in June 2019 using the Google Play Store identified a total of 247 apps in the nutrition field. A comparative analysis of the top 10 apps in the area of nutrition and diet, considering the assessment performed by Kaiser Permanente, is presented in Table 1. This approach allows us to focus on the applications with the greatest impact on the market and to perform a bias-free analysis because the comparative analysis was not performed by the authors and an external credible source was adopted.

The findings allow us to identify many common points between the objectives of these apps. The majority of apps addresses both platforms (i.e., Android and iOS) and is based on the business model of freemium services. This business model offers simultaneously Free and Premium services, and the user chooses which one to fit into. This business model strategy allows those companies to reach more users, that can be initially convinced by the free service and migrate later to Premium (Holm and Günzel-Jensen, 2017). Most of these applications are user-friendliness and offer a responsive design that dynamically adjusts to the various dimensions and resolutions of the devices. One of the main difficulties is the interoperability between the systems that assumes great importance when the user wants to import or export data. Data security is another aspect that is often neglected and it is not possible to accurately assess the security mechanisms offered by each application. Another important aspect is the access of these applications to specific mobile phone functionalities such as cameras or sensors. Access to this information is essential in applications such as Waterlogged, MyPlate Calories Tracker, or Carbs Control. However, despite the high diversity of apps, neither of them has the dual mission of contributing to the avoidance of food waste and the promotion of healthy food habits with the nutritional information associated to each recipe.

MAIN FOCUS OF THE CHAPTER

Cooking can be a necessity, a hobby, a diversion or even a therapy. There are many reasons to take someone to the kitchen, but it's not always easy to decide what to cook or even have all the ingredients available to make a meal. The proposed app makes cooking with the ingredients that a citizen has at home a simple task, suggesting recipes based on the ingredients and taking into account criteria such as food intolerances.

Table 1. Comparative analysis of nutrition and diet apps

App	Platform	Price	Description
HealthyOut[1]	Android and iOS	Free	HealthyOut helps the user to find healthy restaurants. It provides access to menus of local restaurants and matches items on their menu to user's dietary needs and preferences. The app is feature-rich and has a large database of restaurants.
Calorie Counter & Food Diary[2]	Android and iOS	Free but with premium services	Calorie Counter & Food Diary lets users plan meals and monitor adherence. Useful features include the ability to scan supermarket barcodes to get nutritional information that helps users make smart choices while grocery shopping, and the tracking of macronutrients such as carbohydrates, protein, and fat. In fact, the user tracks his/her intake of 45 separate nutrients.
Food Intolerances[3]	Android and iOS	$4,99 for Android and $4.99 for iOS	Food Intolerances is focused on aiding people with allergies and food insensitivities. It's targeted at people with conditions such as histamine intolerance, mastocytosis, fructose malabsorption, sorbitol intolerance, gluten sensitivity, and lactose intolerance. The app contains a database of hundreds of foods and will tell the user whether a particular food is compatible with his/her allergies or food sensitivities.
Waterlogged[4]	iOS	Free but with premium services	Waterlogged helps users to monitor the consumption of water. It takes pictures of the user's drinking vessels to quickly and automatically log user's water intake. The app also set up reminders to drink fluids and can help the user to quickly assess his/her hydration with handy graphs.
Nutrients[5]	iOS	$4.99	Another popular nutrients database and diet tracker is Nutrients. Nutrients app contains the nutritional info for a wide range of foods and a food journal which makes tracking user's food intake simple. One favorite feature is the ability to enter recipes and get an instant nutritional breakdown.
Shopwell[6]	Android and iOS	Free	Shopwell is a standout app that helps users to make healthy choices at the grocery store. The idea is to enter the user's fitness goals, nutritional requirements, and food sensitivities. Then, while shopping, the user can scan the bar-codes of items for information about the nutritional content, added sugar and sodium, and more.
Calorie Counter & Diet Tracker[7]	Android and iOS	Free but with premium services	Calorie Counter & Diet Tracker by MyFitnessPal is oriented toward weight loss and is one of the more popular apps for tracking your food intake. It's got a database of 5,000,000 foods and dishes. The user interface is simple and intuitive.
MyPlate Calories Tracker[8]	Android and iOS	Free but with premium services	MyPlate Calories Tracker is a diet app. It contains a nutritional database of 2 million items and includes the ability to track calories, macronutrients and water intake. It can also generate graphs and charts that help to visualize and assess user's food habits.
Fitocracy Macros[9]	iOS	Free	Macronutrients include carbohydrates, proteins, and fat. Many nutritionists recommend that health-conscious individuals aim for a healthy diet with the right ratio of these "macros". Fitocracy Macros allows users to track the input of these macronutrients and associated caloric intake.
Carbs Control[10]	Android and iOS	$2.99	Carbs Control is designed to help users to monitor their carbohydrates and may be a good choice for diabetics or those on low-carbon diets. Users can track daily carb intake, as well as look at a meal-by-meal breakdown.

(adapted from KP (2018))

The proposed app offers several options that so far have not reached the market in a single application to make life in the kitchen easier. It offers an ingredient search method that helps users to choose their meal according to the ingredients they have at home, thus avoiding wasting food close to the shelf life and also avoiding shopping. The app also allows the user to indicate their allergies and suggests the substitution of ingredients where the user is potentially allergic and presents nutritional information regarding each recipe. Finally, the user has also the possibility to add his/her recipes, comment on other users' recipes, evaluate the recipe, add it to favorites, and also search by type of meal.

Functionalities

A requirement can be defined as the property that software possesses to solve a problem or achieve a goal (Sommerville, 2018). Requirements are one of the primary drivers of software success and are key elements for software estimation, modeling, execution, testing, and maintenance. According to Chakraborty et al. (2012), the requirements are essential throughout the entire life cycle of software. The requirements can typically be grouped into two major groups: functional and non-functional. The functional requirements should specify the functions of how the system should react to specific inputs and how to behave in certain situations (Sommerville, 2018). Table 2 shows the functional requirements offered by the proposed app. In total, seven functional requirements and a total of two actors (i.e., user and administrator) were considered. The user is responsible for registering in the software and interacting with the software, creating recipes, commenting on recipes, searching for recipes among other functionalities. The administrator manages the existing recipes in the software and can edit/remove them as well as add new recipes. Each requirement has a unique identifier to allow its identification throughout the implementation process.

The non-functional requirements are another group of requirements also of great importance in the construction of a software engineering solution. A non-functional requirement aims to meet system requirements that are not functional requirements (i.e., do not refer to business functionalities) but are part of the scope of the system. According to Sommerville (2018), the non-functional requirements place restrictions on the product to be developed, on the development process and external to the product. Furthermore, Shahid and Tasneem (2017) state that it becomes fundamental to consider this type of requirements in an initial phase of engineering projects software, because most of the software problems in operation occur due to the absence of non-functional requirements support. Table 3 presents the non-functional requirements considered in the development of the app. A total of six non-functional requirements were considered due to their relevance for m-health apps in general and to the operation of the proposed application. Three levels of priorities were established (e.g., low, medium, and high). In the exploratory analysis of the top 10 nutrition apps in 2018, the importance of usability becomes clear, which is why this was considered a top priority requirement. Backup is another fundamental requirement to ensure that there is no loss of user information. Performance and safety have medium priority.

Table 2. Functional requirements

ID	Name	Description	Actors
RF1	Register in the app	The user who does not yet have an account will have to register in the application, entering the required data (e.g., Name, Email and Password).	User
RF2	Authenticate in personal account	To authenticate in the account the user or administrator will have to enter his email and password.	User, Administrator
RF3	Manage recipes	The administrator is able to add, edit or remove recipes. The administrator can add nutritional information regarding each recipe.	Administrator
RF4	Manage allergens	The administrator is able to add, edit or remove allergens.	Administrator
RF5	Search recipes	The user can search for recipes based on the name of meals or ingredients. He/she can comment, vote or bookmark any recipe.	User
RF6	Change personal info	The user can change his/her allergies and his/her password.	User
RF7	Personal recipe area	The user can see his/her recipes. He/she can create a new one or remove/edit his/her existing recipes. It is also possible to make comments in a recipe.	User

Security was considered a medium priority requirement because it was considered that the information made available by the user is not critical in case of illegitimate access or data exposure. Finally, the lowest level of priority has been given to scalability and interoperability as they are not critical to the operational functioning of the application.

Architecture

The app was developed to run on the Android operating system. To develop the Android application, we used the Integrated Development Environment (IDE) Android Studio, an Application Programming Interface (API), which has available several tutorials and extensive documentation, thus providing great support and incentive for development. For the database management was used the MySQL system that uses the SQL language. Additionally, PhpMyAdmin was used to manipulate the access to a MySQL database, and XAMPP was used as an independent server. Figure 1 summarizes the app's component diagram. The programming languages included Java and php for the programming and development of the application through the Android System, and the Volley library was also used to establish the communication between the database and the application.

SOLUTIONS AND RECOMMENDATIONS

User Interface

The developed solution promotes healthy food habits through a mhealth application that allows a citizen to take advantage of the ingredients at home to prepare recipes with nutritional value and avoiding risks of potential allergies. The first step in the app is to register a new user. To successfully register a new user, it is necessary to follow a sequence of actions. This process is mandatory to all users without a

Table 3. Non-functional requirements

ID	Name	Description	Priority
RNF1	Usability	The software must be intuitive and easy for any user to use. It must be simple so that the user has greater ease of work and is able to navigate the software without failure, with as few errors as possible.	High
RNF2	Scalability	The software must be created in a way that allows you to easily change and modify the functionalities and add new ones.	Low
RNF3	Performance	The software has several tasks that have to be able to do and, as such, we must make sure that each task is as fast as possible and that it can be executed on any low/medium cost mobile phone without problems.	Medium
RNF4	Security	The software must be created in such a way that the data is stored and protected in the database.	Medium
RNF5	Backup	The software will have an updated backup so that, if the worst happens and we lose data, we can recover the previously saved files, avoiding data loss.	High
RNF6	Interoperability	The software can import and export recipes from/to recipe applications (e.g., Tasty, BigOven). Application adopts open standards to import/export data as suggested by Almeida et al. (2010).	Low

Figure 1. UML component diagram (logical architecture)

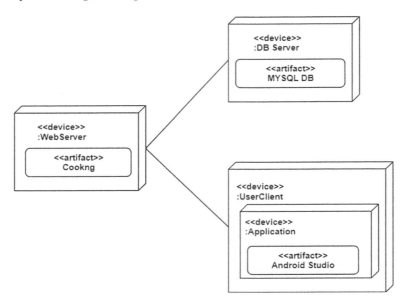

valid account. When arriving at the registration page the user indicates the email, password and user-name for the account that will create, when indicating those data the software sends to the database the data entered and registers the data in the database, the software redirects the user to the login page if the data are entered correctly, if there is an error in the registration the creation of the new registration is not done and an error message is sent to the user so that he can perform the registration again. This process can be easily visualized in Figure 2.

After that, the user can access the login panel as shown in Figure 3. To log in, the user needs to fill in the following fields (username and password) validly so that the login is validated. When logging in incorrectly the software will indicate to the user through the following message "Wrong username/password" or the following message if the user does not fill in one of the fields "Blank username and/or password". In the construction of the login panel two best practices proposed by Babich (2016) were followed, respectively: (i) it is immediately clear the login area in the center of the window; and (ii) the process of "sign-in" and "sign-up" are performed separately. From the login panel, it is still possible to recover the password. For this purpose, a reset password email is sent. In the construction of this email, the recommendations proposed by Dimon (2018) were adopted, respectively: (i) relevant and readable subject and "From" name; (ii) the link to reset the password; (iii) expiration information; (iv) how to contact support; and (v) the IP address that requested the reset. These elements allow us to increase application security and combat potential phishing attacks.

In the "View my recipes" menu, the user can insert a new recipe, where he/she will indicate the name of the recipes, ingredients, a picture of it and instructions on how to make the recipe. Users can also see their recipes, edit/remove some of the recipes that he/she has placed in the software, and add recipes to the favorites. This approach allows the user to easily save his/her favorite recipes and reuse them whenever he/she wants. Each recipe has a brief description, list of ingredients, information about the baking process, nutritional information, and an associated image as shown in Figure 3. In the design of this interface, three fundamental factors were considered. The use of responsive images was fundamental

Figure 2. Sequence diagram of the registration process

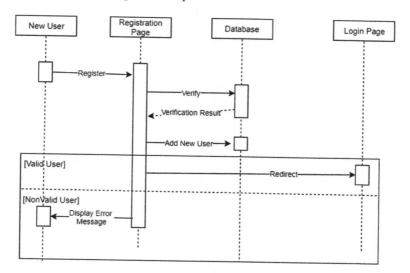

to provide a good navigation experience. According to Wainstein (2018), the adoption of responsive images allows us to have a dynamic image adjustment for the right screen size, improves loading time, and the user experience. The evaluation of the recipe by the user was another aspect considered and, for that, a scale of 5 values was adopted. According to DeCastellarnau (2018), the use of scales' visual presentation based on numbers of fixed reference points from negative-to-positive contributed to a correct assessment of the user, and it also follows the good user interaction practices established by Ali et al. (2014). Finally, the nutritional information is presented according to the food wheel. This ensures the consistency of the information presented for all recipes and adopts terminology familiar to the majority of end-users. This approach contributes to reducing user learning, increases usability, and eliminates confusion (Wong, 2019).

When the user logs into the software the software will return to the main menu where the user can choose between "Search recipe", "My recipe" and "User settings". By selecting the option "Search recipes" the user can choose between searching for recipes, where all existing recipes will be displayed organized by type of meal as shown in Figure 4. Finger-friendly buttons for mobile users were used to choose the type of meal, which simplifies the interaction even with smaller devices and the arrangement of the buttons were ordered according to the traditional process of choosing a meal (Fanguy, 2018).

The user can also choose between searching for recipes by ingredients or by meals. Figure 4 shows a filter search by ingredient. The design of this interface also sought to ensure consistency in the process of choosing ingredients. When meals are listed for the user, the user can comment, vote and add recipes to favorites.

Administrator Interface

When the administrator logs in, he/she finds a menu where he has the following options "Manage Recipe" and "Manage Allergenics". By choosing the "Manage Recipe" option the administrator can view the recipes, add, edit and remove the existing recipes. For example, when adding a new recipe, we have to

Figure 3. Access to login menu and recipe view panel

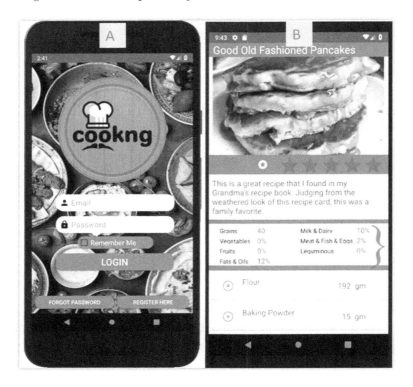

give a name to the recipe, the type of meal, a description and the instructions to make the recipe. We can also add a picture and all the necessary ingredients and their respective measurements as shown in Figure 5. The backend interface intended to follow the same layout patterns as the frontend. This approach is aligned with the recommendations proposed by Hartson and Pyla (2018) that advocate an agile UX design approach to increase the quality of user experience. Furthermore, this approach allows us to provide a consistent experience regardless of the logged-in user (Soegaard, 2019).

In the "Manage Allergenics" option, the administrator can view existing allergens, add, edit or remove any of the existing allergens. After that, when the user searches for a recipe he will receive notification that there are ingredients on which he has an allergy and proposes to replace them with other ingredients. Figure 5 shows this information highlighted in red. It is important to highlight the importance of this window being clearly visible to identify potential ingredients on which the user has an allergy. For this purpose, and following Babich's (2019) recommendations, the red color should be used in the interface with mobile devices to capture the immediate focus of the user and to alert to potential danger or emergency situations.

FUTURE RESEARCH DIRECTIONS

The role of smartphones in the development and expansion of healthcare services is an emerging challenge. A key part of the new phase of promoting innovation in healthcare is the use of mobile devices.

Figure 4. Search by type of meal and filter by ingredient

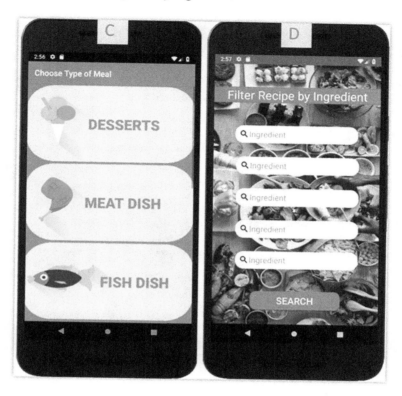

The exponential growth of smartphones among patients and healthcare professionals drives the revolution in healthcare services and products that we are seeing today. Many innovative services have gradually emerged on the market, such as remote patient monitoring, exercise applications, food intake monitoring or real-time cognitive support.

One of the cross-cutting areas of mhealth services is the collection of large amounts of data. Mhealth has a wide range of applications, from passive data extracted in fitness applications, to more critical data such as those collected by smartphones after performing surgical interventions or monitoring newborns. The large amount of data that the mhealth movement will offer to citizens and healthcare professionals provides new points of view and offers the possibility to perform more complex analyses and with more extensive scenarios.

Another relevant area for future mhealth research is the interoperability between the various services. Interoperability is a critical factor in the design of health platforms since the user can interact with health systems through various entities and technological platforms. Genes et al. (2018) advocate that in a context of increasingly shared care provision and multi-stakeholder intervention, interoperability allows the efficient use of existing resources in each organization. Therefore, future research directions in this field should simultaneously consider interoperability in its multiple dimensions. On the technical side, the connectivity of the components should be explored; on the syntactic side, the coherent way in which data are exchanged between the components is explored; on the semantic side, the way in which data are interpreted by different applications is explored (Bhartiya, Mehrotra and Girdhar, 2016).

Figure 5. Add a new recipe and identification of ingredients with allergy

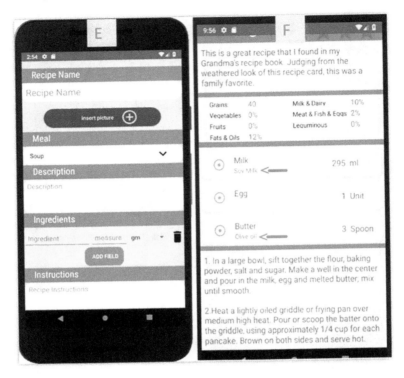

One of the problems with research in the mhealth field relates to the fact that research is continuously evolving, turning mobile systems quickly obsolete before they are fully tested and in an operational environment. For this reason, it is often complicated to develop medium and long-term strategies and the results obtained by mhealth solutions are not consistently and thoroughly evaluated (Idrish et al., 2017). One of the lines of research in this area is the exploration of success factors in the implementation of a mhealth. Research already conducted in this domain by Matthew-Maich et al. (2016), Ahmed et al. (2017) and Handayani et al. (2018) highlight the importance of the organizational environment, the viability of the business model, the added and perceived value of the solution, the ease of use, the interoperability, the privacy, among others. However, there is no complete model that allows a clear assessment of the critical success factors considering the type of services offered by a mhealth solution. This situation is particularly important given the high number and diversity of mhealth platforms and tools.

CONCLUSION

The growth in the use of smartphones and other mobile devices has led to the emergence of mhealth applications based on traditional ehealth applications and the appearance of other innovative solutions that didn't exist in the ehealth services paradigm. In the mhealth are included concepts as diverse as mobile computing, sensors and communication technologies for health care. The mhealth brings numerous benefits to users and healthcare institutions like increased patient safety and efficiency in processes.

In this sense, in recent years a large number of mhealth apps have appeared in the market, particularly for Android devices.

The proposed app is a mobile application for the Android platform and aims to promote healthy food habits through better food management. Therefore, an app was developed for Android devices that encourages the avoidance of food waste and promotes the development of good food practices based on the nutritional value of each recipe and the indication of potential allergies to ingredients. In the latter case, an alert is sent to the user and suggestions are given on how this ingredient can be replaced, without compromising the final quality of the recipe. The design of the application was carried out through the integrated Android Studio environment, also using the Java and php languages in its development process.

The development of the app was based on the best practices of Mobile UX, aiming at an intuitive and fast learning interaction for the user. In this way, it is intended that the content available in the app can be more easily absorbed and contribute to greater retention of users over time. Several models of interfaces were studied during the development period. Some criteria were prioritized, such as the ease of access functionalities of the application, the speed in navigation between screens and a pleasant visual identity for better appreciation of the content. Additionally, other requirements in the design of the application were considered, such as safety, performance, backup or interoperability.

As future work, the authors intend to incorporate new features in the application that will simplify its use and minimize the work of the administrator of the application. One of the proposals is the integration with external recipe apps (e.g., Tasty, BigOven). This will simultaneously increase the quantity and quality of the recipes that the user will have available. It is also important to allow the search for recipes to be carried out also based on their nutritional information. At the moment, nutrition information is already associated with each recipe in the app, but it does not allow searches based on this information. Finally, it would also be challenging to use sensors or to integrate with retail applications that allow in an automated way to know the ingredients that each user has in the house and their expiry dates. This functionality would simplify the use of the platform and contribute to better optimization of the process.

REFERENCES

Abhay, V. (2018). Why Mobile User Experience (UX) is Critical for iOS and Android Apps. Netsolutions. Retrieved from https://www.netsolutions.com/insights/7-reasons-to-customize-mobile-user-experience-for-ios-and-android/

Ahmed, M., Gagnon, M., Hamelin-Brabant, L., Mbemba, G., & Alami, H. (2017). A mixed methods systematic review of success factors of mhealth and telehealth for maternal health in Sub-Saharan Africa. *mHealth*, *3*(22), 1–10. PMID:28293618

Akter, S., Ray, P., & D'Ambra, J. (2013). Continuance of mHealth services at the bottom of the pyramid: The roles of service quality and trust. *Electronic Markets*, *23*(1), 29–47. doi:10.100712525-012-0091-5

Ali, A., Alrasheedi, M., Ouda, A., & Capretz, L. (2014). A study of the interface usability issues of mobile learning applications for smart phones from the user's perspective. *International Journal on Integrating Technology in Education*, *3*(4), 1–16. doi:10.5121/ijite.2014.3401

Almeida, F., & Monteiro, J. (2017). Approaches and Principles for UX Web Experiences. *International Journal of Information Technology and Web Engineering*, *12*(2), 49–65. doi:10.4018/IJITWE.2017040103

Almeida, F., Oliveira, J., & Cruz, J. (2010). Open Standards and Open Source: Enabling Interoperability. *International Journal of Software Engineering and Its Applications*, 2(1), 1–11. doi:10.5121/ijsea.2011.2101

Ater, T. (2017). *Building Progressive Web Apps: Bringing the Power of Native to the Browser*. Newton, MA: O'Reilly Media.

Babich, N. (2016). Designing UX Login Form and Process. UXPlanet. Retrieved from https://uxplanet.org/designing-ux-login-form-and-process-8b17167ed5b9

Babich, N. (2019). Using Red and Green in UI Design. UXPlanet. Retrieved from https://uxplanet.org/using-red-and-green-in-ui-design-66b39e13de91

Batista, M., & Gaglani, S. (2013). The Future of Smartphones in Health Care. *AMA Journal of Ethics*, 15(11), 947–950. doi:10.1001/virtualmentor.2013.15.11.stas1-1311 PMID:24257085

Bhartiya, S., Mehrotra, D., & Girdhar, A. (2016). Issues in Achieving Complete Interoperability while Sharing Electronic Health Records. *Procedia Computer Science*, 78, 192–198. doi:10.1016/j.procs.2016.02.033

Campbell, T., & Jacobson, H. (2014). *Whole: Rethinking the Science of Nutrition*. Dallas, TX: BenBella Books.

Chakraborty, A., Baowaly, M., Arefin, A., & Bahar, A. (2012). The Role of Requirement Engineering in Software Development Life Cycle. *Journal of Emerging Trends in Computing and Information Sciences*, 3(5), 723–729.

Collins, L., & Ellis, S. (2015). *Mobile Devices: Tools and Technologies*. Boca Raton, FL: Chapman and Hall/CRC. doi:10.1201/b18165

DeCastellarnau, A. (2018). A classification of response scale characteristics that affect data quality: A literature review. *Quality & Quantity*, 52(4), 1523–1559. doi:10.100711135-017-0533-4 PMID:29937582

Dimon, G. (2018). Password reset email design best practices. Postmarkapp. Retrieved from https://postmarkapp.com/guides/password-reset-email-best-practices

Dossey, A. (2019). A Guide to Mobile App Development: Web vs. Native vs. Hybrid [Infographic]. Clearbridgemobile. Retrieved from https://clearbridgemobile.com/mobile-app-development-native-vs-web-vs-hybrid/#What_are_Progressive_Web_Apps

Dunaway, J., Searles, K., Sui, M., & Paul, N. (2018). News Attention in a Mobile Era. *Journal of Computer-Mediated Communication*, 23(2), 107–124. doi:10.1093/jcmc/zmy004

Fanguy, W. (2018). A comprehensive guide to designing UX buttons. Invisionapp. Retrieved from https://www.invisionapp.com/inside-design/comprehensive-guide-designing-ux-buttons/

Free, C., Phillips, G., Watson, L., Galli, L., Felix, L., Edwards, P., ... Haines, A. (2013). The Effectiveness of Mobile-Health Technologies to Improve Health Care Service Delivery Processes: A Systematic Review and Meta-Analysis. *PLoS Medicine*, 10(1), 1–26. doi:10.1371/journal.pmed.1001363 PMID:23458994

Genes, N., Violante, S., Cetrangol, C., Rogers, L., Schadt, E., Feng, Y., & Chan, Y. (2018). From smartphone to EHR: A case report on integrating patient-generated health data. *Digital Media*, *23*, 1–6. PMID:31304305

Gonzalez, H., Stakhanova, N., & Ghorbani, A. (2016). Measuring code reuse in Android apps. In *Proceedings of the 14th Annual Conference on Privacy, Security and Trust (PST)* (pp. 187-195). Academic Press. 10.1109/PST.2016.7906925

Gropper, S., Smith, J., & Carr, T. (2017). *Advanced Nutrition and Human Metabolism*. London, UK: Cengage Learning.

Halvorsen, L. (2018). *Functional Web Development with Elixir, OTP, and Phoenix: Rethink the Modern Web App*. Raleigh, NC: Pragmatic Bookshelf.

Handayani, P., Meigasari, D., Pinem, A., Hidayanto, A., & Ayuningtyas, D. (2018). Critical success factors for mobile health implementation in Indonesia. *Heliyon (London)*, *4*(11), 1–26. doi:10.1016/j.heliyon.2018.e00981 PMID:30519665

Harrison, R., Flood, D., & Duce, D. (2013). Usability of mobile applications: Literature review and rationale for a new usability model. *Journal of Interaction Science*, *1*(1), 1–16. doi:10.1186/2194-0827-1-1

Hartson, R., & Pyla, P. (2018). *The UX Book: Agile UX Design for a Quality User Experience*. Burlington, MA: Morgan Kaufmann.

Holm, A., & Günzel-Jensen, F. (2017). Succeeding with freemium: Strategies for implementation. *The Journal of Business Strategy*, *38*(2), 16–24. doi:10.1108/JBS-09-2016-0096

Hussain, M., Al-Haiqi, A., Zaidan, A., Zaidan, B., Kiah, M., Anuar, N., & Abdulnabi, M. (2015). The landscape of research on smartphone medical apps: Coherent taxonomy, motivations, open challenges and recommendations. *Computer Methods and Programs in Biomedicine*, *122*(3), 393–408. doi:10.1016/j.cmpb.2015.08.015 PMID:26412009

Idrish, S., Rifat, A., Iqbal, M., & Nisha, N. (2017). Mobile Health Technology Evaluation: Innovativeness and Efficacy vs. Cost Effectiveness. *International Journal of Technology and Human Interaction*, *13*(2), 1–21. doi:10.4018/IJTHI.2017040101

Iversen, J., & Eierman, M. (2013). *Learning Mobile App Development: A Hands-on Guide to Building Apps with iOS and Android*. Boston, MA: Addison-Wesley Professional.

Johansson, D., & Andersson, K. (2015). Mobile e-Services: State of the Art, Focus Areas, and Future Directions. *International Journal of E-Services and Mobile Applications*, *7*(2), 1–24. doi:10.4018/ijesma.2015040101

Kasinathan, V., Rahman, N., & Rani, M. (2014). Approaching Digital Natives with QR Code Technology in Edutainment. *International Journal of Education and Research*, *2*(4), 169–178.

KP. (2018). 10 nutrition and diet apps for 2018. *Kaiser Permanente*. WA Health. Retrieved from https://wa-health.kaiserpermanente.org/best-diet-apps/

Kumar, A. (2018). *Web Technology: Theory and Practice.* Boca Raton, FL: Chapman and Hall. doi:10.1201/9781351029902

Larson, R. (2018). A Path to Better-Quality mHealth Apps. *JMIR mHealth and uHealth, 6*(7), 1–6. doi:10.2196/10414 PMID:30061091

Loeb, S., Falchuk, B., & Panagos, T. (2009). *The Fabric of Mobile Services: Software Paradigms and Business Demands.* Hoboken, NJ: Wiley-Interscience. doi:10.1002/9780470478240

Machado, J., Abelha, A., Santos, M., & Portela, F. (2017). *Next-Generation Mobile and Pervasive Healthcare Solutions.* Hershey, PA: IGI Global.

Marotz, L. (2014). *Health, Safety, and Nutrition for the Young Child.* London, UK: Cengage Learning.

Matthew-Maich, N., Harris, L., Ploeg, J., Markle-Reid, M., Valaitis, R., Ibrahim, S., ... Isaacs, S. (2016). Designing, Implementing, and Evaluating Mobile Health Technologies for Managing Chronic Conditions in Older Adults: A Scoping Review. *JMIR mHealth and uHealth, 4*(2), 1–29. doi:10.2196/mhealth.5127 PMID:27282195

Mayes, J., & White, A. (2016). How Smartphone Technology Is Changing Healthcare In Developing Countries. *The Journal of Global Health.* Retrieved from https://www.ghjournal.org/how-smartphone-technology-is-changing-healthcare-in-developing-countries/

Meier, R., & Lake, I. (2018). *Professional Android.* Hoboken, New Jersey: Wrox. doi:10.1002/9781119419389

Muoio, D. (2017). New technologies are transforming health, but culture lags behind. Mobile Health News. Retrieved from https://www.mobihealthnews.com/content/new-technologies-are-transforming-health-culture-lags-behind

Nisha, N., Iqbal, M., Rifat, A., & Idrish, S. (2015). Mobile Health Services: A New Paradigm for Health Care Systems. *International Journal of Asian Business and Information Management, 6*(1), 1–17. doi:10.4018/IJABIM.2015010101

Pankomera, R., & Greunen, D. (2018). A model for implementing sustainable mHealth applications in a resource-constrained setting: A case of Malawi. *The Electronic Journal on Information Systems in Developing Countries, 84*(2), 1–12. doi:10.1002/isd2.12019

Sarwar, M., & Soomro, T. (2013). Impact of Smartphone's on Society. *European Journal of Scientific Research, 98*(2), 216–226.

Seguin, R., Aggarwal, A., Vermeylen, F., & Drewnowski, A. (2016). Consumption frequency of foods away from home linked with higher body mass index and lower fruit and vegetable intake among adults: A cross-sectional study. *Journal of Environmental and Public Health, 2016,* 1–12. doi:10.1155/2016/3074241 PMID:26925111

Shahid, M., & Tasneem, K. (2017). Impact of Avoiding Non-functional Requirements in Software Development Stage. *American Journal of Information Science and Computer Engineering, 3*(4), 52–55.

Silva, B., Rodrigues, J., de la Torre Díez, I., López-Coronado, M., & Saleem, K. (2015). Mobile-health: A review of current state in 2015. *Journal of Biomedical Informatics, 56,* 265–272. doi:10.1016/j. jbi.2015.06.003 PMID:26071682

Soegaard, M. (2019). Consistency: More than what you think. Interaction Design. Retrieved from https:// www.interaction-design.org/literature/article/consistency-more-than-what-you-think

Sommerville, I. (2018). *Software Engineering.* New Delhi: Pearson India.

Stremetska, D. (2016). Why mobile development is so expensive. STFalcon. Retrieved from https:// stfalcon.com/en/blog/post/why-mobile-development-is-so-expensive

Tandel, S., & Jamadar, A. (2018). Impact of Progressive Web Apps on Web App Development. *International Journal of Innovative Research in Science, Engineering and Technology, 7*(9), 9349–9444.

Taniar, D. (2008). *Mobile Computing: Concepts, Methodologies, Tools, and Applications.* Hershey, PA: IGI Global.

Van Velthoven, M., & Cordon, C. (2019). Sustainable Adoption of Digital Health Innovations Perspectives From a Stakeholder Workshop. *Journal of Medical Internet Research, 21*(3), 1–8. doi:10.2196/11922 PMID:30907734

Ventola, C. (2014). Mobile Devices and Apps for Health Care Professionals: Uses and Benefits. *P&T, 39*(5), 356–364. PMID:24883008

Verma, N., Kansal, S., & Malvi, H. (2018). Development of Native Mobile Application Using Android Studio for Cabs and Some Glimpse of Cross Platform Apps. *International Journal of Applied Engineering Research, 13*(16), 12527–12530.

Viswanathan, P. (2019). Native Apps vs. Web Apps: What Is the Better Choice? Lifewire. Retrieved from https://www.lifewire.com/native-apps-vs-web-apps-2373133

Wainstein, L. (2018). Why You Should Use Responsive Images. Lab21. Retrieved from https://www. lab21.gr/blog/use-responsive-images

Wong, E. (2019). Principle of Consistency and Standards in User Interface Design. Interaction Design. Retrieved from https://www.interaction-design.org/literature/article/principle-of-consistency-and-standards-in-user-interface-design

World Health Organization. (2016). Disease burden and mortality estimates. Retrieved from https:// www.who.int/healthinfo/global_burden_disease/estimates/en/index1.html

ADDITIONAL READING

Abouelmehdi, K., Beni-Hssane, A., Khaloufi, H., & Saadi, M. (2017). Big data security and privacy in healthcare: A Review. *Procedia Computer Science, 113,* 73–80. doi:10.1016/j.procs.2017.08.292

Azarm, M., Backman, C., Kuziemsky, C., & Peyton, L. (2017). Breaking the Healthcare Interoperability Barrier by Empowering and Engaging Actors in the Healthcare System. *Procedia Computer Science*, *113*, 326–333. doi:10.1016/j.procs.2017.08.341

Dutta, M. J., Kaur-Gill, S., Tan, N., & Lam, C. (2018) mHealth, Health, and Mobility: A Culture-Centered Interrogation. In E. Baulch, J. Watkins, & A. Tariq (Eds.), mHealth Innovation in Asia. Mobile Communication in Asia: Local Insights, Global Implications. Springer.

Hemmat, M., Ayatollahi, H., Makeki, M., & Saghafi, F. (2018). Key Health Information Technologies and Related Issues for Iran: A Qualitative Study. *The Open Medical Informatics Journal*, *12*(1), 1–10. doi:10.2174/1874431101812010001 PMID:29854016

Isterpanian, R., & Woodward, B. (2016). *M-Health: Fundamentals and Applications*. Hoboken, NJ: Wiley. doi:10.1002/9781119302889

Koumpouros, Y., & Georgoulas, A. (2019). The Rise of mHealth Research in Europe: A Macroscopic Analysis of EC-Funded Projects of the Last Decade. In A. Moumtzoglou (Ed.), *Mobile Health Applications for Quality Healthcare Delivery* (pp. 1–29). Hershey, PA: IGI Global. doi:10.4018/978-1-5225-8021-8.ch001

Moumtzoglou, A. (2019). *Mobile Health Applications for Quality Healthcare Delivery*. Hershey, PA: IGI Global. doi:10.4018/978-1-5225-8021-8

Nikou, S., & Bouwman, H. (2017). Mobile Health and Wellness Applications: A Business Model Ontology-Based Review. *International Journal of E-Business Research*, *13*(1), 1–24. doi:10.4018/IJEBR.2017010101

Waegemann, C. P. (2016). mHealth: History, Analysis, and Implementation. In A. Moumtzoglou (Ed.), M-Health Innovations for Patient-Centered Care (pp. 1-19). Hershey, PA: IGI Global.

KEY TERMS AND DEFINITIONS

Application Programming Interface (API): A collection of programming routines and standards for accessing a software application or web-based platform. An API is created when a software company intends for other software developers to develop products associated with its service.

Cascading Style Sheets (CSS): Technology created to complement the HTML language and facilitate the creation and maintenance of the design of web pages through styles, which allows the change of the appearance of all elements of all pages that are related to a certain field of the same style.

EHealth: Broad concept that encompasses all the technological innovations that impact the health area.

HTML5: Last evolution in the pattern that defines the HTML. The term represents two different concepts. This is a new version of the HTML language, with new elements, attributes and behaviors, and a larger set of technologies that allows the creation of websites and Web applications more diverse and powerful.

JavaScript: High-level interpreted programming language, also characterized as dynamic, weakly typified, prototype-based and multi-paradigm.

Macronutrient: Nutrients that help provide energy and the body needs them in large quantities. Water, carbohydrates, grease and protein are classified as macronutrients.

MHealth: A term used to describe the practice of medicine and public health supported by mobile devices.

Smartphone: Mobile phones with advanced technologies that turn possible for anyone to develop programs for them, called applications, and they exist of the most varied types and for the most varied objectives.

Software Development Kit (SDK): A set of software development tools that enable the creation of applications for a given framework.

Unified Modeling Language (UML): Notation and modeling language that is used in software system design process. This language is expressed through diagrams. Each diagram is composed of elements (graphic forms used for drawings) that are related to each other.

User Experience (UX): User experience encompasses all aspects of end-user interaction with the company, its services, and products.

User Interface (UI): User interface aims to create interfaces that are elegant, easy to use and help the end-user complete their tasks and goals.

ENDNOTES

[1]   https://www.healthyout.com

[2]   https://play.google.com/store/apps/details?id=com.fourtechnologies.mynetdiary.ad&hl=en_US

[3]   https://apps.apple.com/us/app/food-intolerances/id419098758

[4]   https://www.waterlogged.com

[5]   https://apps.apple.com/us/app/nutrients-nutrition-facts/id396836856

[6]   https://www.innit.com/shopwell/

[7]   https://play.google.com/store/apps/details?id=com.sparkpeople.androidtracker&hl=pt_PT

[8]   https://play.google.com/store/apps/details?id=com.livestrong.tracker&hl=pt_PT

[9]   https://apps.apple.com/us/app/fitocracy-macros-how-much-should-i-eat-to-lose-weight/id786388273

[10]   http://www.diabeticdiet.health/2017/06/28/carbs-control-carb-tracker/

Chapter 2
Knocking at Alternate Doors:
Survey of Android–Based Smartphone Applications for Alternate Medicines

Rafiullah Khan

ⓘ https://orcid.org/0000-0002-0229-7747

The University of Agriculture, Peshawar, Pakistan

Mohib Ullah

The University of Agriculture, Peshawar, Pakistan

Bushra Shafi

The University of Agriculture, Peshawar, Pakistan

Urooj Beenish Orakzai

Government Girls Degree College, Peshawar, Pakistan

Seema Shafi

Charssada Homeopathic Medical College, Pakistan

ABSTRACT

Despite the extraordinary progression in modern medicines, alternative medicine has always been practiced. Alternative medicine or complementary medicine is a term referring to any practice that aims to achieve healing effects using pseudoscience or without biological explanation. The major drawback of alternative medicine is that these medicines are not scientifically tested as claimed by different studies. Nevertheless, according to the World Health Organization, more than 70% of the population of developing countries prefer alternative medicine systems. In this work, a review of ten most popular Android based smartphone applications that belongs to two most popular alternative medicines systems i.e. Homeopathy and Ayurveda are presented. The apps are selected based on the number of reviews, user rating, and the number of downloads provided by Google's play store. From the reviews of users, it was noted that most of the users are satisfied with the selected smartphone app. Based on this fact, it can be implicitly concluded that these medical systems can effectively solve user health-related issues.

DOI: 10.4018/978-1-7998-2521-0.ch002

1. INTRODUCTION

With the evaluation and development in the societies of different civilizations, the approach to the disease and illness also evolved. The current medical practices are based on the approaches introduced and evolved in different societies such as the concepts of diagnosis and prognosis introduced in India (Wikipedia, n.d.b), medical ethics in Greece (the famous Hippocratic Oath (Hulkower, 2016)), extensive work on human anatomy and surgery by Muslim scholars (Rosenthal, 2015) and many others. Although the invention of the microscope revolutionized the medical practices, still there are still a number of alternative medicines systems are still in practice that follow old healing philosophy. According to one estimate, more than 80% of the population of the developing countries prefer alternative medicines (Bodeker & Kronenberg, 2002). The major reasons behind their preference are faith in the healer, family pressure, religious and spiritual belief, affordable fee and medicine, lack of awareness, proximity, availability, and many others. However, one cannot deny the success stories of some alternative medical systems such as homeopathy and herb-based medicines (Ayurveda, Hakeem, etc.). Since herbs have their own effect on the human body which is verified by scientists. This work presents a review of the major smartphone applications based on alternative medicine practices.

Alternative Medicine or Complementary Medicine is a term referring to any practice that aims to achieve the healing effect using pseudoscience or without biological explanation (contributors). The major drawback of alternative medicine is that these medicines are not scientifically tested as claimed by different studies (contributors). Furthermore, the research in alternative treatments often fails to follow standard scientific experimental protocols. According to some researchers, alternative medicine is usually based on tradition, supernatural energies, pseudoscience, religion, or other unscientific sources (Beyerstein, 2001; Durant, Evans, & Thomas, 1989; Hines, 1988; Sampson, 1995). Yet a survey conducted in the United States reports that 38.3% of adults use alternative medicine in 2007 which was 36% in 2002 (Barnes, Bloom, & Nahin, 2008).

Based on their philosophy and employed methods the National Center on Complementary and Integrative Health classify the complementary or alternative medicine into five major classes (Shorofi & Arbon, 2017): (i) Whole medical systems (e.g. Homeopathy, and Ayurveda), (ii) Mind-body intervention (e.g. cognitive behavioral therapy), (iii) Biology-based practices, (iv) Manipulative and body-based practices, and (v) Energy medicines (e.g. Bio-electromagnetic therapies). In this work, we present the review of most popular Android-based smartphone applications that belongs to the two most popular alternative medicines systems i.e. Homeopathy and Ayurveda.

The rest of the chapter is organized as follows: In Section 2 we present a brief introduction, way of treatment and survey of smartphone apps related to Homeopathic way of treatment. Section 3 gives a brief introduction, way of treatment and survey of smartphone apps related to Ayurvedic way of treatment. While the conclusion is presented in section 4.

2. HOMEOPATHY

In 1796, Samuel Hahnemann created one of the most popular alternative medicine system Homeopathy based on the philosophy, "like cures like" (or in Latin "similia similibus curentur"). More precisely, according to Homeopathic philosophy, a substance that causes the symptoms of a disease in a person can cure similar symptoms in a sick person (Hahnemann, 1833). Originally the concept of "like cures like" was suggested by Hippocrates when he prescribes a small dose of mandrake root to the patient to cure mania (Hemenway, 1894). However, the treatments based on that concept often worsened the symptoms (Kaufman, 1971). Hahnemann rejected the old practice (Singh & Ernst, 2008) and present a lower dose single drug concept. Hahnemann believed in Vitalism theory (Craig, 1998) and according to him, the cause of a disease is the un-tuning of the vital force which expresses itself on the outside of the body by many various symptoms (Hahnemann, 1996). More precisely, diseases are only dynamic disharmonies of human being existence and nature, therefore it is impossible for people to destroy them in any other way than through forces and power, which also have the ability to bring forward dynamic changes of the human existence; that is the diseases will be really and dynamically cured through medicines (Hahnemann, 1996) (Madsen, 2019). He believed that all diseases have physical and spiritual causes (Pray & Worthen, 2003). In his view medicines directly affect the nerves, that is, that part of the body which is in the closest contact with the soul. By diluting medicines their coarse effect is removed on other organs except for the nervous system. After the medicament has been freed of coarse and useless matter what is left is a medicament weaker in material substance but dynamically more effective. He introduced the dynamic potentization methods of drugs to reveal the hidden dynamic healing force from inside the drug (Clarke, 1998; Rowe, 1998). He then performed various experiments and published them with the name "Materia Medica Pura" in 1810 (Hahnemann, 1996).

According to the British Homeopathic Association (BHA) ("What is homeopathy?," 2019), Homeopathy is a holistic kind of treatment that treats the spirit, mind, body and even emotions of the patient. By considering all factors and symptoms, a Homeopathic practitioner will select most appropriate medicine for the patient in order to simulate his/her own healing ability. Although some studies claimed that the philosophy of Homeopathy is scientifically incorrect (Baran, Kiani, & Samuel, 2014; Ladyman, 2013; Smith, 2012; Tuomela, 1987), however BHA claims that homeopathic medicines are safe to use and rarely cause side effects. Their claim is based on the Randomized Controlled Trials (RCTs) reported in more than 100 research articles published in reputed peer-reviewed journals on different medical conditions up to 2014. According to the results, 5% of these RCTs have reported a balance of negative evidence, 41% a balance of positive evidence, and 54% have not been conclusively negative or positive. The medical conditions in which positive RCTs have been reported are rheumatic disease, allergies, vertigo, upper respiratory tract infections, sinusitis, childhood diarrhea, influenza, hay fever, and insomnia. Similarly, a pilot study was conducted over 1602 follow-up patients of five NHS (National Health Service) Homeopathic hospitals in 2008 (Thompson et al., 2008). The study was aimed to examine the patients with different chronic conditions such as menopausal disorder, chronic fatigue syndrome, depression, eczema and depression under homeopathic treatment. The results showed that 34% patients reported improvement in their condition in second appointment. Due to this marvelous reputation of homeopathic way of treatment, more than 200 million people use homeopathy medicines on regular basis worldwide including Pakistan, India, Mexico, United States of America, and some European countries (Prasad, 2007).

2.1 Homeopathic Way of Treatment

For homeopathic treatments, homeopathic practitioners usually prescribe remedies using two references: Materia Medica and Repertories. Materia Medica is a collection of remedies arranged alphabetically according to associated symptoms patterns. While repertory is the collection of symptoms of disease with their associated remedy (Jonas, 2005). The sources of homeopathic remedies are Minerals, Plants,

Animals, Sarcodes, Nosodes, and Imponderabilia. Where Sarcodes are preparation from the secretions of organisms and healthy animal tissues ("List of Sarcode and Nosode remedies in Homeopathy," 2016) such as D.N.A, Aorta, Adrenalin, etc. While Nosodes are prepared from the pathological samples of diseased persons or animals (Crislip, 2010) such as diseased tissue, saliva, blood, urine, or pus (similar to the concept of vaccination). Similarly, Imponderabilia includes natural or artificial energies (Crislip, 2010) such as lunar, magnetic, solar, etc.

One of the major and basic processes in homeopathy drug preparation is "homeopathic dilution". The dilution process is also called "potentiation" process in which the drug source is diluted with distilled water or alcohol to minimize the negative effect of the drug over the human body. The dilution process of each drug is carried out by accruing by three types of scales, Decimal Scale, Centesimal Scale, and Fifty Millesimal Scale (Kayne, 2006; Patil et al., 2019). Then according to the severity of signs and symptoms, treatments are suggested to the patients.

2.2 Smartphone Applications for Homeopathy

For this survey, we have selected the five most popular Android platform apps related to the homeopathic way of treatment. The apps are selected based on the number of reviews, user rating and the number of downloads provided by Google's play store. Among those 5 apps, 3 belongs to the general category that provides general-purpose homeopathic therapy. Whereas the remaining two apps are for pocket prescribing references i.e. Materia Medica and Repertory. Table 1 gives the statistics of each selected app based on reviews, ratings, and number of downloads. The review of each app is given below.

2.2.1 Materia Medica Lite

Materia Medica Lite is an offline pocket reference guide that allows the user to search homeopathic remedies by either Materia Medica or by remedies. The current version of this application is the collection of six well-known Materia Medicas including Materia Medicas by Boericke (Boericke, 2001), Lectures On Homeopathic Materia Medica By J.T. Kent (Kent, 1904), Keynotes on Materia Medica by Allen (Allen, 2002), Materia Medica by Nash (Dubey, 1975), Materia Medica by Clarke (Clarke, 1902), and Seven hundred Redline symptoms. Apart from the collection of Materia Medica, this app also has Organon 6th edition (one of the basic books of homeopathy), and Facts about homeopathy.

According to the user perspective and reviews, the offline search engine feature is considered to be the best feature of this app. Similarly, most of the users agreed that the vast collection of famous Materia Medicas gives a better idea about remedy selection. Apart from the positive aspects, most of the users

Table 1. Homeopathic selected Application

Name	Reviews	Rating	Downloads
Materia Medica Lite	4594	4.4	100,000+
Homeo Guide	5026	4.3	100,000+
Shifa Repertory Homoeopathy	682	4.1	50,000+
Select Remedy	966	4.5	10,000+
Theory of Acutes	1133	4.6	10,000+

complained about its user interface, annoying advertisements and lack of updates in new drugs. Overall 10 Million plus download shows that this app is one of the favorite homeopathic apps.

2.2.2 Homeo Guide

Homeo Guide app is a general-purpose app that suggests homeopathic medicines for different common diseases such as allergies, flu, cough, cold, gastroenteritis, etc. This app provides a short description of the diseases with a suggested homeopathic remedy. Although the app lacks the facility of local search however, the list of drugs and list of symptoms are alphabetically arranged to find the information of desired drug or symptoms. This app also allows the user to mark a symptom or a drug as favorites in order to get a quick reference. Additionally, this app also provides some extra downloadable material and information such as reference books about basic homeopathy, downloadable link to their other apps like homeopathy treatment for children and homeopathy treatment for pets.

The users' perspective about this app is positive, as the average rating of this app is 4.3 out of 5. Many users found it fast, easy to use and helpful even for non-homeopathic practitioners. However, most of the users recorded complaints about annoying advertisements, small buttons, limited disease lists, and a lack of drug potency suggestion features. Moreover, some users' complaints that this app sends the user's location to the app publisher that might breach the location privacy of the user.

2.2.3 Shifa Repertory Homoeopathy

Shifa Repertory Homoeopathy is a comprehensive homeopathic app that can help homeopathic doctors, students, patients, or even the general public. It have efficient patients management system, online discussion forum, chat facility with the specialist, private messaging service, abbreviation glossary, well known Repertories (Kent, 1992), Boenninghausen (Boger, 1995), and Boger (Boger & von der Lieth, 2004) and Materia Medica (Kent, 1992), Allen (2002), and Boericke (2001), reversed repertory feature, Organon and many other notable features. Shifa Repertory Homoeopathy is a good application for offline use, with better user interface, local search facility, and quick remedy reference facility. Moreover, this application is also available for Apple's iOS platform.

With over 50 thousand downloads and 4.1 rating, this application makes remarkable progress in the users' community. Most of the users gave a 5-star rating to this app however, most of the items in this app are not free due to which some the users prefer Materia Medica Lite. Moreover, some users complaints that this application is too slow and consumes too much memory.

2.2.4 Select Remedy

Select Remedy app is based on the homeopathic repertory book "Select Your Remedy" (Das, 1981) written by Dr. Bishambar Das (Rai Bahadur). This app provides a list of despises organized according to the anatomy of the human body such as diseases related to eyes and vision, nose, throat pharynx and larynx, ears and hearing, etc. This app also provides an offline local search facility to find the treatment of specific symptoms and also gives a brief introduction of the drug with its usage and follow up guidance. Moreover, users can also share specific medicine with its symptoms on social media.

According to the users' perspective, the user interface of this app is easy and efficient. Additionally, due to consistent updates and a local search facility, this application gets a 4.5 average rating. Some of the homeopathic practitioners recommend it to the young physicians and even for common people due to its simplicity. However, one of the major shortcomings identified by the users of this app is that potency of the recommended medicine is not included.

2.2.5 Theory of Acutes

This app is based on the book titled "Theory of Acutes" (Vijayakar, 1999) written by Dr. Prafull Vijaykar. The book contains simplified methods to approach acute cases. The book contains thumb rules, flowcharts, pointers, and scientific explanations for efficient prescription and acute diseases. In the app, users can not only search for the remedy of the symptoms or vice versa but also add their own remedies for future reference. Users can also maintain patients and history and can share it with other users through email.

The user rating of this app is 4.6 based on the reviews of 1133 users. Most of the users found this app very helpful and handy in case of acute diseases. Most of the users recommend it for students and even some of them found it useful. However, some of the user complaints about the failure of the chat feature and automatic uninstall problem.

3. AYURVEDA

Ayurveda is another well-known kind of alternative medicine that was developed in the Indian sub-continent (Meulenbeld, 1999) and still, it is in practice in India and countries beyond India. Ayurvedic treatment is based on the ancient holy text "Sushruta Samhita" (Bhishagratna, 1911) in Sanskrit on surgery and medicine written by "Sushruta" in 6th century BC (Hoernle, 1907). Ayurveda is one of the early medicine systems which is still widely in practice (Wujastyk & Smith, 2013). Although the origin of Ayurveda has traced back 6 century BC (in the form of Vedas), however some of the concepts have existed since Indus valley civilization (3300 BC – 1300 BC) (Svoboda, 1992). Word Ayurveda is the combination of two Sanskrit words "Ayur" means life and "Veda" means science or knowledge (it is also referred to as a religious text in Hinduism). Hindus believed that "Dhanvantari" (god of Ayurveda) taught medicine to the Sushruta while he incarnated himself as a king of Varanasi and thought the knowledge of medicine to a group of human physicians (Britannica, 1993). According to Narayanaswamy, Ayurveda is the discipline of "Upaveda" (part of Veda) and also mentioned in "Atharvaveda" (Narayanaswamy, 1981). Ancient Ayurveda text is about surgical techniques such as extraction of kidney stones or foreign objects (Raju, 2003), however, the therapies evaluated from the last two millennia (Selin, 2002). During the Vedic period (1500 BCE- 1100 BCE), Ayurveda developed significantly which also inspired other religions such as Buddhism and Jainism (Gupta, Sharma, & Sharma, 2014).

There are three major texts on Ayurveda are available, the Charaka Samhita, the Sushruta Samhita, and the Bhela Samhita (6th century BC). The text is then adopted and updated by Buddhist scholars in the 2nd century AD. During 5th and 8th century AD, the text is translated into Chinese (Wujastyk, 2012), Arabic and Persian languages (Selin, 2013). In 12th century AD, after the translation into Arabic language, the Ayurveda eventually reached Europe. During the colonial era, in favor of modern medicine the Ayurvedic practice was ignored. However, Ayurveda again becomes popular after Indian independence in 1947. Today Ayurveda is the part of Indian National health care system in state hospitals (Bodeker & Ong, 2005).

Currently, most of the Ayurvedic medicines are composed of minerals, metals, and complex herbal compounds. However, besides medicines, Ayurveda emphasizes the improvement in person's lifestyle practices for good health and prevention and treatment of illness. These practices are massage, meditation, yoga, and dietary changes (Team, 2017). Despite the fact that herbal compounds might be beneficial for the human body, yet they are not tested scientifically. Moreover, some of the drugs contain toxic metal such as arsenic, mercury, and lead which are fatal for human health (Saper et al., 2008). Even though the fact that Ayurvedic way of treatment is not scientifically tested, yet 80% of the Indian population uses Ayurvedic (Piane & Eggleston, 2016).

3.1. Ayurveda Way of Treatment

Ayurvedic medicine is holistic, which means viewing the body and mind as a whole. Ayurveda not only treats a person's physical complaints, but it also changes lifestyle practices to help maintain or improve health. According to the concepts of Ayurveda, bodily substances are composed of five elements, water, ether, air, fire, and earth (Underwood & Rhodes, 2008). Apart from the previous five elements, there are other three bodily bio-elements "Kapha", "Vata", and "Pitta" (Patwardhan, Warude, Pushpangadan, & Bhatt, 2005) which are also called as "Doshas" as shown in Figure 1. According to Ayurveda, the imbalance of these Doshas results in disease while the balance in these Doshas is required for optimal health.

- **Kapha:** Represents the water and earth element that governed the physical structure and immune system of the human body. Kapha also represents the watery element in the body and charac-

Figure 1. Representation of five elements and three Doshas of Ayurveda (Wikipedia, n.d.a)

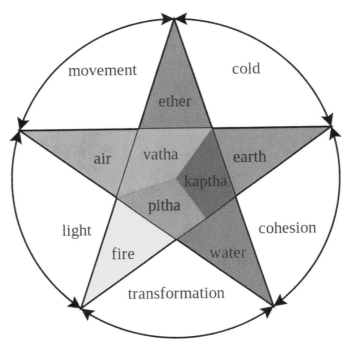

terized by slowness, heaviness, lubrication, tenderness, coldness, and the carrier of nutrients. Moreover, Kapha is also responsible to control human emotions such as love, calmness, greed, and forgiveness (Susruta, 1963).

- **Vata:** Represents the ether and air element that controls all the movement and the part related to the movement of the body such as breathing, joint, and muscle, heartbeat etc. Vata is characterized by cold, minute, dry and movements and it also controls the different functions of nervous system such as pain, fear, anxiety, etc (Susruta, 1963).
- **Pitta:** Represents the water and fire element that controls the body related functions such as intelligence, metabolism, digestion, skin color, etc. Pitta is characterized by sourness, heat, liquidity, heat, and sharpness and it controls the emotions of jealousy, hate, and anger (Susruta, 1963).

The Doshas are also related to the human's physical appearance, for example, the person with Kapha makeup usually has well developed and bigger body structure as compere to Vata based who are small and thin build. While Pitta builds persons are muscular and medium build. Usually every person's body is considered to have a combination of Doshas, with one Dosha is usually being predominant.

Ayurvedic medicines in are divided into eight major components according to the earlier classical work i.e. general medicine (Kayachikitsa), Children medicine (Kaumara-bhrtya), extraction of foreign object and surgical techniques (Salyatantra), ENT treatment (Shalakyatantra), pacification of sprits (Bhuta-vidya), Toxicology (Agadatantra), intellect, strength and life span increasing tonics (Rasayantantra), and treatment for increasing sexual pleasure and viability of semen (Vajikaranatantra) (Bhishagratna, 1911; Fields, 2014). For diagnosis, Ayurvedic practitioners use pulse, urine, stool, tongue, speech, touch, vision and appearance of the patient (Mishra, Singh, & Dagenais, 2001). Usually, Ayurveda recommends that a person should attain vitality by building a healthy metabolic system and maintaining good digestion and excretion (Shapiro, 2006). For that purpose, Ayurvedic practitioners recommend meditation, yoga, and exercise with better hygiene (Wikipedia, n.d.a).

The usual source for Ayurvedic medicines is part of plants including, seeds, fruits, roots, bark, and leaves. However, animal products (such as milk, gallstones, fats, and bones) and minerals (such as arsenic, copper, gold, lead, etc.) are also prescribed as medicine or use as a component of the medicine (Gyamfi, 2019). Sometimes alcoholic products are also used to balance the Doshas (Sekar, 2007).

3.2 Smartphone Applications for Ayurveda

For this survey, we have selected the 5 most popular Android platform apps related to the Ayurvedic way of treatment. The apps selection criteria kept the same as for homeopathic app selection. The apps are selected based on the number of reviews, user rating and the number of downloads provided by Google's play store. The statics of each selected app is given in Table 2. The review of each app is given below:

3.2.1 Ayurvedic Treatments (Ayurveda)

Ayurvedic Treatments is one of the most popular apps that provides several therapies, medicines, treatments, and tips in the Hindi language. This app provides Ayurvedic treatments and therapies of Diabetes mellitus, kidney stones, sexual disorder, and hormone therapies, gas, acidity and constipation treatments, and other common diseases. Moreover, this app also provides different types of diet plans such as weight gain, weight loss, etc. and different types of beauty tips for hairs, skin and other body parts.

Table 2. Ayurvedic selected application

Name	Reviews	Rating	Downloads
Ayurvedic Treatments (Ayurveda)	3368	4.3	500,000+
101 Natural Home Remedies Cure	1908	4.3	100,000+
Ayurveda Products and Ayurveda Tips	2165	4.4	100,000+
Ayurveda	804	4.1	100,000+
Ayurveda - Cures n Remedies	995	4.3	50,000+

With over 500k downloads and more frequent updates, this app is among the most successful apps of the Google play store. Most users have given positive reviews for this app, however, the major downside of this app is its language. For the users who know Hindi, this app may be more than useful but the English version of this app might increase the popularity of this app in other countries. Also, this app lacks the local search feature.

3.2.2 101 Natural Home Remedies Cure

This smartphone app is a perfect application for finding naturals and Ayurvedic homemade remedy for common symptoms efficiently and quickly. The symptoms and diseases are organized in alphabetical order with a local search facility. This app provides a remedy for common health issues such as asthma, burns, cough, skin, wart, sore throat and many more.

Many users shared their success stories regarding the effective treatment of their illness using this app. Most of the users liked this app due to cost-effective and natural items used as medicine. More than 100k downloads and 4.3 user-rating (average), this app can be one of the best instant access handbook for the user. Apart from so many good features some users complaint about the limited information about remedies and annoying advertisements.

3.2.3 Ayurveda Products and Ayurveda Tips

This app provides a wide variety of Ayurvedic products that the user can order for home delivery. Their products include pure ghee (clarified butter), honey, medicinal fruit juices, and health drinks, beauty products, such as bathing soaps and shampoos, different kinds of oils, toothpaste, face creams and other variety of Ayurvedic products and medicines. Users can search their desired products and brands using the inbuilt search engine. Users can also compare and order their desired product. Apart from Ayurvedic products, this app also provides different tips on a daily basis to the users.

The user rating of this app is 4.4 based on the reviews of 2165 users. Most of the users appreciated the homed livery system of Ayurvedic products, product search, and comparison feature, and "tip of the day" feature. The user interface of this app is easy to use. However, the home delivery feature is only available in India which is one of the major drawbacks of the app due to which some of the users prefer Amazon's app.

3.2.4 Ayurveda

This app provides a brief overview, history, philosophy, and treatment approaches of Ayurveda. Using this app, the user can also find Ayurvedic treatment according to his/her customized Doshas and mental constitution. User can also find a list of common health problem connected with each Doshas with explanation and cure, guideline about nutrients, Ayurvedic terms glossary, exercises, diet plans, list of incompatible food products, methods for meditation, purification and detoxification, recommendation of massage oils, various kinds of diagnostics methods, tips, therapies and many other things in paid version.

According to users' reviews, the app is very easy and useful for even for non-practitioners however, most of the content of the app is available only in the paid version which is very nominal (around 1.5 US$). Some of the users also suggested adding more features to the app such as more recipes, Ayurvedic books, etc. Over 100k downloads and 4.1 user ratings show that this app is among the popular apps among Ayurvedic fans.

3.2.5 Ayurveda - Cures n Remedies

This app provides Ayurvedic remedies and cure for common and rare diseases such as aids, anemia, cough, body heat, asthma, and many others using herbs and other items that can be found in the garden and kitchen. The app provides 2-3 Ayurvedic remedies for every disease or symptom. Furthermore, this app also provides "Ask to Expert" feature that allows the user to get an expert's opinion on any disease, symptom, and remedy.

According to the user perspective, navigation is not user-friendly, too many annoying advertisements and the symptoms are not sorted alphabetically. The success stories shared by the users show the importance of this app.

4. CONCLUSION

The statistics released WHO[1] and NCCIH[2] by the clearly support the fact that more than 80% population of developing countries rely on alternative medicine systems. For centuries, people use variety of alternative medicine systems which are based on their religion, faith, tradition. In this work, we present the review of most popular smartphone applications belongs to two most popular alternative medicines systems i.e. Homeopathy and Ayurveda with their way of treatment. During the analysis of the users' review, it was noted that most of the users are satisfied with the smartphone app. Based on this fact we can implicitly conclude that these medical systems can effectively solve users' health-related issues. Although most of the alternative medicine systems are reportedly not tested using standard scientific procedures, yet there are many success stories of these medicine systems. Besides that, most of the herbal-based medicines in different alternate medicine systems are scientifically proved beneficial for human health. Moreover, the scientific methods applied to test the medicines might need to be upgraded by the time and should according to the philosophy of the alternative medicine systems.

5. FUTURE WORK

This work presents the review of ten most popular Android-based smartphone applications belongs to two most popular alternative medicines systems i.e. Homeopathy and Ayurveda are presented. However, there are other very important areas which need to be investigated and introduced in future. In future the chapters can be written on other alternative medicine systems. Similarly, as the major competitor of android, iOS (Apple) and Windows (Microsoft), based smartphones are also famous. Therefore, future chapters can also be written from this perspective as well.

REFERENCES

Allen, H. C. (2002). *Keynotes and Characteristics with Comparisons of some of the Leading Remedies of the Materia Medica with Bowel Nosodes.* B. Jain Publishers.

Baran, G. R., Kiani, M. F., & Samuel, S. P. (2014). *Science, Pseudoscience, and Not Science: How Do They Differ? In Healthcare and Biomedical Technology in the 21st Century* (pp. 19–57). Springer.

Barnes, P. M., Bloom, B., & Nahin, R. L. (2008). Complementary and alternative medicine use among adults and children; United States, 2007. CDC Stacks Public Health Publications.

Beyerstein, B. L. (2001). Alternative medicine and common errors of reasoning. *Academic Medicine,* *76*(3), 230–237. doi:10.1097/00001888-200103000-00009 PMID:11242572

Bhishagratna, K. L. (1911). *An English translation of The Sushruta Samhita: based on original Sanskrit text* (Vol. 2). author.

Bodeker, G., & Kronenberg, F. (2002). A public health agenda for traditional, complementary, and alternative medicine. *American Journal of Public Health, 92*(10), 1582–1591. doi:10.2105/AJPH.92.10.1582 PMID:12356597

Bodeker, G., & Ong, C.-K. (2005). *WHO global atlas of traditional, complementary and alternative medicine* (Vol. 1). World Health Organization.

Boericke, W. (2001). *New manual of homoeopathic materia medica and repertory.* B. Jain Publishers.

Boger, C. M. (1995). *Boenninghausen's Characteristics Materia Medica and Repertory. Indian Reprint Edition.* New Delhi: B. Jain Publishers.

Boger, C. M., & von der Lieth, B. (2004). *General Analysis.* Von der Lieth.

Britannica, E. (1993). *Encyclopædia britannica.* Chicago: University of Chicago.

Clarke, J. H. (1902). *A dictionary of pratical materia medica*: homoeopathic publishing Company.

Clarke, J. H. (1998). *The Prescriber: How to Practice Homoeopathy*: B. Jain Publishers. contributors, W. Alternative medicine. Retrieved from https://en.wikipedia.org/w/index.php?title=Alternative_medicine&oldid=906879807

Craig, E. (1998). *Routledge encyclopedia of philosophy: questions to sociobiology* (Vol. 8). Taylor & Francis.

Crislip, M. (2010). Homeopathic Vaccines. *Science-Based Medicine.* Retrieved from https://science-basedmedicine.org/homeopathic-vaccines/

Das, B. (1981). *Select your remedy.* Vishwamber Free Homeo Dispensary.

Dubey, S. (1975). *Textbook of Materia Medica.* Dubey.

Durant, J. R., Evans, G. A., & Thomas, G. P. (1989). The public understanding of science. *Nature, 340*(6228), 11–14. doi:10.1038/340011a0 PMID:2739718

Fields, G. P. (2014). *Religious therapeutics: Body and health in yoga, ayurveda, and tantra.* SUNY Press.

Gupta, P., Sharma, V. K., & Sharma, S. (2014). *Healing traditions of the Northwestern Himalayas.* Springer. doi:10.1007/978-81-322-1925-5

Gyamfi, E. T. (2019). Metals and metalloids in traditional medicines (Ayurvedic medicines, nutraceuticals and traditional Chinese medicines). *Environmental Science and Pollution Research International,* 1–12. PMID:31004267

Hahnemann, S. (1833). *The Homœopathic Medical Doctrine: Or," Organon of the Healing Art."* WF Wakeman.

Hahnemann, S. (1996). Materia medica pura (Vol. 2). B. Jain Publishers.

Hemenway, H. B. (1894). Modern Homeopathy And Medical Science. *Journal of the American Medical Association, 22*(11), 367–377. doi:10.1001/jama.1894.02420900001001

Hines, T. (1988). *Pseudoscience and the paranormal: A critical examination of the evidence.* Prometheus Books.

Hoernle, A. F. R. (1907). *Studies in the medicine of ancient India: Osteology, or the bones of the human body.* Clarendon Press.

Hulkower, R. (2016). The history of the Hippocratic Oath: Outdated, inauthentic, and yet still relevant. *The Einstein Journal of Biology and Medicine; EJBM, 25*(1), 41–44. doi:10.23861/EJBM20102542

Jonas, W. B. (2005). Dictionary of complementary and alternative medicine. *Journal of Alternative and Complementary Medicine, 11*(4), 739–740. doi:10.1089/acm.2005.11.739

Kaufman, M. (1971). *Homeopathy in America: The rise and fall of a medical heresy.* The Johns Hopkins Press.

Kayne, S. B. (2006). *Homeopathic pharmacy: theory and practice.* Elsevier Health Sciences.

Kent, J. T. (1904). *Lectures on homeopathic materia medica with new remedies. New Dehli: B.* Jain Publishers.

Kent, J. T. (1992). *Repertory of the homoeopathic materia medica.* B. Jain Publishers.

Ladyman, J. (2013). Toward a demarcation of science from pseudoscience. In *Philosophy of pseudoscience: Reconsidering the demarcation problem* (pp. 45-59). Academic Press.

List of Sarcode and Nosode remedies in Homeopathy. (2016). Homeobook. Retrieved from https://www.homeobook.com/list-of-sarcode-and-nosode-remedies-in-homeopathy/

Madsen, R. (2019). Characteristics of Contemporary Methodologies of Classic Homeopathy. *Homœopathic Links, 32*(1), 18-22.

Meulenbeld, G. J. (1999). *A history of Indian medical literature* (Vol. 3). E. Forsten Groningen.

Mishra, L.-c., Singh, B. B., & Dagenais, S. (2001). Healthcare and disease management in Ayurveda. *Alternative Therapies in Health and Medicine, 7*(2), 44–51. PMID:11253416

Narayanaswamy, V. (1981). Origin and development of ayurveda:(a brief history). *Ancient Science of Life, 1*(1), 1. PMID:22556454

Patil, A. D., Chinche, A. D., Singh, A. K., Peerzada, S. P., Barkund, S. A., Shah, J. N., & Jadhav, A. B. (2019). Ultra high dilutions: A review on in vitro studies against pathogens.

Patwardhan, B., Warude, D., Pushpangadan, P., & Bhatt, N. (2005). Ayurveda and traditional Chinese medicine: A comparative overview. *Evidence-Based Complementary and Alternative Medicine, 2*(4), 465–473. doi:10.1093/ecam/neh140 PMID:16322803

Piane, G. M., & Eggleston, B. M. (2016). Complementary, Alternative, And Integrative Health Approaches Among West Asian American Communities. *Complementary, Alternative, and Integrative Health, Multicultural Perspectives*, 305.

Prasad, R. (2007). Homoeopathy booming in India. *Lancet, 370*(9600), 1679–1680. doi:10.1016/S0140-6736(07)61709-7 PMID:18035598

Pray, W. S., & Worthen, D. B. (2003). *A history of nonprescription product regulation.* CRC Press.

Raju, V. (2003). Susruta of ancient India. *Indian Journal of Ophthalmology, 51*(2), 119. PMID:12831140

Rosenthal, F. (2015). *The physician in medieval Muslim society. In Man versus Society in Medieval Islam* (pp. 1026–1042). BRILL.

Rowe, T. (1998). *Homeopathic Methodology: Repertory, Case Taking, and Case Analysis: an Introductory Homeopathic Workbook.* North Atlantic Books.

Sampson, W. (1995). Antiscience Trends In The Rise of The "Alternative Medicine' movement. *Annals of the New York Academy of Sciences, 775*(1), 188–197. doi:10.1111/j.1749-6632.1996.tb23138.x PMID:8678416

Saper, R. B., Phillips, R. S., Sehgal, A., Khouri, N., Davis, R. B., Paquin, J., ... Kales, S. N. (2008). Lead, mercury, and arsenic in US-and Indian-manufactured Ayurvedic medicines sold via the Internet. *Journal of the American Medical Association, 300*(8), 915–923. doi:10.1001/jama.300.8.915 PMID:18728265

Sekar, S. (2007). Traditional alcoholic beverages from Ayurveda and their role on human health.

Selin, H. (2002). A History of Indian Medical Literature.

Selin, H. (2013). *Encyclopaedia of the history of science, technology, and medicine in non-westen cultures*. Springer Science & Business Media.

Shapiro, H. (2006). *Medicine across cultures: history and practice of medicine in non-western cultures* (Vol. 3). Springer Science & Business Media.

Shorofi, S. A., & Arbon, P. (2017). Complementary and alternative medicine (CAM) among Australian hospital-based nurses: Knowledge, attitude, personal and professional use, reasons for use, CAM referrals, and socio-demographic predictors of CAM users. *Complementary Therapies in Clinical Practice, 27*, 37–45. doi:10.1016/j.ctcp.2017.03.001 PMID:28438278

Singh, S., & Ernst, E. (2008). *Trick or treatment: The undeniable facts about alternative medicine*. WW Norton & Company.

Smith, K. (2012). Homeopathy is unscientific and unethical. *Bioethics, 26*(9), 508–512. doi:10.1111/j.1467-8519.2011.01956.x PMID:22506737

Susruta, S. (1963). *An English translation of the Sushruta samhita, based on original Sanskrit text* (Vol. 30). Рипол Классик.

Svoboda, R. (1992). *Ayurveda: Life, health and longevity*. Penguin Books India.

HCD Team. (2017). Ayurveda. *Health Topics* Retrieved from https://www.healthlinkbc.ca/health-topics/aa116840spec

Thompson, E. A., Mathie, R. T., Baitson, E. S., Barron, S. J., Berkovitz, S. R., Brands, M., ... Mercer, S. W. (2008). Towards standard setting for patient-reported outcomes in the NHS homeopathic hospitals. *Homeopathy, 97*(03), 114–121. doi:10.1016/j.homp.2008.06.005 PMID:18657769

Tuomela, R. (1987). *Science, protoscience, and pseudoscience. In Rational Changes in Science* (pp. 83–101). Springer.

Underwood, E., & Rhodes, P. (2008). History of medicine. In *Encyclopaedia Brittanica*. Chicago, IL: Encyclopaedia Brittanica.

Vijayakar, P. (1999). *Predictive Homoeopathy*. Preeti Publishers.

What is homeopathy? (2019). *Homeopathy*. Retrieved from https://www.britishhomeopathic.org/homeopathy/what-is-homeopathy/

Wikipedia. (2019b). History of medicine. Retrieved from https://en.wikipedia.org/w/index.php?title=History_of_medicine&oldid=905929535

Wikipedia. (n.d.a). Ayurveda.

Wujastyk, D. (2012). *Well-mannered medicine: Medical ethics and etiquette in classical ayurveda*. Oxford University Press. doi:10.1093/acprof:oso/9780199856268.001.0001

Wujastyk, D., & Smith, F. M. (2013). *Modern and global Ayurveda: pluralism and paradigms*. Suny Press.

ADDITIONAL READING

Annigeri, N. M., & Sunagar, P. (2018). Ayurveda Upachara-An Android app. *International Journal of Advanced Research in Computer Science*, 9(1), 354–356. doi:10.26483/ijarcs.v9i1.5301

Baharum, A., Ismail, R., Fabeil, N. F., Fatah, N. S. A., Hanapi, R., & Zain, N. H. M. (2018). Sabah Traditional Medicine Database and Application: SabahTMed. *Advanced Science Letters*, 24(3), 1834–1838. doi:10.1166/asl.2018.11171

Bonizzoni, G., Caminati, M., Ridolo, E., Landi, M., Ventura, M. T., Lombardi, C., ... Gani, F. (2019). Use of complementary medicine among patients with allergic rhinitis: An Italian nationwide survey. *Clinical and Molecular Allergy*, 17(1), 2. doi:10.118612948-019-0107-1 PMID:30804711

Foley, H., Steel, A., Cramer, H., Wardle, J., & Adams, J. (2019). Disclosure of complementary medicine use to medical providers: A systematic review and meta-analysis. *Scientific Reports*, 9(1), 1573. doi:10.103841598-018-38279-8 PMID:30733573

Foroughi, N., Zhu, K. C. Y., Smith, C., & Hay, P. (2019). The perceived therapeutic benefits of complementary medicine in eating disorders. *Complementary Therapies in Medicine*, 43, 176–180. doi:10.1016/j.ctim.2019.01.025 PMID:30935527

Gray, A. C., Diezel, H., & Steel, A. (2019). The use of learning technologies in complementary medicine education: Results of a student technology survey. In Advances in Integrative Medicine. Academic Press.

Huber, B. M., von Schoen-Angerer, T., Hasselmann, O., Wildhaber, J., & Wolf, U. (2019). Swiss paediatrician survey on complementary medicine. *Swiss Medical Weekly*, 149(2324). PMID:31203577

Kaur, J., Hamajima, N., Yamamoto, E., Saw, Y. M., Kariya, T., Soon, G. C., ... Sharon, S. H. (2019). Patient satisfaction on the utilization of traditional and complementary medicine services at public hospitals in Malaysia. *Complementary Therapies in Medicine*, 42, 422–428. doi:10.1016/j.ctim.2018.12.013 PMID:30670278

Mills, P. J., Peterson, C. T., Wilson, K. L., Pung, M. A., Patel, S., Weiss, L., ... & Chopra, D. (2019). Relationships among classifications of ayurvedic medicine diagnostics for imbalances and western measures of psychological states: An exploratory study. *Journal of Ayurveda and Integrative Medicine, 10*, 198-202.

Mookherjee, A., Mulay, P., Joshi, R., Prajapati, P. S., Johari, S., & Prajapati, S. S. (2019). Sentilyser: Embedding Voice Markers in Homeopathy Treatments. In Interdisciplinary Approaches to Information Systems and Software Engineering (pp. 181-206). Hershey, PA: IGI Global.

Nedungadi, P., Jayakumar, A., & Raman, R. (2018). Personalized health monitoring system for managing well-being in rural areas. *Journal of Medical Systems*, 42(1), 22. doi:10.100710916-017-0854-9 PMID:29242996

Panda, B., Mohapatra, M. K., Paital, S., Kumbhakar, S., Dutta, A., Kadam, S., ... Manchanda, R. K. (2019). Prevalence of afebrile malaria and development of risk-scores for gradation of villages: A study from a hot-spot in Odisha. *PLoS One*, 14(9), e0221223. doi:10.1371/journal.pone.0221223 PMID:31490940

Parvathamma, N. (2018). Use of Information Resources and Services in Ayurvedic Medical College Libraries in Karnataka State India: A Study.

Sherly, S. I., Ramya, B., & Dhinesh, D. (2019). Android Mobile Application for Disease Diagnosis System. *Engineering Reports*, 2(1), 86–90.

Van Galen, L. S., Xu, X., Koh, M. J. A., Thng, S., & Car, J. (2019). Eczema apps conformance with clinical guidelines: A systematic assessment of functions, tools and content. *British Journal of Dermatology*. PMID:31179535

KEY TERMS AND DEFINITIONS

Alternate Medicine: Alternate or alternative medicine term is refer to the medicine system, theories and practices that are scientifically untested and lacks the biological plausibility instead they rely on pseudoscience and some supernatural phenomena. While according to the definition of United States National Center for Complementary and Integrative Medicine (NCCIH), a group of products, practices, and health care systems that are not generally considered as part of conventional medicines are called Alternative Medicine Systems.

Android: Android is open source Linux kernel based operating mobile platform based smart gadgets such as tablets, phones etc. Apart from mobile platform, variants android operating systems are also available for other electronic devices such, smart TV, PC, cameras, gaming consoles, wearable devices etc.

Ayurveda: Ayurveda or Ayurvedic medicine system is classified as complementary or Alternate Medical system by United States National Center for Complementary and Integrative Medicine (NCCIH). Ayurveda is one of the oldest medical system originate from Indian subcontinent in 6th century BC and still popular in India and other countries.

Complementary Medicine (CM): A kind of alternative medicine used together with other functional treatment with the belief to improve the effect of functional medicine is called Complementary Medicine. It is also abbreviated as CAM (Complementary and Alternative Medicine).

Google Play: Google play is official online market for android based apps or software. Google Play allows users to browse and download different android based application. Google Play also provide a large variety of apps for other electronic android based devices such as smart TV, digital camera, gaming consoles etc.

Holistic Medicine: Holistic Medicine is another kind of Alternative Medicine that claim to take into account a "whole person" including body, mind, and spirit, as compare to the supposed reductionism of medicine. Similarly, according to American Holistic Health Association (AHHA) holistic medicines integrates alternative and conventional therapies to prevent and treat disease as well as to promote optimal health.

Homeopathic: Homeopathy or Homoeopathic is medical system classified as complementary or Alternate Medical system by United States National Center for Complementary and Integrative Medicine (NCCIH). This system was created by Samuel Hahnemann in 1796 and its philosophy is based on phrase *"like cure like"*.

Integrative Medicine (IM): Integrative Medicine is healing oriented medicine system that consider whole person including his/her lifestyle. Integrated or Integrative Medicine (IM) is also known as Complementary Medicine (CM).

Materia Medica: Materia Medica is a collection of reliable, pure, and real methods of action of a simple medicinal substances in Homeopathy way of treatments". In other words, Materia Medica is an encyclopedia of purported therapeutic properties of each Homeopathic medicine.

Medical App: Medical app is a smart phone application software or program that is designed to give medical related information to the user such suggestions of therapies and medicine, information about condition and diseases, new medical research etc.

Smartphone App: Smart phone app is a mobile phone application software or computer program that is designed to run on mobile devices to perform some specific task. These apps are usually available at online store operated by owner of mobile phone operating system.

Repertory: Homeopathic repertory is an index of symptoms, listed in an order with their associated remedies. It is also defined as the logically and systematically arranged index to the Homeopathic Materia Medica that also contains the information collected from clinical experience and research. It is also known as the link between diseases and Materia Medica.

Vedas: According to the Hindu religion, Vedas (singular "Veda") are a collection religious text composed in Sanskrit. Hindus belief that Vedas are authorless in fact Veda are revelations seen by ancient sages after meditation. There are four collections of Vedas, the Rigveda, the Yajurveda, the Samaveda, and the Atharvaveda.

ENDNOTES

[1]   https://www.who.int/traditional-complementary-integrative-medicine/en/

[2]   https://nccih.nih.gov

Chapter 3
Healthcare Gets Smarter:
Smart and Digital Technology Usage by Maternal and Neo-Natal Healthcare Providers

Theodora Dame Adjin-Tettey
University of Professional Studies, Accra, Ghana

ABSTRACT

There is the emerging use of smart and digital (modern) technologies, such as smart TVs, Internet of Things-connected devices, mobile devices, Big Data software and analytics in healthcare practice and administration. The deployment of such technologies is meant to provide quality, prompt, accurate, tangible information and other critical resources for patients. At a national level, drone technology is being used in African countries like Ghana and Rwanda to deliver critical medications and blood supplies to hospitals difficult to reach because of poor road infrastructure. This chapter of the book explores what technologies are being deployed at institutional levels to provide efficient medical care to patients. Fifteen maternal and neonatal health care practitioners in Accra, Ghana, were interviewed on their use of modern technologies in healthcare administration and delivery and what their challenges are. The study also explored what technologies they currently do not have that they think will be of benefit to their practice.

1. INTRODUCTION

Healthcare providers are leveraging smart technologies, such as smart TVs, Internet of Things-connected-devices, mobile devices, big data software and analytics to provide quality, prompt, accurate, tangible information and other important resources for clients or patients (Foley, 2017). These newer models of healthcare delivery thrive on collaborative efforts by different caregivers, as well as patients and are largely being facilitated by mobile technologies (Nasi, Cucciniello, & Guerrazzi, 2015). Under this circumstance, it requires that caregivers proactively deploy technology to track patients' wellbeing and also use technology and information to better engage patients and meet or exceed their expectations.

DOI: 10.4018/978-1-7998-2521-0.ch003

Digital and smart technologies are used for disease surveillance, treatment support, epidemic outbreak tracking and chronic disease management by healthcare practitioners. It is in the light of this that Kahn, Yang, and Kahn (2010) advanced that:

Innovative applications of mobile technology to existing health care delivery and monitoring systems offer great promise for improving the quality of life. They make communication among researchers, clinicians, and patients easier, and as chronic disease becomes more prevalent, mobile technologies offer care strategies that are particularly suited to combating these conditions (Kahn et al., p. 254).

In essence, while the technologies facilitate easy accessibility to patient records and offer more efficient diagnosis, patients are able to use the technologies to access relevant educational content related to their health and to manage their lives health wise.

Essentially, smart and digital technologies, be it portable or otherwise, are transforming health care systems, as they help provide accurate information about diagnosis and medications, clinical scoring and also facilitate access to healthcare resources. In this chapter, all digital or smart technologies and applications are operationalised as modern technologies. This is because they are emergent technologies that are constantly being updated and improved.

2. CONTEXTUAL BACKGROUND

In the management of non-communicable diseases like diabetes, there is evidence that technology is a great asset. Ghana is ranked sixth in sub-Saharan Africa and counts over seven million people with diabetes in the country. Among countries within the sub-Saharan African region, there are approximately 13.6 million people living with diabetes (Daily Guide, 2017). Among diabetics, there has been reported complications and reduced quality of life in certain parts of the world and Ghana is not likely an exception. This is as a result of poor self-management skills, lack of personalized education and clinical inertia, leading to grave complications (Goyal & Cafazzo, 2013).

There have been constant improvements in technologies that are used in hospital settings to offer healthcare, especially, in the area of medical diagnosis. During the Ebola outbreak, many health facilities in Ghana started using smart thermometers. These technologies, unlike the mercury-filled ones, do not need to have physical contact with human body in order to determine temperature of patients, aside the fact that they determine human body temperature within a relatively shorter time.

Also, there is the common usage of the digital pulsometer (called the fingertip pulse oximeter) which is placed at the fingertips to digitally measure the pulse of patients. This is a digital mobile device which is easy to operate. This smart digital technology measures pulse strength and pulse rate in a few seconds and displays it conveniently on a digital LED display. Yet is the use of the digital sphygmomanometer (blood pressure device). Unlike the manual instrument which requires listening while slowly releasing the pressure in the cuff that comes with the device, this digital sphygmomanometer eliminates disruptions during the listening stage that can impede proper detection of the blood pressure of a patient. The digital instrument, although uses a cuff which may be placed around the upper arm or wrist just like the manual meter, in this case, requires minimal human effort and intervention while using it.

Technology usage for healthcare delivery and management is not only at the individual and institutional levels. On a much higher level, the regulatory institution for health services in Ghana, the Ministry of Health, at the beginning of 2019 started deploying drone technology to deliver healthcare in some public hospitals in Ghana. This is to allow for vital medical supplies, such as blood, to be delivered to remote areas which typically have underdeveloped or poorly maintained roads that link them to major cities where medical supplies are found. Rwanda, an East African country, earlier in 2016 started using similar technology to deliver blood from the service base to regional hospitals.

The World Health Organization (WHO) has found that severe bleeding (usually after childbirth) is the most common cause of maternal mortality in Africa. This contributes to around 75% of all maternal deaths in Africa (WHO, 2018). These maternal deaths are largely accounted for because of shortage or late arrival of blood supply to health facilities during critical moments in health delivery. However, the use of drone technology in Rwanda is said to have cut down blood delivery time from four hours to just 15 minutes, contributing to a significant reduction in child and maternal mortality in the country (Cheruto, 2019).

Seeing the noteworthy strides made in the area of medical delivery through the use of drones chalked by Rwanda, Ghana bought into the idea. In the Ghanaian context, it has been projected that the drones will be able to travel to 500 health facilities within an 80-kilometer-range from their centre which is stocked with vaccines, emergency blood, blood products and medicines. By using this technology, it is hoped that there will be a reduction in the incidence of wastage of medical products which comes about on account of overstocking in hospitals (Cheruto, 2019).

Modern technologies are used to enhance healthcare delivery and so are intended to be purpose-driven. So, technology manufacturers must, of necessity, look out for the professional needs of healthcare providers as well as patient needs and provide relevant solutions for them. On the other hand, it is worthy to note that most of the technologies developed to enhance medical care and healthy lifestyles are produced in the global north. Less is heard or seen of Ghanaians going into the production of digital smart technologies and applications. Without understanding the cultural, social and economic contexts of target users, it is most likely technologies will be rendered unusable to potential users.

Bearing this observation in mind, it is important that digital and smart technologies and applications developers know the unique circumstances of target users before technologies are developed for them. Since healthcare technologies find their way to different parts of the world, sometimes, through aid or donation, it is important to understand the different contexts under which technologies may be used so they become usable in diverse contexts. This is because it has been found that software developers (by extension medical technologies developers) face the challenge of offering products and services that potential users hardly can easily afford or operate aside other challenges faced in certain parts of the world (Murugesan, 2013), rendering products and services unbeneficial.

An application developer should consider the context within which product is going to be used or better still, customise it to suit the needs of users in various contexts. This also goes for any other digital and smart technologies developed for the medical practice or healthcare delivery. What may work in western countries may not necessarily work in Africa and what may be useful in Africa may not be useful in western countries. Owusu and Chakraborty (2009) have proffered that "understanding user requirements is a fundamental part of information systems design and is key to the success of interactive systems" (p. 386). It is therefore important to consider factors such as ease of use, usefulness and affordability when developing digital and smart technologies. It is also vital to have cross-cultural interface designs to ensure products and services are usable and will consequently result in high acceptance rate (Rau, Plocher & Choong, 2012).

Developing a functional smart or digital health technology or application also requires the involvement of the potential user and the application of human-centered design methodologies. But the reality, according to Owusu & Chakraborty (2009) is that mHealth applications [and possibly other smart and digital technologies] are faced with usability challenges in relation to usefulness, owing to the non-inclusion of the end user during the design process. This chapter, therefore, has the intent of contributing to the suggested data gathering prerequisite needed to design and develop targeted smart health technologies which aid medical delivery.

For this reason, a critical set of end users (i.e., healthcare providers) shed light on how they are using these technologies; how the technologies are assisting them in their practice and what challenges they are faced with using smart and digital technologies. Another important area explored was the technologies currently unavailable to practitioners that they reckon will help improve service delivery in their areas of practice.

3. LITERATURE REVIEW

Smart and digital healthcare technologies may come in the form of personalized mobile/smart phone applications that are meant to enhance personal wellbeing as well as monitor one's health status at any given time. Some are in the form of gaming applications. An example is "Time to Eat", a mobile phone-based game, which is meant to motivate children to make healthy choices about food by caring for a virtual pet. In order to score high points for the game, players are to send pictures of food their pets consume throughout the day. The healthiness of the food determines the score they get and the final outcome of the game.

Undoubtedly, when a child scores high points for making healthy choices for a pet, they are likely motivated to make healthy choices for themselves too. And as Pollak, Gay, Byrne, Wagner, Retelny & Humphreys (2010) found, this game provides reliable proof for the prospect mobile phones have in deploying health games which can result in healthy living.

There are also smart and digital fitness trackers, such as the *S-Health* and wearables such as *Samsung Gear S Watch*, to track personal health status. The *S-Health* app, which seems to be popular among youthful Ghanaians, is able to monitor one's heartbeat, stress levels, weight and calories burnt over a period of time. Users are, thus, able to effectively manage their lifestyles to stay healthy.

Subscription to certain short messaging services, enabled by mobile phone technology, is also another way of enhancing wellbeing. Results of a study conducted among 30 patients diagnosed of Type 2 diabetes revealed that most of the patients had their health statuses improved with the use of internet and cell phones. Such patients received daily messages informing them to improve their diabetic self-care behaviour, which positively resulted in better wellbeing (Faridi et al., 2008). The use of mhealth technologies and their associated platforms seems to be a game changer in healthcare delivery, access and management. According to Goyal and Cafazzo (2013):

Recent evidence suggests that mobile health (mHealth) applications (apps) may be used to effectively deliver health services and self-management tools while overcoming certain barriers to provider access. A significant potential lies in the ability to communicate with individuals in real-time, be able to capture data, and provide decision support. mHealth apps may be targeted for patient use, the care provider, or both, promoting communication, sharing of information and decision-making (p. 1067).

There is evidence to suggest that many hospitals (especially in advanced countries) have taken interest in using highly sensitive wearable health devices/sensors. These Wearable Health Devices (WHDs) allow for the "ambulatory acquisition of vital signs and health status monitoring over extended periods (days/weeks) and outside clinical environments" (Dias & Paulo Silva Cunha, 2018, p. 1). The devices can be attached to the human skin or integrated with textiles, to remotely monitor human body temperature, as well as other vital signs, usually during the early stages of diagnosis (Yao, Swetha & Zhu, 2018). Statista (2017) projected that the fast-growing world-wide wearable devices market would reach $34 billion in 2019, a significant increase from $26 billion in 2017.

In neonatal care, Goyal et al. (2019) proposed using non-contact smartphone-based screening system in retinopathy of prematurity (ROP). This involves using a smartphone and +40D, +28D, or +20D indirect non-contact condensing lenses which functions as an indirect ophthalmoscope by using the coaxial light source of the phone and creating a digital image of the fundus. After using that technology to screen 228 eyes of 114 infants, it was found that the image quality was good in close to 90% of infants. The researchers concluded that this smartphone-guided imaging for ROP has a great potential as an efficient tool for teleophthalmology. This is aside the fact that it is of low cost, light weigh, portable, user friendly and has simple power sources.

Realising the importance of monitoring vital signs to aid early detection of diseases among infants and newborns so as to reduce mortality, Ali, Tahir, and Ali (2018) also suggested a system that could lessen the burden on hospitals and parents. The suggested system is also meant to enable direct intervention for unserious conditions and facilitate early intervention for serious conditions. The system is a combination of a number of functions in one single device and analyses data from sensors to diagnose conditions. This integrated system uses technology for existing medical practices, carry out real-time monitoring and provide special treatment and assistance for newborns (Ali et al., 2019).

In prenatal and maternal care the use of smart technologies is also becoming common. Alotaibi, Albalawi, and Alwakeel (2018) have developed a technological system that they believe will facilitate communication between pregnant women and healthcare providers, increase interactions amongst pregnant women, as well as motivate them to get involved in physical activities. The system offers remote monitoring of mothers and their foetuses using the smartphone and the Internet of Things (IoT) technologies. It was specially developed for pregnant women in remote areas in Saudi Arabia. Alotaibi et al. argue that their system is an all-inclusive system offering a combination of all functionalities available through individual pregnancy monitoring systems, making it a unique mhealth system.

The system architecture includes smart phone, wristband and a kick belt. It records the number of steps the pregnant woman walked during the day, counts baby kicks and offers remote care through physician follow-up, social networking and the sharing of educational content by physicians connected to the network. Information on pregnant women gleaned from the system is stored through Wi-fi in a database and made available to healthcare providers through the cloud technology.

To assess the practicability of using the smart wristband to collect continuous activity, sleep and heart rate data from the beginning of the second trimester until one month postpartum, Grym et al. (2019) recruited 20 pregnant women for an experiment. Each participant used the smart wristband for an average of 182 days throughout the seven-month study. Participants who were unable to wear smart wristbands at work used the device 300 min less each day compared to those who used it limitlessly and eight participants stopped wearing the devices or rarely wore them after giving birth. Nineteen participants held that the smart wristband did not have long-lasting consequences on their behaviour. Reasons for not using the smart wristbands ranged from "problems with charging and synchronizing the devices, perceiving the devices as uncomfortable, or viewing the data as unreliable, and the fear of scratching their babies with the devices" (Grym et al., 2019, p. 1). The researchers found the wristband to be practicable for the continuous tracking, monitoring and transmission of personal health metrics in real time as part of maternity care. However, the daily use decreased after birth. There were also challenges related to pregnant women being prohibited from wearing the device at work as well as some technical problems encountered during usage.

These are just but a few studies revealing how effectively technology can be deployed in healthcare, especially in the area of maternal and neonatal care. It is in this light that this study sought to enquire from practitioners the smart technologies available to them for their daily practice. Another area explored was whether they recommend mhealth or self-care technologies to their clients and what the general reaction of patients/clients is to such recommendation.

This chapter of the book holds the potential to serve as a valuable reference for developers of smart technologies and gadgets for individuals, health care practitioners and hospitals, especially those who target Ghana specifically and Africa at large.

4. CHAPTER OBJECTIVES

The specific objectives of this chapter were to find out:

1. The smart technologies available to maternal and neo-natal healthcare practitioners for their daily practice.
2. What smart technologies they currently do not have which they believe could enhance their practice.
3. The challenges healthcare practitioners face while using smart/digital (modern) technologies for healthcare delivery.

5. DATA GATHERING PROCESSES

Data collection and analysis followed qualitative techniques. Participants were purposively selected. The criteria for selecting participants of the study were as follows: respondent must be a healthcare practitioner in the field of pre-natal, post-natal (maternal) and neo-natal care; may have a specialized area of practice and must be using smart/digital technologies in their practice. A total of 15 maternal and neonatal healthcare practitioners were interviewed. The choice of this group of practitioners was premised on the fact that they deliver a very critical service which is considered one of the essential quality improvement goals for most healthcare organizations (Premier Inc., 2019). In-depth interviews were used as data collection method because the researcher wanted to delve deep into practitioners' experiences with smart/digital technologies and establish individual challenges that they faced in the use of the technologies. Practitioners were interviewed at their preferred time and location.

Each interview lasted a minimum of 30 minutes. Some of the questions posed included: How valuable are smart technologies to your practice?; What smart technologies do you regularly use in your practice as a healthcare practitioner?; What would you say is the general reaction of patients to using smart technologies in healthcare delivery?; What technologies or apps do you believe will help improve service delivery in your area of practice?; How is the hospital you work for embracing the use of smart gadgets, apps and software in service delivery?; To what extent do you think the hospital you work for is ready to invest in smart technologies to deliver healthcare?; What health apps have you ever recommended to your client?; why that recommendation?

As a qualitative study, the intention was not to generalise results, but to explore how selected healthcare practitioners are using smart technologies in healthcare delivery, the challenges they encounter while using them and how valuable it is to their practice. With that in mind, data obtained were transcribed and analysed thematically by following Bryman's (2016) recommendation for thematic analysis. The researcher made the themes emerge from the qualitative data by reading through the transcripts of open-ended questions/comments, identifying the basic codes, and combining such codes to build more composite codes or categories that were related to the study interests. The researcher also tried to understand how participants valued the use of smart technologies in their practice and whether there were any challenges associated with their usage and what technologies are currently not present in their practice that they wish to have.

In presenting results of the study, actual names of participant are not disclosed. This is in the spirit of complying with ethical standards of qualitative data analysis. Therefore, where there are direct quotations, the names used are only pseudonyms but the content of the quotes are accurate reflection of what participants said. Table 1 is a breakdown of respondents and their areas of practice.

6. RESULTS

This section presents results of the study. They are discussed under the major themes obtained from data collection.

Table 1. Details of respondents

S/N	Pseudonym	Area of Practice
1	Aba	General nurse
2	Kofi	Neo-natal intensive care nurse
3	Dan	Maternal healthcare nurse
4	Sally	General Nurse
5	Maame	Midwife
6	Akua	Maternal care nurse
7	Kuukua	Neo-natal care nurse
8	Selina	Maternal care nurse
9	Kay	Neo-natal intensive care nurse
10	Alina	Midwife
11	Mary	Neo-natal care nurse
12	May	Neo-natal intensive care nurse
13	Oforiwaa	General Nurse
14	Gifty	Midwife
15	Mercy	General nurse

6.1. Technologies Used in Daily Practice

The healthcare practitioners were familiar with smart/digital technologies in their areas of practice. Most of them expressed satisfaction and ease at using digital technologies in their practice. In terms of technologies used on daily basis, most respondents said they had technologies that were important to their practice at their disposal. They included fetoscopes, digital thermometers, ultrasound machine, blood pressure machine, stethoscope, pulse oximeters, incubator, nebulizer, suction system (Machine), ambubag ventilator, feeding tubes, photo therapy lights and maternal monitor. They, however, recognized the fact they lacked more advanced technologies, such as smart inhalers, robotics surgery and health wearables, which they believed would enhance maternal, neo-natal and general healthcare.

For administrative aspect of health delivery, all respondents mentioned using computer database systems for record-keeping, specifically, the Electronic Health Records (EHRs) database system. Respondents had a positive attitude towards using technology for record-keeping rather than manual record-keeping routines. Most of them were of the view that it facilitated their work and helped track records of patients in order to deliver better services to them. Table 2 (which is below) shows the predominant themes that emerged from data analysis:

6.2. How Practitioners Value Modern Technologies for Healthcare Delivery

Practitioners considered smart/digital (modern) technologies as very vital to their practice, without which they would be ineffective, imprecise with diagnosis and involved in time-wasting ventures. They alluded to the fact that digital technologies did not only aid their practice but resulted in better service delivery to their clients. As a result, practitioners said clients sometimes expressed their delight to them

Table 2. Technologies used, technologies unavailable to practitioners and benefits of using automated systems for record-keeping

Technologies Currently Available to Practitioners	Technologies Not Yet Available to Practitioners	Technologies Used for Administrative Part of Healthcare Delivery	Benefits of Using Automated Systems for Healthcare Administration (Computer Database)
Fetal Monitor Digital thermometer Baby warmers Neonatal Incubator Feeding tubes Photo therapy lights Maternal monitor Weighing scale Blood pressure machine Incubator Nebulizer Electronic Suction system (Machine) Ambubag ventilator Pulse Oximeter Digital Sphygmomanometer Glucometers Electronic beds	Smart inhalers Robotic Surgery Health wearables Wireless brain sensors Artificial organs Tele health Virtual health reality	Computer database system I.e., Electronic Health Records (EHRs)	It has helped to track and reduce appointment and no-show rates It eases workflow. It has also improved public health care. Better and safer data storage. It has helped to identify high-risk patients, enhancing services provided to them Enhanced communication and information-sharing about these patients across the care team. Access to big data. Easy to store and track data Ease of access to patient's history Enhanced data transfer to doctors for consultation

when they are served promptly and efficiently with the utility of technology. Here are some quotes from interview with practitioners to that effect:

"They are highly valuable both to patients and health personnel. It saves time and is more convenient", Dan.

"They are highly valuable because it makes work much faster and easier", May.

Technologies have become live-saving as practitioners, with the support of technology, are able to diagnose diseases faster and offer the right advice and support to cure sicknesses in a swift manner. The maternal monitoring system, for example, was mentioned as one of the valuable tools for post-partum healthcare. Until practitioners had it, it was difficult to monitor mothers comprehensively after delivery. In situations where there were a lot of mothers on the ward at the same time, it was hard monitoring their progress without encountering difficulty and restrictions due to human limitations and barriers. But the machines have come in handy to make monitoring easier and to offer fast and efficient healthcare to aid quick recovery. Some of the respondents had this to say:

"It's improving quality of life as it is one of the main benefits of integrating new technologies into medicine [smiles] Technologies like minimally invasive surgeries, better monitoring systems and more comfortable scanning equipment are allowing patients to spend less time in recovery", Gifty.

"Through modern technologies lives have been saved. It has improved healthcare delivery and contributed to sustainable healthcare, that is diagnostic devices", Selina

"These modern technologies help in efficient, quality and fast delivery of healthcare to improve and save lives", Kofi.

6.3. Training of Practitioners on How to Use Modern Technologies for Healthcare Delivery

Most of the practitioners said there were no specific times set aside for training them on how to use the technologies when they are procured. This is because of their schedules and the fact that the technologies are procured when they are critically needed and so must be used almost immediately. In most cases, they learn how to use technologies by reading the accompanying manuals or learning from a practitioner who has successfully used them. Sometimes, in the process of using the technologies, they learn from their mistakes and re-adjust where necessary. For more complicated technologies, time is spent on training practitioners on how to operate them. The following quotes from the interviews buttress this point:

"Workshops are held to train medical practitioners on new health delivery technologies that are a little complicated to use. Most of the time, we learn on the job. We just need to know what it is used for and read the manual a bit", Alina.

"There are no specific times or days involved in training on how to use the technologies but it depends on the type of technology and one is trained verbally if possible [pauses]... practical, that is theoretical and practical", Akua.

"There are no specific time or days involved in training. It mainly depends on the type of technology introduced", Kofi.

6.4. Challenges Faced with Using Modern Technologies

There are a number of challenges faced while using modern technologies for healthcare. These challenges can be counted as both operational and technical challenges. Challenges ranged from bad internet network while using the database systems for health administration which becomes an impediment to retrieving patient records when needed. There were challenges related to faulty equipment, especially computers. Practitioners also harboured the fear of losing records of patients as a result of hacking. Respondent's challenges and reservations are resonated in the following quotes:

"There is the risk of medical records of patients being hacked", Kay.

"We face network problems, especially when using computer", Kofi.

"Sometimes we have faulty computers, especially the ones that are donated by certain groups to us", Mary

"One of our greatest fears is information security of patients including data privacy and storage", Maame.

Some respondents also felt because they deal with patients who may have contagious diseases, the computers they use could be infected and become conduit of infection, should they have some form of contact with patients while serving them. This puts practitioners at risk of them being infected if they are negligent or do not adhere to safe medical procedures like wearing of gloves, handwashing or disinfecting hands. A respondent had this to say:

"Infections [Pauses]. An example is using the computer to collect patient information, sometimes during this process you have to touch the patient and if the patient has a contagious disease and proper handwashing is not done immediately, the healthcare provider might pass it unto the computer. The next person who uses the computer might be infected with the disease", Oforiwaa.

6.5. Healthcare Practitioners' Recommendation of Modern Technologies to Clients, Reason for Recommendation and General Reaction of Patients to the Use of Modern Technologies in Healthcare Delivery

Patients are generally delighted when modern technologies are used to provide healthcare for them. This is because the assurance of being provided with efficient, reliable and speedy service delivery is enough to put them at ease. Practitioners also sometimes recommend certain technologies that they believe will be of benefit to clients for clients' personal use. Such technologies are able to help them track their progress with treatment and general wellbeing. These technologies are also characteristically easy to operate. One such technology that is regularly recommended by practitioners is the Electronic Sphygmomanometer which is meant for constant checking of blood pressure of hypertensive patients. Respondents' thoughts about patients' reactions towards using modern technologies in healthcare delivery are captured in the quotes below:

"Patients are happy to be using modern technologies because it is highly accessible for diagnosis of diseases", Kuukua.

"Patients really appreciate the use of modern technologies because it is efficient, more reliable and less costly", Selina.

"Patients are happy because it is helping people live longer, reducing wait times and making it easier for doctors to diagnose and treat diseases" Dan.

"Patients feel safe and secured since it makes the delivery of healthcare to be fast to prevent them from wasting time at the facility", Maame.

6.6. Health Facilities' Assent to the Use of Modern Technologies in Healthcare Delivery

Respondents were of the opinion that managers of health facilities recognize how useful the use of modern technologies is to healthcare delivery. Their appreciation of the value of healthcare technologies makes them not to drag their feet when the need arises to invest in such technologies. Their responses are testament to this:

"My health facility is highly embracing modern technologies because they are ready to invest more", Mercy.

"... About 90% ready to invest in acquiring modern technologies because of its efficiency", Kuukua.

7. DISCUSSION OF FINDINGS

Smart/digital (modern) technologies have evidently improved healthcare delivery. This is reflected in responses given by participants. Because of their usefulness in medical practice healthcare practitioners have a positive attitude towards them. This study has shown that practitioners have access to basic essential technologies that help them in their practice. However, they do not have access to more advanced technologies. Technologies such as tele-medicine and health wearables and other IoT-enabled technologies that are gaining grounds in medical practice in the global west are yet to be entrenched in Ghana. This may not be surprising as the study by Scott Kruse et al. (2018) showed that a lot of the literature on telemedicine is from USA, Europe, Australia, respectively. There seem to be a dearth in literature from Africa, the Middle East and India, a possible indicator of the low presence of such technologies in medical practice in these parts of the world.

These advanced, cutting-edge technologies are meant to offer "near flawless" healthcare delivery by providing close-to-perfect diagnoses, stress-free medical screenings as well as providing access to big data to make practitioners customise healthcare delivery. Telemedicine has proven to successfully decrease the geographical and time barriers associated with traditional healthcare with similar or greater efficacy (Scott Kruse et al., 2018). Delivering care through telemedicine saves the patient an average of 145 miles and 142 minutes per visit, according to a study carried out in the US Department of Veterans Affairs (Russo, McCool, & Davies, 2016). This is because this technology-aided service is offered with special emphasis on accurate and timely interventions. In order to match up to global trends, it is important to invest in such innovative technologies at healthcare institutional levels to deliver more timely, accurate and efficient healthcare.

Major challenges encountered while using technologies available to maternal and neonatal healthcare practitioners were bad internet network, which impedes the retrieval of patient records and faulty equipment. These challenges may not be peculiar to these practitioners as Grym et al. (2019) found similar challenges in relation to even more personal technologies such as the smart wristbands. There was also the fear of losing records of patients as a result of hacking. This can be avoided when data is stored in the cloud as in the case of the technological system developed by Alotaibi et al. (2018). The cloud storage will defy any hardware breakdown and will for allow data retrieval in spite of location and time.

The self-care technology recommended by practitioners is the digital or electronic Sphygmomanometer. There were no indication that neonatal and maternal healthcare practitioners who participated in this study recommend mhealth or other self-care technologies to clients or patients, although they admit that patients are delighted when modern technologies are used in healthcare delivery. Nunes, Andersen and Fitzpatrick (2019) argue that mhealth technologies have the prospect to improve the agency of patients and healthcare practitioners. Practitioners can therefore, be more efficient if they encourage patients or clients to use such technologies. This is because the collaborative platform provided for patients and healthcare provider disrupt the traditional power and control in healthcare delivery and put patients at the centre so they will bring useful insights and actively be involved in building better quality of health (Berwick, 2009).

8. CONCLUSION

This study has shown that maternal and neonatal practitioners interviewed have access to basic essential technologies that help them in their practice. They, however, do not have access to very advanced technologies, such as, tele-medicine and health wearables and other IoT-enabled technologies. Practitioners also hardly recommend mhealth technologies to their clients.

9. RECOMMENDATIONS

With the pervasive use of mobile technologies in Ghana, health facilities should consider institutionalising mhealth as part of their service delivery as well. Practitioners, in consultation with appropriate actors in healthcare organisations, can commission the development of relevant mobile health applications that will make them track clients' recovery progress and their conformity with recommended treatment and lifestyles outside of the hospital environs. Practitioners can also recommend suitable applications that clients can fall on to improve their health. This requires that practitioners themselves are up to speed with mhealth and other health technologies.

One of the risks involved in using computer systems for record-keeping is the danger of losing records, as a result of hacking or system breakdown. This is why it is important to put in appropriate online and offline security measures to deal with such risks. System administrators could consider backing up data in the cloud and/or using external storage devices to backup data. These devices are to be kept safely away for use when need be. Where internet technologies are relied upon to gain access to database, it is important to provide reliable and efficient internet service to allow for effective workflow.

It is not a good idea to work with faulty computers and equipment. When equipment meant to do diagnosis is faulty, the results it produces can be only left to one's imagination. The best way out of it is for management of health facilities to invest in good computer systems and equipment that will not cause disruptions in service delivery as a result of them being faulty.

It is hard for anyone to discount the usefulness of digital and smart technologies in healthcare delivery. This is because there is a lot of evidence to attest to their usefulness and instrumentality for the practitioner as well as the client. Health facilities should, therefore, continue to invest in these technologies.

10. FUTURE WORK

This study looked at smart technologies usage among neonatal and maternal healthcare practitioners. It is recommended that a similar study be conducted among practitioners who have specialised in other areas of healthcare delivery. A study that focuses on the response or reaction to smart healthcare among patients is also recommended.

REFERENCES

Ali, M. A., Tahir, N. M., & Ali, A. I. (2018). *Monitoring Healthcare System for Infants: A Review. Paper presented at the 2018 IEEE Conference on Systems, Process and Control* (pp. 44–47). IEEE Press. Retrieved from https://ieeexplore.ieee.org/abstract/document/8704143

Alotaibi, M., Albalawi, M., & Alwakeel, L. (2018). A Smart Mobile Pregnancy Management and Awareness System for Saudi Arabia. *International Journal of Interactive Mobile Technologies*, *12*(5), 112–125. doi:10.3991/ijim.v12i5.9005

Berwick, D. M. (2009). What 'patient-centered' should mean: confessions of an extremist: A seasoned clinician and expert fears the loss of his humanity if he should become a patient. *Health Affairs*, *28*(1), 555–565. doi:10.1377/hlthaff.28.4.w555

Bryman, A. (2016). *Social research methods*. United Kingdom: Oxford university press.

Cheruto, V. (2019, July 1). Rwanda and Ghana: Drones delivering medical supplies. *MSN News*. Retrieved from https://www.msn.com/en-za/news/other/rwanda-and-ghana-drones-delivering-medical-supplies/ar-AADJpCD

Daily Guide. (2017, November 17). Ghana ranks 6th on diabetes table in Africa. *Myjoyonline*. Retrieved from https://www.myjoyonline.com/lifestyle/2017/november-17th/ghana-ranks-6th-on-diabetes-table-in-africa.php

Dias, D., & Paulo Silva Cunha, J. (2018). Wearable health devices—Vital sign monitoring, systems and technologies. *Sensors (Basel)*, *18*(8), 12–18. doi:10.339018082414 PMID:30044415

Faridi, Z., Liberti, L., Shuval, K., Northrup, V., Ali, A., & Katz, D. L. (2008). Evaluating the impact of mobile telephone technology on type 2 diabetic patients' self-management: The NICHE pilot study. *Journal of Evaluation in Clinical Practice*, *14*(3), 465–469. doi:10.1111/j.1365-2753.2007.00881.x PMID:18373577

Foley, T. (2017). Transforming the patient experience through "Smart Room" technologies: Tablets, flat-screen TVs and educational resources help engage patients in their healthcare during and after a hospital stay. *Health Tech Magazine*. Retrieved from https://healthtechmagazine.net/article/2017/01/transforming-patient-experience-through-smart-room-technologies

Goyal, A., Gopalakrishnan, M., Anantharaman, G., Chandrashekharan, D. P., Thachil, T., & Sharma, A. (2019). Smartphone guided wide-field imaging for retinopathy of prematurity in neonatal intensive care unit–a Smart ROP (SROP) initiative. *Indian Journal of Ophthalmology*, *67*(6), 840. doi:10.4103/ijo.IJO_1177_18 PMID:31124499

Goyal, S., & Cafazzo, J. A. (2013). Mobile phone health apps for diabetes management: Current evidence and future developments, *QJM. International Journal of Medicine*, *106*(1), 1067–1069. doi:10.1093/qjmed/hct203 PMID:24106313

Grym, K., Niela-Vilén, H., Ekholm, E., Hamari, L., Azimi, I., Rahmani, A, Liljeberg, P., Loyttyniemi, E. & Axelin, A. (2019). Feasibility of smart wristbands for continuous monitoring during pregnancy and one month after birth. *BMC pregnancy and childbirth*, *19*(1), 34. doi:10.118612884-019-2187-9

Kahn, J. G., Yang, J. S., & Kahn, J. S. (2010). Mobile'health needs and opportunities in developing countries. *Health Affairs*, *29*(2), 252–258. doi:10.1377/hlthaff.2009.0965 PMID:20348069

Murugesan, S. (2013). Mobile apps in Africa. *IT Professional*, *15*(5), 8–11. doi:10.1109/MITP.2013.83

Nasi, G., Cucciniello, M., & Guerrazzi, C. (2015). The role of mobile technologies in health care processes: the case of cancer supportive care. *Journal of medical Internet research*, *17*(2), e26. doi:10.2196/jmir.3757

Nunes, F., Andersen, T., & Fitzpatrick, G. (2019). The agency of patients and carers in medical care and self-care technologies for interacting with doctors. *Health Informatics Journal*, *25*(2), 330–349. doi:10.1177/1460458217712054 PMID:28653552

Owusu, E., & Chakraborty, J. (2019). User requirements gathering in mHealth: Perspective from Ghanaian end users. In *Proceedings of the International Conference on Human-Computer Interaction* (pp. 386-396). Springer. 10.1007/978-3-030-22577-3_28

Pollak, J., Gay, G., Byrne, S., Wagner, E., Retelny, D., & Humphreys, L. (2010). It's time to eat! Using mobile games to promote healthy eating. *IEEE Pervasive Computing*, *9*(3), 21–27. doi:10.1109/MPRV.2010.41

Premier Inc. (2019, September 06). How health systems are prioritizing maternal and infant health. [Blog post]. Retrieved from https://www.premierinc.com/newsroom/blog/how-health-systems-are-prioritizing-maternal-and-infant-health

Rau, P. L., Plocher, T., & Choong, Y. Y. (2012). *Cross-cultural design for IT products and services*. CRC Press. doi:10.1201/b12679

Russo, J. E., McCool, R. R., & Davies, L. (2016). VA telemedicine: An analysis of cost and time savings. *Telemedicine Journal and e-Health*, *22*(3), 209–215. doi:10.1089/tmj.2015.0055 PMID:26305666

Scott Kruse, C., Karem, P., Shifflett, K., Vegi, L., Ravi, K., & Brooks, M. (2018). Evaluating barriers to adopting telemedicine worldwide: A systematic review. *Journal of Telemedicine and Telecare*, *24*(1), 4–12. doi:10.1177/1357633X16674087 PMID:29320966

World Health Organisation. (2018). Maternal mortality: Key facts. Retrieved from https://www.who.int/news-room/fact-sheets/detail/maternal-mortality

Yao, S., Swetha, P., & Zhu, Y. (2018). Nanomaterial-Enabled wearable sensors for healthcare. *Advanced Healthcare Materials*, *7*(1), 1–27. doi:10.1002/adhm.201700889 PMID:29193793

ADDITIONAL READING

Bloch, L. R., & Lemish, D. (1999). Disposable love: The rise and fall of a virtual pet. *New Media & Society*, *1*(3), 283–303.

Brejcha, J. (2015). *Cross-cultural human-computer interaction and user experience design: a semiotic perspective*. CRC Press. doi:10.1201/b18059

Canhoto, A. I., & Arp, S. (2017). Exploring the factors that support adoption and sustained use of health and fitness wearables. *Journal of Marketing Management*, *33*(1-2), 32–60. doi:10.1080/0267257X.2016.1234505

Chau, P. Y., & Hu, P. J. H. (2002). Investigating healthcare professionals' decisions to accept telemedicine technology: An empirical test of competing theories. *Information & Management*, *39*(4), 297–311. doi:10.1016/S0378-7206(01)00098-2

Clim, A., Zota, R. D., & Tinica, G. (2019). Big Data in home healthcare: A new frontier in personalized medicine. Medical emergency services and prediction of hypertension risks. *International Journal of Healthcare Management*, *12*(3), 241–249. doi:10.1080/20479700.2018.1548158

Katwa, U., & Rivera, E. (2018). Asthma management in the era of smart-medicine: Devices, gadgets, apps and telemedicine. *Indian Journal of Pediatrics*, *85*(9), 757–762. doi:10.100712098-018-2611-6 PMID:29524089

Kumar, A. K., & Sherkhane, M. S. (2018). Assessment of gadgets addiction and its impact on health among undergraduates. *International Journal of Community Medicine And Public Health*, 5(8), 3624–3628. doi:10.18203/2394-6040.ijcmph20183109

Lin, J. J., Mamykina, L., Lindtner, S., Delajoux, G., & Strub, H. B. (2006, September). Fish'n'Steps: Encouraging physical activity with an interactive computer game. In *Proceedings of the International conference on ubiquitous computing* (pp. 261-278). Springer. 10.1007/11853565_16

Mair, F., & Whitten, P. (2000). Systematic review of studies of patient satisfaction with telemedicine. *BMJ (Clinical Research Ed.)*, 320(7248), 1517–1520. doi:10.1136/bmj.320.7248.1517 PMID:10834899

Mathew, C. M., Wanjari, A. K., Varghese, B., Singh, U., Acharya, S. P., & Shukla, S. A. (2019). Smart phones for medical undergraduates: Friend or foe? *International Journal of Advances in Medicine*, 6(1), 135. doi:10.18203/2349-3933.ijam20190119

Piwek, L., Ellis, D. A., Andrews, S., & Joinson, A. (2016). The rise of consumer health wearables: Promises and barriers. *PLoS Medicine*, 13(2), e1001953. doi:10.1371/journal.pmed.1001953 PMID:26836780

Verma, R. (2019). Smart Internet of Things (IoT) Applications. In Handbook of Research on Implementation and Deployment of IoT Projects in Smart Cities (pp. 33-42). Hershey, PA: IGI Global.

KEY TERMS AND DEFINITIONS

Ambubag Ventilator: It is a self-inflating bag resuscitator that helps patients get oxygen and ventilation until they are able to breath on their own.

Baby Warmers: They are used to direct heat to an infant in order to keep them warm.

Digital Technologies: They are equipment or machinery that function (generate, store and process data) using numeric of binary code or logic. This allows for the storage of large amounts of data, media files and other documents and data to be stored in small spaces or devices. In the context of healthcare such technologies are very intelligent, can store large amounts of data and rely on to provide diagnosis and other interventions in a fast, reliable manner.

Electronic Bed: An electronic bed has a motor control system that is able to raise the head, foot and height of a bed frame just at the push of a button.

Electronic Suction System (Machine): It is an electronic equipment or machine used to extract nasal secretions and other fluids from babies.

Fetal Monitor: It is a machine, tool or equipment used to track the heartbeat of a fetus in the womb, especially when a mother is in labour. It is also used during routine visits of a pregnant woman to the health facility. It tracks the fetal heart patterns and helps healthcare practitioners decide to provide some interventions or not.

Glucometer: It a portable device used to monitor the blood sugar (glucose) level in one's body.

Incubator: It is an equipment or apparatus with a special chamber to offer a controlled environmental condition for the care and protection of a premature or sick infant.

Maternal Healthcare Providers: They are healthcare practitioners who seek to the health and well-being of pregnant women and new mothers. They, essentially, take care of the health needs of women during pregnancy and post-partum.

Maternal Monitor: It is a machine used to track the heart rate, blood pressure and other vitals of a pregnant woman.

Nebulizer: It is a device used to administer medication in the form of mist which is inhaled into the lungs. It is usually used to administer asthma medications to infants when they find it difficult to use asthma inhaler.

Neo-natal Healthcare Providers: They are healthcare practitioners who provide healthcare to new-born babies who are usually critically ill and need special medical attention.

Neonatal Incubator: It is a machine that heats the air around a newborn (neonate), usually a premature infant, in order to ensure the ideal environment for the infant as well as protect the infant against infection, too much noise, allergic substances and light levels that can cause harm. It also regulates oxygen levels and air humidity for the infant to easily breath. This is to create an environment similar to what is found in the natural growing environment of a fetus. It is also fitted with special lights to treat neonatal jaundice.

Photo Therapy Lights: They are special lights used for the treatment of skin diseases.

Pulse Oximeter: It is a small, light device attached or clipped to the fingertip to check for the pulse rate or the amount of oxygen carried in one's body.

Smart Technologies: They are technologies that provide users with remote access, control and interaction through the internet. Because of their ability to adjust to the needs of the user, they are considered very intelligent technologies.

Chapter 4
Virtual Reality in Medical Education

Ahmet B. Ustun
ⓘ https://orcid.org/0000-0002-1640-4291
Bartin University, Turkey

Ramazan Yilmaz
Bartin University, Turkey

Fatma Gizem Karaoglan Yilmaz
Bartin University, Turkey

ABSTRACT

The aim of this research is to examine student acceptance and use of virtual reality technologies in medical education. Within the scope of the research, a questionnaire consisting of 4 sub-dimensions and 21 items was developed by the researchers. This questionnaire consists of sub-dimensions of performance expectancy, effort expectancy, facilitating conditions, and social influence. The study was conducted on 421 university students who participated in courses and activities related to the use of virtual reality applications in medical education. The findings of the research demonstrated that the students' acceptance and use of virtual reality applications were high in medical education. Various suggestions were made for researchers and educators in accordance with the findings.

INTRODUCTION

Although Virtual Reality (VR) has been used in a few fields such as some sectors in the military since the 1970s, technological advances have recently made the accessibility of VR affordable and the use of it prevalent now (Beheiry et al., 2019). While the affordability of it has increased its usage among prospective customers, it has evolved to become a sophisticated technology that immerses a user in a virtual environment that is getting similar to reality, which even draws non-consumer attention towards

DOI: 10.4018/978-1-7998-2521-0.ch004

this technology. It can be seen as a technological revolution that leads to the triumph of 3-D environments. Therefore, it is widely used in fields such as healthcare, military and education.

The popularity of VR increases in the realm of medicine. Many researchers emphasize the use of VR in healthcare as a potentially effective tool that provides innovative techniques for clinical practice settings. Morel, Bideau, Lardy, and Kulpa (2015) state that standardization, reproducibility and stimuli control are the benefits of the VR system in clinical assessment and rehabilitation. The use of VR technology offers a standardized virtual environment in which stimuli can be controlled to accurately evaluate the balance recovery of patients and their progression, and this standardized environment can be reproducible to make comparisons among patients in the same condition or between the trials of patients (Morel et al., 2015). Also, the accessibility and affordability of VR technologies are easier with the commencing mass production of low-cost devices so rehabilitation can be continued anywhere, anytime in motivating and entertaining virtual environments (Morel et al., 2015; Riener, & Harders, 2012).

Rose, Nam and Chen (2018) indicate that VR technologies have been employed in treatments of physical impairments as an emerging rehabilitation technology for those who suffer from "stroke (Jack et al., 2001), cerebral palsy (Reid, 2002), severe burns (Haik et al., 2006), Parkinson's disease (Mirelman et al., 2010), Guillain-Barré syndrome (Albiol-Pérez et al., 2015), and multiple sclerosis (Fulk, 2005) among others" (p. 153). This aligns with the comprehensive systematic review study conducted by Ravi, Kumar and Singhi (2017) who state that the utilization of VR technologies in therapeutic interventions for children and adolescents suffering from cerebral palsy is a promising intervention in order to make improvement in balance and overall motor capabilities. VR technology can also be used in psychotherapy. The use of VR applications has been proved as an effective treatment for phobias through the processes of habituation and extinction (Riva, 2005). In the VR treatment of phobias, patients are exposed to controlled, fear-provoking stimuli to gradually alleviate the anxiety in the realistic environment.

While VR has been gained popularity in the use of interventions for balance assessment, rehabilitation and psychotherapy in the medical field, De Luca et al. (2019) point out that it is commonly cited as a valuable educational tool used in many fields of study such as medical and dental sciences. When VR is employed in medical education, it offers a safe environment where students gain fun, engaging, interactive and cost-effective experiences by eliminating the risk factors (de Ribaupierre et al., 2014). These situation-based experiences including specifically surgical experiences generated by VR technologies represented to students enable them to practice how to perform surgery for knowledge and skill acquisition without suffering possibly life-changing consequences. When the promise and potential of VR are considered in medical education, it can be seen that there are few numbers of research. It is important to increase current knowledge and diversity of research on this subject. Therefore, the aim of the study is to investigate the students' acceptance and use of VR technologies in healthcare education.

BACKGROUND

Brief History of VR

Although VR can be seen as a new phenomenon because of recent technological advancements that support the development of today's VR systems, the early roots for VR emerged in the 1920s. In 1920, Edwin Albert Link began working on a flight simulator for flight training and the first flight simulator was presented in 1929. Link later launched a company that produced flight simulators for flight training in the early 1930s (Page, 2000). The evolutionary origins of the VR system can be traced back to the 1960s when Cinematographer Morton Heilig created a multi-sensorial simulator "Sensorama" that stimulates the senses through wind and scent emitter, vibratory sensation, audio and a colorful 3D display (Pelargos et al., 2017). In the mid of 1960s, Ivan Sutherland, a head of computer graphics, developed the "Sword of Damocles" that was the first VR systems equipped with head-mounted displays (HMDs), which enabled users to be able to view the virtual world and interact with objects (Drummond, Houston & Irvine, 2014). In 1975, Myron Krueger developed the first interactive VR platform, video place, that captures the users' image to allow them to see their computer-generated silhouettes imitating their own movements in 2D screens (Krueger & Wilson, 1985). Besides, VCASS developed by Thomas Furness in 1982 was for a better flight simulator than previous ones and VIVED – Virtual Visual Environment Display developed by NASA in 1984 was for their astronauts. Over the last decade, there were many other advancements in the developments of VR systems such as DataGlove (1985), HMD (1988), BOOM (1989), CAVE (1992) and Augmented Reality (1990s). In spite of the endeavours of these early researchers and companies, the technological improvements in computer efficiency were not sufficient to support VR systems that could be widely appealing until the year 2010 (Pelargos et al., 2017). VR systems including Augmented Reality (AR) have therefore been utilized in a variety of fields and worldwide sales of products and services of VR systems by the Oculus Rift from Oculus VR and Facebook, HTC Vive from HTC and Valve Corporation, PlayStation VR from Sony Corporation, Samsung Gear VR from Samsung Electronics, and HoloLens from Microsoft Corporation are expected to increase more than $162 billion in 2020 (Gaggioli, 2017).

Definition and Description of VR

Zhang et al. (2018) define VR as "a computer-generated simulation of a 3-D environment that users can interact with in a seemingly real or physical way using special electronic equipment, such as a helmet with a screen inside or gloves fitted with sensors" (p. 138). Sacks, Perlman and Barak (2013) define (VR) as "a technology that uses computers, software and peripheral hardware to generate a simulated environment for its user" (p. 1007). As understood from the definitions, the VR system aims to provide a sense of being within a simulated environment. Users can experience a generated artificial environment that is exhibited to them by means of electronic equipment in such a way as to persuade their brain to perceive this artificial environment as a real environment. Due to this reason, those who viewed this artificial computer-generated environment for the first time depict their experience as a surprise or "wow effect" (Beheiry et al., 2019).

It is important to describe VR/AR and how both differ from each other. AR can be categorized as a subset of VR (Sharif, Ansari, Yasmin, & Fernandes, 2018). Although these technologies have similarities, there are major differences between them to individually provide a distinguished experience. Klopfer and Squire (2008) define AR as "a situation in which a real-world context is dynamically overlaid with coherent location or context sensitive virtual information" (p. 205). According to the definition, virtual objects are integrated into the real world (Durak, Karaoglan, & Yilmaz, 2019). Therefore, users can simultaneously experience the blending of the real world and virtual objects instead of being fully immersed in a virtual world (Pelargos et al., 2017). However, the idea behind VR is the creation of a simulated three-dimensional world that can be similar to or totally different from the real-world. The users are completely immersed in this simulated reality in which they can interact by holding, pushing, pulling and throwing virtual objects. In this sense, VR and AR systems have their own advantages and disadvantages to create a safe and simulated setting and therefore; there are concrete differences between the use of VR and AR systems in medical (Lee & Wong, 2019). On the one hand, the AR system allows a surgeon to see the surgical field as a real-life structure and at the same time artificial elements such as digital images of the surgical field and patient's other vital information (Murthi & Varshney, 2018). In this surgery, one of the distinguished benefits of AR is to enable the surgeon to see the patient's multiple interpreted information without breaking his concentration by looking away from the patient to obtain this information from multiple different displays (Murthi & Varshney, 2018). On the other hand, VR system can be used to fully immerse a mental illness patient in a crafted, virtual conditions where the patient encounters his fear to treat and cure phobia such as a fear of spiders, flying or being in a small space (Riener & Harders, 2012, p. 5). In this type of treatment, VR applications can be used to gradually expose the patient to the phobic condition and the treatment of the VR session can instantly be terminated if necessary.

Virtual Reality in Education

The use of VR technology in education and training has widely attracted attention because of its capability to create a virtual environment in which learners are steered toward achieving targeted tasks in order to acquire a variety of new skills. These tasks can be designed to captivate and engage learners in the learning process (Norris, Spicer & Byrd, 2019). This system mostly uses head-mounted displays with headphones and hand controllers as electronic devices to engage their multiple senses. Engaging multiple senses increases learners' attention and focus, and fosters meaningful learning experiences to develop new knowledge or skills in an immersive environment. Gadelha (2018) states that VR is a state-of-the-art technology product that enables learners to make connections with the instructional material in a way that has never been possible before by eliminating external distractions in the classroom.

According to Gadelha (2018), VR technology has changed how teachers teach and how learners learn. It has the potential to help shift from the traditional teacher-centered approach to a student-centered approach. The Multimedia Cone of Abstraction (MCoA) based on Dale's Cone of Experience (CoE) explicating learners retain more information when they learn by doing demonstrates that learners become active learners by interacting with a purposeful virtual environment in which they learn by doing targeted tasks (Baukal, Ausburn, & Ausburn, 2013). Basically, the researchers put the VR technology in place of the base of the CoE that is "Direct Purposeful Experiences" the least abstract level, which means that VR provides very realistic simulations of things that learners can interact with and learn best by doing.

Under appropriate conditions such as providing immediate feedback and enough time to allow learners to progress at their own pace, individual students achieve mastery of the task or materials (Bloom, 1974). The use of VR technology gives the opportunity for learners to practice what they have learned regardless of the number of repetitions until they carry out the targeted tasks. Its use also intrinsically motivates them to keep striving to successfully practice (Sánchez-Cabrero et al., 2019). In other words, its use encourages them to perform to their own capacities until mastering a skill or task instead of giving up repeating instructional sessions. Besides, they can receive immediate feedback on their current level of mastery in a virtual learning environment. The instant feedback helps them realize what they need to do better to achieve a skill or task and initiates the visual programming to recreate a virtual learning environment to be tailored (Norris, Spicer, & Byrd, 2019).

VR technology provides safe learning environments that learners can experience damaging, risky, dangerous or harmful situations while never putting their safety in jeopardy. Not only safe virtual situations that are hazardous in reality such as operating medical devices in healthcare training and combat training in the military can be created by VR for learners, but also can possibly be personalized according to each learner's need by simulating countless scenarios (Norris, Spicer, & Byrd, 2019). While infinite virtual instructional scenarios that are only limited by imagination and knowledge can be generated, Zhang et al. (2018) point out that the creation of these scenarios consumes very few natural and social resources in comparison with a real one.

Virtual Reality in Healthcare Education

Particularly, several studies have shown simulation training as an effective approach to improve knowledge acquisition and skills in healthcare education (Bracq, Michinov, & Jannin, 2019). VR training enables healthcare professionals to educate medical students by eliminating potential risks resulting in an adverse outcome in a patient. VR technology is not only considered as interactive and effective experiential learning for medical students to develop skill and confidence needed when they encounter in a real-life situation, but it is also seen as a cost-effective learning approach to repeatedly practice number of simulated clinical scenarios in healthcare (King et al., 2018). Therefore, the utilization of VR gives opportunities for medical learners to rehearse without being anxious about making mistakes and facing any grave results and to be prepared for recognizing the symptoms of a disease and even conducting complicated operations.

The utilization of VR simulations eliminates the need for the use of cadavers or animals to acquire professional knowledge and develop essential practical skills by providing a realistic method of training in the field of medicine. VR system also provides surgery training and rehearsal for inexperienced trainees to gain surgical skills in a variety of surgery operations such as endoscopic surgery, laparoscopic surgery, neurosurgery and epidural injections. Vaughan, Dubey, Wainwright and Middleton (2016) highlight the importance of attaining practice skills before operating theatre scenarios in real life and indicate that surgeons have great chance to develop and enhance their operative and decision-making skills in a controlled, risk-free realistic operating room through the utilization of orthopedic VR training simulations. Thus, the use of these VR simulations can be seen as suitable training opportunities for surgeons who have a lack of surgical experience to practice key skills in orthopedic and other types of surgeries.

Traditional forms of education like a verbal presentation of information and conveying written material may not be appropriate to teach complicated medical information for patients and their primary caregivers (Hoffmann & McKenna, 2006). Specifically, language proficiency, cultural and socioeconomic backgrounds, levels of education and understanding and language or cognitive impairment should be taken into consideration in stroke cases where risk factors and causes vary greatly from person to person in stroke survivors (Thompson-Butel et al., 2019). In this sense, it is a demand to tailor education according to the stroke survivor's needs for providing relevance and comprehensible information (Eames, Hoffmann, Worrall, & Read, 2010). A study was conducted by Thompson-Butel et al. (2019) who developed guided and personalized VR education sessions to prevent recurrent stroke and maximize rehabilitation for stroke survivors and their primary caregivers and explored the use of these VR sessions in delivering post stroke education to find out its effectiveness. They revealed that the use of VR provides safe and individualized educational experiences for participants who were highly satisfied with the education sessions and "demonstrated varied improvements in knowledge areas including brain anatomy and physiology, brain damage and repair, and stroke-specific information such as individual stroke risk factors and acute treatment benefits" (p.450).

Roy, Bakr and George (2017) explored the current situation of VR simulations and evaluated the value of VR simulations in dental education. According to them, VR devices that are employed in dental education offer great possibilities for flexible learning and self-learning. Learners can play an active role in their learning. For instance, the features of VR devices enable them to practice simulations in the form of VR when and where they want and assess their work after completing practices by storing and replaying. Besides, the use of VR technology also alleviates anxiety and boredom of a classroom setting and makes the learning process engaging and effective. The rapid technological advances in VR provide more effective and efficient realistic pre-clinical dental experiences for students in all disciplines of dentistry (Roy et al., 2017).

Purpose of the Study

The use of VR to train medical learners for the acquisition of clinical skills has several advantages including but not limited to offering safe and reliable clinical learning environments, facilitating self-directed learning and providing personalized learning (Ruthenbeck & Reynolds, 2015). Riener and Harders (2012) articulate the aim of the VR system in healthcare as enhanced quality of the education and long and efficient training sessions through motivating and exciting realistic simulations. Seymour (2008) indicates that training in a VR environment improves learning outcomes in clinical settings when taking advantage of the advancing capabilities of VR simulation. A study conducted by Gunn et al. (2018) who assessed the effect of using VR simulation on the first-year medical imaging students' technical skills by comparing their technical skill acquisition via the traditional laboratory-based simulation and the medical imaging VR simulation revealed that the use of VR simulation improved their technical skill acquisition better than the use of the traditional laboratory-based simulation. However, VR system has limitations including the latency, "the delay between the actions of the immersed patient with input devices and the reaction of the virtual environment" and "the underestimation of perceived distance in virtual environments compared to real situations" (Morel et al., 2015, p.324). These limitations may hinder the delivery of effective learning content or make the learning process difficult. Also, educators' self-perception of inadequate technological skills might hinder the use of VR technology. For example, VR technology is considered in some instances as a technology that requires a high level of technological knowledge and skills in order that learners are able to use (Warburton, 2009). Also, Sanchez-Cabrero et al. (2019) point out that VR as a learning tool "is a relatively unexplored area in its beginnings that urgently needs to deepen its application in the classroom" (p. 2). In addition, Gunn et al. (2018) indicate that there are limited scholarly documentations in the realm of undergraduate medical education in spite of the growing popularity of using VR technologies in healthcare. Taking full advantage of using the VR system as an educational tool depends ultimately on medical students' acceptance of VR (Huang, Liaw, & Lai, 2016). In this sense, it is vital to widen existing knowledge and a variety of research on the use of VR technologies in medical education. Thus, the purpose of the study is to explore the students' acceptance and use of VR technologies in medical education.

METHOD

This section includes information about the research design, participants, data collection tool and data analysis.

Research Design and Participants

Within the scope of the research, a survey model was used to examine the university students' opinions about the use of VR technology in medical education. The participants were university students studying at a public university and taking the anatomy course that is taught by using VR technologies. Accordingly, this study was carried out on 421 university students. This study was conducted on undergraduate students studying at a public university in Turkey. When the distribution of students was examined according to their gender; it was determined that 46.8% (n = 197) are female and 53.2% (n = 224) are male. The students who participated in the research studied in diverse departments including health sciences (f = 111, 26.4%), physical education and sports (f = 91, 21.6%), coaching (f = 63, 15%), recreation (f = 81, 19.2%) and sports management (f = 75, 17.8%). The reason why the research was carried out on students studying at different departments was that an anatomy course was taught in these departments. It was attempted to contribute to the generalizability of the results by including students studying at different departments in this research. The students were in the 18-25 age range. More than half (61%) of the students were freshmen and the rest of them (39%) were sophomores. They were enabled to experience VR technologies within the scope of their anatomy course At the end of the research process, a questionnaire was completed by students to determine their acceptance and use of VR technologies in healthcare education.

Data Collection Tools

The data were obtained by a questionnaire developed by the researchers in this study. In the first phase of the development process of the questionnaire, the problem situation was determined and then the appropriate themes were composed in accordance with this problem situation by carefully examining the related literature (Sezer & Yilmaz, 2019; Yilmaz, Karaoglan Yilmaz, & Ezin, 2018). These sub-themes were 'Performance Expectancy', 'Effort Expectancy', 'Facilitating Conditions', 'Social Influence'. The sub-themes were developed by taking into account the Unified Theory of Acceptance and Use of Technology (UTAUT) model, which is one of the technology Acceptance models. Technology acceptance is a structure consisting of cognitive and psychological variables underlying the use of technology (Venkatesh, Morris, Davis, & Davis, 2003). The aim of this structure is to explain the acceptance of individuals to use a particular technology and the factors that affect this acceptance. Many models (TAM, TAM 2, UTAUT, UTAUT2, etc.) have been proposed in technology acceptance studies (Schepers & Wetzels, 2007). The aim of all these models elucidates the factors that affect the effective use of technology. Venkatesh et al. (2003) believe that it would be inadequate to explain a complicated structure consisting of cognitive and psychological variables like technology acceptance with a single model. Because of this reason, they expressed that this complicated structure should be examined in a multidimensional way and formulated the Unified Theory of Acceptance and Use of Technology (UTAUT) (Venkatesh et al., 2003). UTAUT model is consisted of four essential elements including "performance expectancy", "effort expectancy", "facilitating conditions" and "social influence" (Venkatesh et al., 2003). The graphic representation of the model is given in Figure 1.

As shown in Figure 1; Performance expectancy pertains to the belief that performance increases with the use of technology. Effort expectancy pertains to the belief that the related technology is easy to use. Social influence pertains to the belief and attitudes of influential individuals (teachers, successful students, etc.) towards the use of the related technology. The positive belief and attitudes of these indi-

Figure 1. Unified theory of acceptance and use of technology
(Source: Venkatesh et al., 2003, p.447)

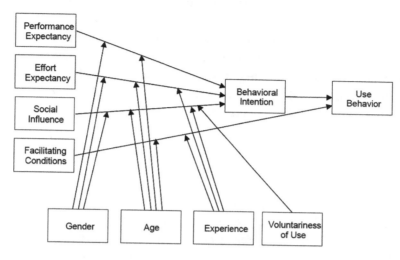

viduals create a positive social impact on other individuals to use that technology. Facilitating conditions are related to whether or not various facilitating elements exist to support the use of technology for the individual (Venkatesh et al., 2003). Within the scope of this research, UTAUT model was taken into consideration in order to investigate the acceptance and use of VR technologies in healthcare education and a measurement instrument consisting of sub-dimensions of 'Performance Expectancy', 'Effort Expectancy', 'Facilitating Conditions', 'Social Influence' was developed.

After the determination of the sub-themes, a pool of 55 items based on the information extracted from the literature review was created. 35 items that were picked to suit the draft of the opinion form were selected from the item pool and a pre-application form was created with a Likert-type rating. In order to discuss the appropriateness of the pre-application form, three experts working in the field of Turkish language and literature, instructional technologies and health sciences were consulted on. The linguist evaluated the items in terms of intelligibility, expression and grammar. The experts in the field of instructional technology and health sciences assessed the items in terms of scope, criteria, structure and appearance validity. Modifications were carried out to the questionnaire in accordance with the feedback from the experts. Subsequently, the pilot test of the questionnaire was conducted on 95 university students who were excluded in the main study and the questionnaire items were revised and finalized by evaluating the questionnaire in terms of criteria such as language validity, clarity and appropriateness. Thus, the final version of the student evaluation form prepared for the investigation into the use of VR technologies in medical education was structured as a five-point Likert type scale consisting of four sections and 21 items.

Data Analysis

The value of factor loading for the developed data collection tool, KMO (Kaiser-Meyer-Olkin Measure of Sampling Adequacy) coefficient value to determine the suitability of the sample for measurements, Bartlett test to determine the consistency of inter-items, and Cronbach α reliability coefficient to estimate the reliability were used. The values of factor loading for 21 items ranged from .91 to .95. KMO value was .89. As the KMO value comes close to 1, factor analysis becomes more significant. KMO value between .50 and .70 is considered to be a medium level, between .71 and .80 is considered to be a good level and between .81 and .90 is considered to be a very good level and .91 and above is considered to be a great level (Field, 2005). Therefore, the sample was sufficient that data analysis could be conducted. It was found that the result of Bartlett's test was significant (Chi-square = 2329.147, p < 0.01). When the reliability of the questionnaire was examined, it was found that Cronbach's alpha reliability coefficient was .91. These findings confirmed that the data collection tool was reliable. Frequency and percentage values were used in the analysis of the collected data.

FINDINGS

Particular themes were found out in the process of preparing the data collection tool. These themes were Performance Expectancy', 'Effort Expectancy', 'Facilitating Conditions', 'Social Influence'. The findings related to the analysis of the first theme, "Performance Expectation" are given in Table 1.

Table 1 discusses the statistics in regard to the questions of "Performance Expectancy". The vast majority of students stated that the use of VR technologies in medical education enables the work to be done faster, enhances their performance, boosts their productivity and motivation, makes doing the assignments and practices easier, enhances the quality of the work done by them, and makes their learning process more effective and efficient. Based on these results, the students' performance expectancies

Table 1. Performance expectancy

Items		Strongly Disagree --- Strongly Agree					Total
		1	2	3	4	5	
1. Using Virtual Reality applications help me do my work more quickly in my courses.	f	18	26	78	197	102	421
	%	4.3	6.2	18.5	46.8	24.2	100.0
2. Using Virtual Reality applications improves my performance in my courses.	f	12	31	70	203	105	421
	%	2.9	7.4	16.6	48.2	24.9	100.0
3. Using Virtual Reality applications increases my productivity in my courses.	f	16	18	74	193	120	421
	%	3.8	4.3	17.6	45.8	28.5	100.0
4. Using Virtual Reality applications increases my motivation in my courses.	f	14	19	72	200	116	421
	%	3.3	4.5	17.1	47.5	27.6	100.0
5. Using Virtual Reality applications makes it easier for me to do my assignments in my courses.	f	10	30	76	192	113	421
	%	2.4	7.1	18.1	45.6	26.8	100.0
6. Using Virtual Reality applications improves the quality of my work in my courses.	f	10	30	74	191	116	421
	%	2.4	7.1	17.6	45.4	27.6	100.0
7. I find the use of Virtual Reality applications beneficial in my courses.	f	10	25	77	187	122	421
	%	2.4	5.9	18.3	44.4	29.0	100.0
8. Using Virtual Reality applications enables the learning process to be effective in my courses.	f	14	21	82	184	120	421
	%	3.3	5.0	19.5	43.7	28.5	100.0

regarding the use of VR technologies in medical education were high. This finding can be interpreted as facilitating students' acceptance and use of VR technologies in medical education.

The findings related to the analysis of the second theme, "Effort Expectancy" are given in Table 2.

Table 2 discusses the statistics in regard to the questions of "Effort Expectancy". The vast majority of students pointed out that learning the use of VR technologies in medical education is easy, they are effortlessly able to VR applications, the use of VR applications is not challenging and time-consuming, they feel comfortable while using VR applications, and they can easily do everything with VR applications. Based on these results, the students' effort expectancy regarding the use of VR technologies in medical education was low. In other words, students thought that they can easily utilize VR technologies by making a little effort. This finding can be interpreted as facilitating students' acceptance and use of VR technologies in medical education.

The findings related to the analysis of the third theme, "Facilitating Conditions" are given in Table 3.

Table 3 discusses the statistics in regard to the questions of "Facilitating Conditions". The vast majority of students indicated that they have the required knowledge to use VR technologies in medical education, there are persons whom they can get help when they have difficulty in using VR technologies in medical education, the use of VR applications is similar to the use other computer systems, they know persons whom they can get help in solving the problems that they encounter while using VR applications, and the help that they get will be sufficient to solve the problems they face. Based on these results, students have facilitating conditions related to the use of VR technologies in medical education. This finding can be interpreted as facilitating students' acceptance and use of VR technologies in medical education.

The findings related to the analysis of the fourth theme, "Social Influence" are given in Table 4.

Table 3 discusses the statistics in regard to the questions of "Facilitating Conditions". The vast majority of students indicated that people around them think it is important to effectively use VR technologies in medical education, the effective use of VR technologies increases their eminence among their schoolmates in medical education, and the effective use of VR technologies increases their respectability among their friends in medical education. Based on these results, it is concluded that students have social influence

Table 2. Effort expectancy

Items		Strongly Disagree --- Strongly Agree					Total
		1	2	3	4	5	
9. It is easy for me to learn to use Virtual Reality applications.	f	10	25	102	183	101	421
	%	2.4	5.9	24.2	43.5	24.0	100.0
10. I can easily use Virtual Reality applications.	f	12	24	97	189	99	421
	%	2.9	5.7	23.0	44.9	23.5	100.0
11. It takes less time to complete a task when I use Virtual Reality applications	f	12	28	107	170	104	421
	%	2.9	6.7	25.4	40.4	24.7	100.0
12. I feel comfortable while using Virtual Reality applications.	f	11	21	88	186	115	421
	%	2.6	5.0	20.9	44.2	27.3	100.0
13. I can do anything I want to do with Virtual Reality applications.	f	16	40	111	167	87	421
	%	3.8	9.5	26.4	39.7	20.7	100.0

Table 3. Facilitating conditions

Items		Strongly Disagree --- Strongly Agree					Total
		1	2	3	4	5	
14. I have the essential knowledge to use Virtual Reality applications effectively.	f	15	32	134	154	86	421
	%	3.6	7.6	31.8	36.6	20.4	100.0
15. There are persons whom I can get help when I have difficulty in using Virtual Reality applications.	f	11	23	87	183	117	421
	%	2.6	5.5	20.7	43.5	27.8	100.0
16. Using Virtual Reality applications is similar to using other computer applications.	f	13	29	122	171	86	421
	%	3.1	6.9	29.0	40.6	20.4	100.0
17. I know persons whom I can get help in solving the problems that I encounter while using Virtual Reality applications.	f	14	21	98	179	109	421
	%	3.3	5.0	23.3	42.5	25.9	100.0
18. The help service of Virtual Reality applications is enough to solve the problems I face.	f	15	30	105	181	90	421
	%	3.6	7.1	24.9	43.0	21.4	100.0

conditions related to the use of VR technologies in medical education. This finding can be interpreted as facilitating students' acceptance and use of VR technologies in medical education.

CONCLUSION

This study explored university student acceptance and use of VR technologies in medical education. The study was conducted with a sample of 421 university students who participated in courses and activities related to the use of VR applications in medical education. A questionnaire consisting of 4 sub-dimensions and 21 items developed by the researchers was administered to the students. This questionnaire consisted of sub-dimensions of 'Performance Expectancy', 'Effort Expectancy', 'Facilitating Conditions' and 'Social Influence'. The results demonstrated in general that the students' acceptance and use of VR technologies are high in medical education.

Table 4. Social influence

Items		Strongly Disagree --- Strongly Agree					Total
		1	2	3	4	5	
19. People around me think it's important that I use Virtual Reality applications effectively.	f	15	25	116	176	89	421
	%	3.6	5.9	27.6	41.8	21.1	100.0
20. The fact that I use Virtual Reality applications effectively increases my prestige among my schoolmates.	f	18	41	123	152	87	421
	%	4.3	9.7	29.2	36.1	20.7	100.0
21. My friends who effectively use Virtual Reality applications have more respectability.	f	25	38	130	137	91	421
	%	5.9	9.0	30.9	32.5	21.6	100.0

When the results related to the performance expectancy sub-dimension were examined, the majority of the students indicated that the use of VR applications helps make tasks faster, increase their performance, productivity and motivation in the courses, do assignments easily, improve the quality of assignments and lectures, and make the learning process more effective. Beheiry et al. (2019) state that tasks can easily be divided into virtual manageable tasks through the adoption of VR technologies, which boosts knowledge acquisition and makes knowledge transfer faster and they also state that the use of VR applications helps close knowledge gaps between experts and novices, which enables an inexpert to maintain and promote interest and motivation in healthcare.

When the results related to the effort expectancy sub-dimension were probed, the majority of the students remarked that the use of VR applications is easy to learn, that they can easily use these technologies and applications, and that they feel comfortable while using these applications. For these reasons, it can be claimed that the use of VR technologies is simple to operate for students. In other words, they can use VR technologies without making much effort. This result supported the claim that VR applications are easy to use (Huang et al., 2016).

When the results related to the facilitating conditions sub-dimension were looked into, the majority of the students pointed out that they have the required knowledge to use the VR applications effectively, that they know individuals whom they can get help around them when they have difficulty in using these applications and technologies, and that the use of VR applications is similar to the use of other computer systems. Therefore, these findings showed that students have facilitating conditions for using VR technologies, which increases their acceptance and use of VR technologies in medical education. This aligns with the study conducted by Sanchez-Cabrero et al. (2019) who explored users' interest in the use of VR technologies as a learning tool. They revealed that the desire to utilize VR as a learning tool is higher than the current use of VR although they didn't just focus on the interest in the use of VR in healthcare settings.

When the results related to the social influence sub-dimension were investigated, the majority of the students stated that the people around them think it is important to effectively use VR technologies in medical education and that the effective use of these technologies increases the prestige and respect among their friends. Based on these results, students have social influence for the use of VR technologies, which increases their acceptance and use of VR technologies in medical education. After Lee, Kim and Choi (2019) administered a survey with 350 people from South Korea, they reached a similar result that social interactions have a great effect on the intention to use VR technologies.

Based on these results, it can be asserted that university students are highly prone to accept and use VR technologies in medical education. Similar studies have shown that medical students have high acceptance and use of technology in medical education (Sezer & Yilmaz, 2019). These results of studies have a significant implication in terms of integrating VR technologies into courses and laboratory applications in medical education. A variety of instructional design models can be used in the VR integration process. Specifically, one of the instructional design models is ASSURE Model that can be used by instructors to design and develop an appropriate learning environment in medical education (Sezer, Yilmaz, & Karaoglan Yilmaz, 2013). Also, when the integration of VR technologies into a medical class is properly done, it potentially provides interactive and effective virtual learning experiences in which medical students can learn the subjects that are difficult to understand and practice the burdensome tasks that result likely in adverse outcomes. Thus, it will be possible to improve student performance, learning process and outcomes.

FUTURE RESEARCH DIRECTIONS

This study has some limitations. First, the students' acceptance and use of VR technologies in medical education is limited to data collected from the students through a questionnaire developed by researchers within the framework of UTAUT Model. Data from the questionnaire were described as item-based frequency and percentage values and the survey results were interpreted in the study. In future studies, students' acceptance and use of VR technologies in medical education would be examined according to other technology acceptance model in the literature. Besides, instead of item-based analysis of questionnaire items, students' acceptance and use of VR technologies in medical education would be investigated by using a questionnaire tested through exploratory factor analysis and confirmatory factor analysis in future studies. In this research, the students' acceptance and use of VR technologies in medical education were explored within the scope of an anatomy course. In order to increase the generalizability of the results of the study, students' acceptance and use of VR technologies would be compared by conducting similar studies within the scope of different courses in other specialties such as physiology, public health, emergency medicine, psychiatry. The acceptance and use of VR technologies in medical education were discussed in the view of the students in this study. The acceptance and use of VR technologies in medical education would be examined from the faculty perspective in future research. Therefore, it would be possible to gain insight into their opinions of utilizing VR technologies. Lastly, this study is limited to explore the acceptance and use of VR technologies in medical education. In future studies, the acceptance and use of VR technologies in different fields of higher education would be investigated.

REFERENCES

Baukal, C. E., Ausburn, F. B., & Ausburn, L. J. (2013). A Proposed Multimedia Cone of Abstraction: Updating a Classic Instructional Design Theory. *Journal of Educational Technology*, *9*(4), 15–24.

Bloom, B. S. (1974). Time and learning. *The American Psychologist*, *29*(9), 682–688. doi:10.1037/h0037632

Bracq, M. S., Michinov, E., & Jannin, P. (2019). Virtual reality simulation in nontechnical skills training for healthcare professionals: A systematic review. *Simulation in Healthcare*, *14*(3), 188–194. doi:10.1097/SIH.0000000000000347 PMID:30601464

De Luca, R., Manuli, A., De Domenico, C., Voi, E. L., Buda, A., Maresca, G., ... Calabrò, R. S. (2019). Improving neuropsychiatric symptoms following stroke using virtual reality. *Case Reports in Medicine*, *98*(19), e15236. PMID:31083155

de Ribaupierre, S., Kapralos, B., Haji, F., Stroulia, E., Dubrowski, A., & Eagleson, R. (2014). Healthcare training enhancement through virtual reality and serious games. In *Virtual, Augmented Reality and Serious Games for Healthcare 1* (pp. 9–27). Berlin: Springer. doi:10.1007/978-3-642-54816-1_2

Drummond, K. H., Houston, T., & Irvine, T. (2014). *The rise and fall and rise of virtual reality*. Vox Media.

Durak, A., & Karaoglan Yilmaz, F. G. (2019). Artirilmiş gerçekliğin eğitsel uygulamalari üzerine orta-okul öğrencilerinin görüşleri [Opinions of secondary school students on educational practices of augmented reality]. *Abant İzzet Baysal Üniversitesi Eğitim Fakültesi Dergisi, 19*(2), 468–481. doi:10.17240/aibuefd.2019.19.46660-425148

Eames, S., Hoffmann, T., Worrall, L., & Read, S. (2010). Stroke patients' and carers' perception of barriers to accessing stroke information. *Topics in Stroke Rehabilitation, 17*(2), 69–78. doi:10.1310/tsr1702-69 PMID:20542850

El Beheiry, M., Doutreligne, S., Caporal, C., Ostertag, C., Dahan, M., & Masson, J. B. (2019). Virtual Reality: Beyond Visualization. *Journal of Molecular Biology, 431*(7), 315–321. doi:10.1016/j.jmb.2019.01.033 PMID:30738026

Field, A. (2005). *Discovering statistics using SPSS*. London: Sage Publications.

Gadelha, R. (2018). Revolutionizing Education: The promise of virtual reality. *Childhood Education, 94*(1), 40–43. doi:10.1080/00094056.2018.1420362

Gaggioli, A. (2017). An open research community for studying virtual reality experience. *Cyberpsychology, Behavior, and Social Networking, 20*(2), 138–139. doi:10.1089/cyber.2017.29063.csi

Gunn, T., Jones, L., Bridge, P., Rowntree, P., & Nissen, L. (2018). The use of virtual reality simulation to improve technical skill in the undergraduate medical imaging student. *Interactive Learning Environments, 26*(5), 613–620. doi:10.1080/10494820.2017.1374981

Hoffmann, T., & McKenna, K. (2006). Analysis of stroke patients' and carers' reading ability and the content and design of written materials: Recommendations for improving written stroke information. *Patient Education and Counseling, 60*(3), 286–293. doi:10.1016/j.pec.2005.06.020 PMID:16098708

Huang, H. M., Liaw, S. S., & Lai, C. M. (2016). Exploring learner acceptance of the use of virtual reality in medical education: A case study of desktop and projection-based display systems. *Interactive Learning Environments, 24*(1), 3–19. doi:10.1080/10494820.2013.817436

Karaoğlan Yılmaz, F. G., & Yılmaz, R. (2019). Examining the opinions of prospective teachers about the use of virtual reality applications in education [Sanal gerçeklik uygulamalarının eğitimde kullanımına ilişkin öğretmen adaylarının görüşlerinin incelenmesi]. In *Proceedings of the International Congress on Science and Education*. Academic Press.

King, D., Tee, S., Falconer, L., Angell, C., Holley, D., & Mills, A. (2018). Virtual health education: Scaling practice to transform student learning: Using virtual reality learning environments in healthcare education to bridge the theory/practice gap and improve patient safety. *Nurse Education Today, 71*, 7–9. doi:10.1016/j.nedt.2018.08.002 PMID:30205259

Klopfer, E., & Squire, K. (2008). Environmental detectives: The development of an augmented reality platform for environmental simulations. *Educational Technology Research and Development, 56*(2), 203–228. doi:10.100711423-007-9037-6

Krueger, M. W., & Wilson, S. (1985). VIDEOPLACE: A report from the artificial reality laboratory. *Leonardo, 18*(3), 145–151. doi:10.2307/1578043

Lee, C., & Wong, G. K. C. (2019). Virtual reality and augmented reality in the management of intracranial tumors: A review. *Journal of Clinical Neuroscience, 62*, 14–20. doi:10.1016/j.jocn.2018.12.036 PMID:30642663

Morel, M., Bideau, B., Lardy, J., & Kulpa, R. (2015). Advantages and limitations of virtual reality for balance assessment and rehabilitation. *Neurophysiologie Clinique [Clinical Neurophysiology], 45*(4-5), 315–326. doi:10.1016/j.neucli.2015.09.007 PMID:26527045

Mukkamala, S. R., & Madhusudhanan, M. (2016). *U.S. Patent Application No. 14/478,277.*

Murthi, S., & Varshney, A. (2018). How Augmented Reality Will Make Surgery Safer. *Harvard Business Review.* Retrieved from https://hbr.org/2018/03/how-augmented-reality-will-make-surgery-safer

Norris, M. W., Spicer, K., & Byrd, T. (2019). Virtual Reality: The New Pathway for Effective Safety Training. *Professional Safety, 64*(06), 36–39.

Page, R. L. (2000). Brief history of flight simulation. In *SimTecT 2000 Proceedings* (pp. 11-17). Academic Press.

Pelargos, P. E., Nagasawa, D. T., Lagman, C., Tenn, S., Demos, J. V., Lee, S. J., ... Bari, A. (2017). Utilizing virtual and augmented reality for educational and clinical enhancements in neurosurgery. *Journal of Clinical Neuroscience, 35*, 1–4. doi:10.1016/j.jocn.2016.09.002 PMID:28137372

Ravi, D. K., Kumar, N., & Singhi, P. (2017). Effectiveness of virtual reality rehabilitation for children and adolescents with cerebral palsy: An updated evidence-based systematic review. *Physiotherapy, 103*(3), 245–258. doi:10.1016/j.physio.2016.08.004 PMID:28109566

Riener, R., & Harders, M. (2012). *Virtual reality in medicine.* Springer Science & Business Media. doi:10.1007/978-1-4471-4011-5

Riva, G. (2005). Virtual reality in psychotherapy [review]. *Cyberpsychology & Behavior, 8*(3), 220–240. doi:10.1089/cpb.2005.8.220 PMID:15971972

Rose, T., Nam, C. S., & Chen, K. B. (2018). Immersion of virtual reality for rehabilitation-Review. *Applied Ergonomics, 69*, 153–161. doi:10.1016/j.apergo.2018.01.009 PMID:29477323

Roy, E., Bakr, M. M., & George, R. (2017). The need for virtual reality simulators in dental education: A review. *The Saudi Dental Journal, 29*(2), 41–47. doi:10.1016/j.sdentj.2017.02.001 PMID:28490842

Ruthenbeck, G. S., & Reynolds, K. J. (2015). Virtual reality for medical training: The state-of-the-art. *Journal of Simulation, 9*(1), 16–26. doi:10.1057/jos.2014.14

Sacks, R., Perlman, A., & Barak, R. (2013). Construction safety training using immersive virtual reality. *Construction Management and Economics, 31*(9), 1005–1017. doi:10.1080/01446193.2013.828844

Sánchez-Cabrero, R., Costa-Román, Ó., Pericacho-Gómez, F. J., Novillo-López, M. Á., Arigita-García, A., & Barrientos-Fernández, A. (2019). Early virtual reality adopters in Spain: Sociodemographic profile and interest in the use of virtual reality as a learning tool. *Heliyon (London), 5*(3), e01338. doi:10.1016/j.heliyon.2019.e01338 PMID:30923768

Seymour, N. (2008). VR to OR: A review of the evidence that virtual reality simulation improves operating room performance. *World Journal of Surgery*, *32*(2), 182–188. doi:10.100700268-007-9307-9 PMID:18060453

Sezer, B., & Yilmaz, R. (2019). Learning management system acceptance scale (LMSAS): A validity and reliability study. *Australasian Journal of Educational Technology*, *35*(3), 15–30. doi:10.14742/ajet.3959

Sezer, B., Yilmaz, R., & Karaoglan Yilmaz, F. G. (2013). Integrating technology into classroom: The learner-centered instructional design. *International Journal on New Trends in Education and Their Implications*, *4*(4), 134–144.

Sharif, M., Ansari, G. J., Yasmin, M., & Fernandes, S. L. (2018). Reviews of the Implications of VR/AR Health Care Applications in Terms of Organizational and Societal Change. *Emerging Technologies for Health and Medicine: Virtual Reality, Augmented Reality, Artificial Intelligence, Internet of Things, Robotics Industry*, *4*(0), 1–19.

Thompson-Butel, A. G., Shiner, C. T., McGhee, J., Bailey, B. J., Bou-Haidar, P., McCorriston, M., & Faux, S. G. (2019). The Role of Personalized Virtual Reality in Education for Patients Post Stroke— A Qualitative Case Series. *Journal of Stroke and Cerebrovascular Diseases*, *28*(2), 450–457. doi:10.1016/j.jstrokecerebrovasdis.2018.10.018 PMID:30415917

Vaughan, N., Dubey, V. N., Wainwright, T. W., & Middleton, R. G. (2016). A review of virtual reality based training simulators for orthopaedic surgery. *Medical Engineering & Physics*, *38*(2), 59–71. doi:10.1016/j.medengphy.2015.11.021 PMID:26751581

Venkatesh, V., Morris, M. G., Davis, G. B., & Davis, F. D. (2003). User acceptance of information technology: Toward a unified view. *Management Information Systems Quarterly*, *27*(3), 425–478. doi:10.2307/30036540

Warburton, S. (2009). Second Life in higher education: Assessing the potential for and the barriers to deploying virtual worlds in learning and teaching. *British Journal of Educational Technology*, *40*(3), 414–426. doi:10.1111/j.1467-8535.2009.00952.x

Yilmaz, R., Karaoglan Yilmaz, F. G., & Ezin, C. C. (2018). Self-directed learning with technology and academic motivation as predictors of tablet PC acceptance. In Handbook of Research on Mobile Devices and Smart Gadgets in K-12 Education (pp. 87-102). Hershey, PA: IGI Global. doi:10.4018/978-1-5225-2706-0.ch007

Zhang, M., Zhang, Z., Chang, Y., Aziz, E. S., Esche, S., & Chassapis, C. (2018). Recent developments in game-based virtual reality educational laboratories using the Microsoft Kinect. *International Journal of Emerging Technologies in Learning*, *13*(1), 138–159. doi:10.3991/ijet.v13i01.7773

ADDITIONAL READING

Harders, M. (2008). *Surgical scene generation for virtual reality-based training in medicine*. Springer Science & Business Media. doi:10.1007/978-1-84800-107-7

Kyaw, B. M., Saxena, N., Posadzki, P., Vseteckova, J., Nikolaou, C. K., George, P. P., ... Car, L. T. (2019). Virtual reality for health professions education: Systematic review and meta-analysis by the Digital Health Education collaboration. *Journal of Medical Internet Research*, *21*(1), e12959. doi:10.2196/12959 PMID:30668519

Layona, R., Yulianto, B., & Tunardi, Y. (2018). Web based augmented reality for human body anatomy learning. *Procedia Computer Science*, *135*, 457–464. doi:10.1016/j.procs.2018.08.197

Munzer, B. W., Khan, M. M., Shipman, B., & Mahajan, P. (2019). Augmented Reality in Emergency Medicine: A Scoping Review. *Journal of Medical Internet Research*, *21*(4), e12368. doi:10.2196/12368 PMID:30994463

Nicholson, D. T., Chalk, C., Funnell, W. R. J., & Daniel, S. J. (2006). Can virtual reality improve anatomy education? A randomised controlled study of a computer-generated three-dimensional anatomical ear model. *Medical Education*, *40*(11), 1081–1087. doi:10.1111/j.1365-2929.2006.02611.x PMID:17054617

Riener, R., & Harders, M. (2012). *Virtual reality in medicine*. Springer Science & Business Media. doi:10.1007/978-1-4471-4011-5

Roland, J. (2018). *Virtual reality and medicine*. Reference Point Press.

Sezer, B., & Sezer, T. A. (2019). Teaching communication skills with technology: Creating a virtual patient for medical students. *Australasian Journal of Educational Technology*, *35*(5), 183–198.

Uppot, R. N., Laguna, B., McCarthy, C. J., De Novi, G., Phelps, A., Siegel, E., & Courtier, J. (2019). Implementing virtual and augmented reality tools for radiology education and training, communication, and clinical care. *Radiology*, *291*(3), 570–580. doi:10.1148/radiol.2019182210 PMID:30990383

KEY TERMS AND DEFINITIONS

Acceptance of Augmented Reality: Students' behavioral status of acceptance and adaptation with regard to usage of augmented reality technologies with the educational purpose.

Acceptance of Virtual Reality: Students' behavioral status of acceptance and adaptation with regard to usage of virtual reality technologies with the educational purpose.

Augmented Reality: Augmented reality is a set of technologies that superimpose a computer-generated image(s) on the physical world, therefore providing a simultaneously mixed experience of virtual objects and the real world.

Effort Expectancy: The degree of ease associated with the use of the system (Venkatesh et al., 2003, p. 450).

Facilitating Conditions: The degree to which an individual believes that an organizational and technical infrastructure exists to support use of the system (Venkatesh et al., 2003, p. 453).

Performance Expectancy: The degree to which an individual believes that using the system will help him or her to attain gains in job performance (Venkatesh et al., 2003, p. 447).

Simulation: A simulation is an imitation of a real-world process in a controlled environment.

Social Influence: The degree to which an individual perceives that important others believe he or she should use the new system (Venkatesh et al., 2003, p. 451).

UTAUT Model: UTAUT Model is the Unified Theory of Acceptance and Use of Technology that is used for explanation of user perception and acceptance behavior. (Venkatesh et al., 2003).

Virtual Reality: Virtual reality is computer-generated simulations of three or more dimensions created by modelling of real objects or environments. Users can interact with these computer-generated simulations through their senses such as vision, hearing and touch and experience realistic objects by controlling them (Karaoğlan Yılmaz & Yılmaz, 2019).

Virtual Reality Immersion: Virtual reality immersion is the perception of being physically present in a non-physical world (Mukkamala & Madhusudhanan, 2016)

Virtual World: A virtual world is a computer-based simulated environment.

Chapter 5
QoS–Aware Data Dissemination Mechanisms for Wireless Body Area Networks

Javed Iqbal Bangash
ⓘ https://orcid.org/0000-0002-5622-0796
The University of Agriculture, Peshawar, Pakistan

Abdul Waheed Khan
FAST, National University of Computer and Emerging Sciences, Pakistan

Adil Sheraz
Abasyn University, Pakistan

Asfandyar Khan
The University of Agriculture, Peshawar, Pakistan

Sajid Umair
ⓘ https://orcid.org/0000-0002-6798-8426
The University of Agriculture, Peshawar, Pakistan

ABSTRACT

To reduce healthcare costs and improve human well-being, a promising technology known as wireless body area networks (WBANs) has recently emerged. It is comprised of various on-body as well as implanted sensors which seamlessly monitor the physiological characteristics of the human body. The information is heterogeneous in nature, requires different QoS factors. The information may be classified as delay-sensitive, reliability-sensitive, critical, and routine. On-time delivery and minimum losses are the main QoS-factors required to transmit the captured information. Various researchers have work to provide the required QoS, and some have also considered the other constraints due to the characteristics and texture of the human body. In this research work, we have discussed the communication architecture of

DOI: 10.4018/978-1-7998-2521-0.ch005

WBANS along with the various challenges of WBANS. Furthermore, we have classified and discussed the existing QoS-aware data dissemination mechanisms. In the end, a comparative study of existing QoS-aware data dissemination mechanisms highlights the pros and cons of each mechanism.

1. INTRODUCTION

Rapid increase in population of elderly people living with chronic diseases is inevitable in years to come which requires round the clock monitoring of such patients (Movassaghi et al., 2013). According to World Population Ageing 2017, the worldwide elderly population (60+ aged people) is predictable to be increased from 962 million to 2100 million between 2017 & 2050 and 3100 million in 2100 (World Population Ageing, 2017). Similarly, as per report of World Health Organization (WHO), the world's population of 60+ aged people between 2015 and 2050 will be almost doubled (12% - 22%) (World Health Organization (WHO) - Ageing and Health, 2017). Besides the people suffering from chronic diseases, the patients inside the hospital also require different level of monitoring ranging from a couple of times a day to continuous monitoring. The continuous and on-and-off health monitoring requires a huge amount of additional medical and health-care cost (World Health Organization (WHO) - Gobal Health Observatory, 2018). The aforementioned statistics ask for major change towards proactive and more affordable management to prevent or detect the diseases at an early stage (Movassaghi et al., 2014). The merger of pervasive computing, wireless sensor technologies and bio-medical engineering has led to the emergence of a promising technology called as Wireless Body Area Networks (WBANs), as shown in Figure 1. WBANs provide continuous and unsupervised vital-signs monitoring of human body. It can be utilized in various monitoring applications, such as medical assistance and health-care, sports, entertainments and rehabilitation systems.

WBANs offer the paradigm change towards proactive arrangements and early detection of the different diseases. In WBANs, with the help of various on-body, on-cloths (wearable) and/or implanted sensors (Ullah et al., 2010) like temperature[1], heartbeat[2], electromyography (EMG)[3], pH-level[4], blood pressure[5], electrocardiogram (ECG)[6], electroencephalogram (EEG)[7], respiration rate[7] data collection and analysis is performed thereby reducing the health-care cost. Such sensors are commonly known as Bio-Medical Sensor Nodes (BMSNs). Different BMSNs are shown in Figure 2 where upon sensing and locally processing, the vital signs information is further reported to a Body Coordinator (BC), located locally near the human body or on the human body.

Various types of data packets are generated by the heterogeneous natured BMSNs which require different QoS parameters among which latency and reliability are of key importance (Monowar et al., 2014). Certain data packets can tolerate some losses but require delivery within certain time-frame and others might require shortest delay and highest reliability. There may be some data packets that should be delivered with highest reliability while others may not any such constraints.

2. COMMUNICATION ARCHITECTURE OF WBSNs

The communication architecture of WBSNs is consisting of three tiers as shown in Figure 3.

2.1 Tier 1 – Intra-WBAN

It is the local body area network of various BMSNs where they report the sensory data of patients to the Body Coordinator (BC) which is the base station located locally.

2.2 Tier 2 – Inter-WBAN

It is the segment of the network where different BCs process, aggregate and forward the received vital-signs information towards the sink(s).

Figure 1. Building blocks of WBANs

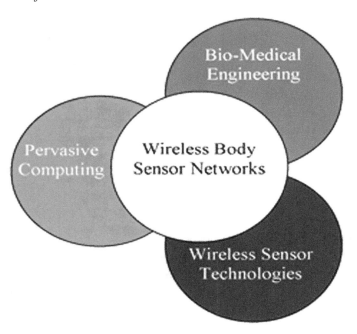

Figure 2. (a) Wearable BMSNs (b) Implanted BMSNs and (c) Deep brain stimulator (Yang, 2014)

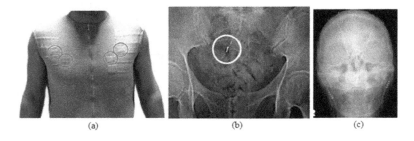

Figure 3. Communication architecture of WBSNs

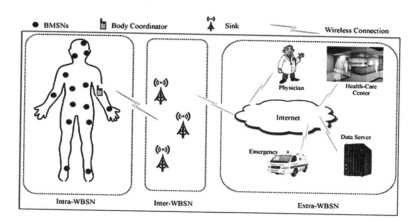

2.3 Tier 3 – Extra-WBAN

It is the long-range network where the sink(s) report the collected data towards the point of interest which may be medical center or database via regular infra-structure such as fixed network or internet, for monitoring and/or storage purposes.

3. ISSUES AND CHALLENGES IN WBANs

Being a subset of WSNs, WBANs inherent all the constraints of WSNs. Moreover, there are some other unique constraints and challenges of WBANs that need to be addressed. Unlike traditional applications of WSNs, where homogeneous types of sensor nodes are used, different types of BMSNs are used in WBANs. These BMSNs differ from each other in terms of data generation rates, energy consumption, storage capacity and computation (Ullah et al., 2012). The use of various types of BMSNs operating at various frequencies results in compatibility issues. The algorithms and systems designed for WBANs need to address the compatibility problem. Similarly, the data generation rate is high in WBANs and need efficient data gathering and processing methods (Darwish & Hassanien, 2011). In some cases, for example to detect heart-related diseases, several BMSNs are required and result in generation of large amount of data.

In addition to stringent resources in terms of computation, storage and radio transceiver, the low bandwidth of BMSNs may be fluctuated because of the variation in noise along with other types of interferences (Ullah et al., 2012). Proper deployment of BMSNs and their topology is of high significance for WBANs (Ullah et al., 2012). Other than aforementioned stringent resources, heterogeneity of BMSNs as well as postural movements of body affects the performance of the system in all aspects.

Security and privacy of WBANs is also of paramount importance. The patient's vital-signs information becomes vulnerable if the security issue is not being considered (Xiao et al., 2006; Dagtaş et al., 2008). Any leakage of the patient's vital-signs information may have physiological impact if he/she is suffering from any embarrassing disease (Kumar and Lee, 2012). The conventional security and privacy techniques cannot be directly adopted in WBANs due to inherent limitations of BMSNs (Lee et al.,

2013). Therefore, security and privacy related problems of the patient's vital-signs data should also be taken into consideration while designing algorithms and systems for WBANs.

WBANs aim to provide continuous observation of vital-signs information of the human body and giving freedom of movement. Mobility is not a new concept in WSNs but WBANs require applications that support mobile users. Mobility of users necessitates multi-hop networks with location awareness (Darwish & Hassanien, 2011). Moreover, the different BMSNs need to be synchronized so that to avoid any conflicts in reporting sensory data to body coordinator. Finally, the different implanted and wearable BMSNs are different in terms of resources, data rates and frequency they use, thereby need to be integrated that demands for improvements in the modular based approaches (Darwish & Hassanien, 2011).

4. ISSUES AND CHALLENGES RELATED TO DATA DISSEMINATION IN WBANs

Design and development of efficient data dissemination mechanisms in WBANs is a difficult job due to the unique constraints implied by the nature of human tissues, behavior of human body and the QoS requirements of the heterogeneous natured sensory data. The traditional WSNs' research does not address the unique constraints of WBANs (Honeine et al., 2011). The different issues and challenges related to data dissemination in WBANs are identified and briefly discussed in the succeeding sub-sections.

4.1 Desired QoS Provisions Based on Nature of Vital Signs

Heterogeneous natured sensor nodes generate various kinds of data packets containing the vital-signs information and require different QoS provisions. Djenouri and Balasingham (2009), Razzaque et al. (2011) and Monowar et al. (2014) have categorized the sensory vital-signs information into non-constrained data, reliability-constrained data, latency-constrained data and critical data (both latency and reliability constrained). Some of the QoS-aware data dissemination mechanisms, discussed later in this chapter, have addressed the issue of the heterogeneous nature of sensory data. The proposed data dissemination mechanisms need to be aware of the desired QoS provisions based on the nature of the vital signs.

4.2 Radiation Absorption and Overheating

The electromagnetic waves generated when BMSNs communicate with each other wirelessly are absorbed by the human tissues as they are saline-water in nature. Energy consumption of sensor node's circuitry and absorption of antenna radiation are the two main factors contribute to the temperature rise issue of BMSNs (Tang et al., 2005). This temperature rise will affect the human tissues (Tang et al., 2005), which are heat sensitive organs and may damage some tissues (Bag and Bassiouni, 2008), if continued for long period of time. The main goal of the temperature-aware data dissemination mechanism is that the temperature of the BMSNs needs to be under the threshold value to avoid overheating. Researchers should minimize the overheating phenomenon of BMSNs thereby designing temperature-aware data dissemination mechanisms for WBANs.

4.3 High and Dynamic Path Loss

The path loss models designed for traditional wireless networks characterized by free-space and multipath fading effects are not really appropriate for WBANs which implies higher and dynamic on and in-body path loss (Quwaider et al., 2010). The reasons behind the dynamic and high path loss in WBANs are the human body's postural movements and the in-body wireless communication (in case of implanted BMSNs) (Lin et al., 2014; Khan et al., 2010; Reusens et al., 2009; Sayrafian-Pour et al., 2009). Therefore, researchers should take care of the high and dynamic path loss while designing data dissemination mechanisms for WBANs.

4.4 Energy Efficiency

Energy efficiency not only covers the individual nodes' energy consumption but also that of the overall network's lifetime. For implanted BMSNs, replacement of power source may not be feasible whereas for wearable BMSNs it might results in discomfort of patients. Energy consumption is relatively high for communication in comparison to other tasks of sensor nodes such as processing and sensing, (Kandris et al., 2009). Instead of overwhelming the energy resource of a single node thereby repeatedly selecting the same node as next-hop should be avoided thereby alternating among a set of different paths and/or nodes during data dissemination (Anisi et al., 2012). Quwaider and Biswas (2009) defines the network life as elapsed time till the first node depletes its energy. Due to inconvenience of battery replacement for implanted BMSNs, the network's lifetime is of crucial importance for WBANs (Boulis et al., 2012).

5. CLASSIFICATION OF DATA DISSEMINATION MECHANISMS FOR WBANs

During last decade, data dissemination in WBANs has gained the attention of the research community and industry. Different types of data dissemination mechanisms have been proposed. This section covers the state-of-the-art data dissemination mechanisms are discussed. The existing data dissemination mechanisms may be categorized as QoS-aware, postural-movement-based, temperature-aware, cross-layered and cluster-based data dissemination mechanism, as given in Figure 4.

6. OVERVIEW Of QoS-AWARE DATA DISSEMINATION MECHANISMS

The different QoS-aware and energy-aware data dissemination mechanisms designed for WSNs (Nazir & Hasbullah, 2013; Su et al., 2013; Ben-Othman & Yahya, 2010), wireless multimedia sensor networks (Kandris et al., 2011; Li & Chuang, 2013; Shen et al., 2013) and MANETs (Srinivasan & Kamalakkannan, 2012; Charu, 2013), cannot be directly used due to unique constraints of WBANs. However, with due customization according to the dynamics and requirements of WBANs they can be incorporated. Different QoS-aware data dissemination mechanisms for WBANs are discussed below and shown in Figure 5.

Figure 4. Classification of data dissemination mechanisms for WBANs

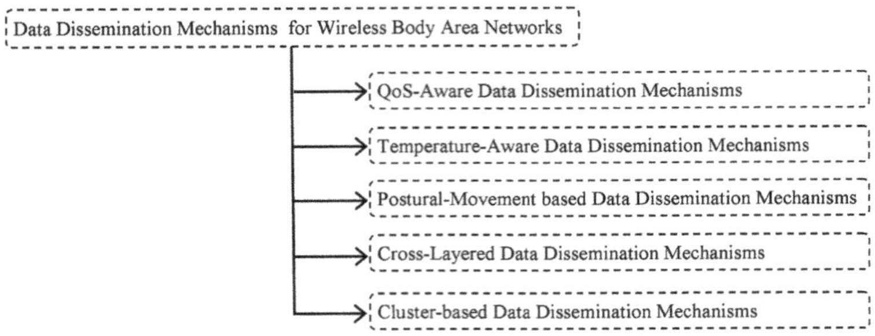

6.1 QoS-Aware Routing Service Framework (QoS-ARSF)

To cater QoS support to users and priority-based routing, QoS-ARSF is proposed in (Liang and Balasingham, 2007). Wireless channel status, user specific QoS requirements, nodes' willingness to behave as router and priority levels of the data packets, are considered as QoS metrics. There are four modules in the architecture: Routing Service Module (RSM), Application Programming Interfaces (APIs) module, Packet Queuing and Scheduling Module (PQSM) and System Information Repository Module (SIRM). The functionalities of APIs module include interfacing the user application with RSM. The APIs module is further divided into four sub modules: QoS-metrics selection which considers packet succes ratio, power consumption, and end-to-end latency. Packet sending/receiving sub module gets data packets from user application and directs it toward next node which may be sink node. Data packets are prioritized by packet priority level setting sub module. Admission control and service level control sub module is responsible for network condition feedback to user application. Eight different level priority is being defined fro both Data and Control packets, where control packets are assigned with highest priority level as compared to other data packets. RSM maintains and updates the routing table according to neighbor's status information. Due to network congestion if sensor node is unable to access the wireless channel, and the buffer reaches to a pre-assigned threshold, then PQSM intimates the user application to minimize willingness level and service level to behave as a router, to avoid packet losses. SIRM includes Routing Willingness (RW) table and Link State (LS) table. The status of the link in accordance with end-to-end latency, average packet success ratio and channel bandwidth is maintained by the LS table. The RW table maintains the information of all nodes to behave as forwarding node or router.

6.2 Reinforcement Learning Based Routing Protocol with QoS Support (RL-QRP)

In (Balasingham, 2008) a RL-QRP is proposed having QoS support, and it uses distributed Q-learning algorithm and geographic information in which optimal routes can be observed and noted using experience and achievements. The small bio-medical sensor nodes that are fixed either with the body or inside the body sense the data and forward to the sink nodes that are installed at fixed places. After sink nodes collect the data packets from BMSNs, forward that collected data to medical center and/or data center for further analysis in real time. The major QoS metrics in this approach are end-to-end latency and success ratio of packets. Each sensor node in Q-learning algorithm gathers a reward which may be either

Figure 5. QoS-Aware data dissemination mechanisms for WBANs

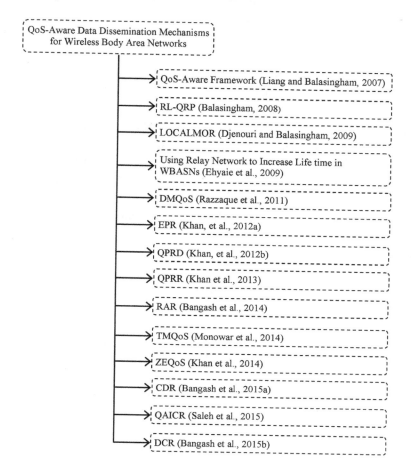

negative or positive after sending the collected data to its neighbor. Future decisions will be based on the Q-value of the BMSN, as in Q-learning algorithm it gets reward and expected future reward from its neighbor nodes. Optimal routes are made final and known once sensor nodes Q-values are exchanged with its neighbors on one hop distance. Expected future reward is predicted by sensor nodes using Q-value information of the neighbor sensor nodes. Routing table is formed in the each sensor node by considering its list of Q-values.

For the mobile nodes, the authors have suggested to use RWMM (Random Waypoint Mobility Model), in which the BMSNs can only shift to the destinations which are randomly predefined and remain there for certain time. However, in RL-QRP, Q-values of the neighbors are used to get the optimal paths and energy level as one of big constraints in WBANs is overlooked.

6.3 QoS and Geographic Routing (LOCALMOR)

In (Djenouri & Balasingham, 2009), LOCALMOR is proposed to fulfill QoS needs that rely on type of data like reliability, latency and energy efficiency so that system could be assisted. The proposed technique categorizes data of the patient into different types of traffic like, critical (adverse), delay sensitive, reliability sensitive and regular traffic. Data in the raw form from sensors is gathered by the body sensor node that is also known as coordinator, and after necessary processing and aggregation data is finally sent to the sink node. One or more than one patients that may be fixed or mobile can be covered and protected by each fixed sink node. Two types of sink nodes have been presented in the proposed protocol i.e. Primary and Secondary Sinks. A similar copy of each message is gathered by all the individual sinks.

In this approach, four different modules are used i-e neighbor manager, delay sensitive, reliability sensitive and energy/power efficiency module. The responsibility of Neighbor Manager (NM) module is to gather and forward Hello packets and updates about neighbor's information. Latency sensitive data packets are being routed and forwarded by delay sensitive module using Pocket Velocity Approach as in (Chipara et al., 2006). The duty of the reliability sensitive module is to acquire the desired reliability for the data packets by taking all data packets to the destination (Primary and Secondary sinks). The responsibility of power/energy efficiency module is to deal with the data packets of the regular traffic and ensures the efficient utilization of the data related metrics that can be used by other modules. This energy efficiency can be obtained by taking both the residual and transmission energy and taking minimum and maximum approaches as in (Coello, 2000).

6.4 Using Relay Nodes to Increase Lifetime in WBANs

Ehyaie et al. (2009) have proposed a QoS-aware data dissemination mechanism to improve the energy consumption as well as the network lifetime using special types of nodes called as relay nodes. Three types of nodes: BMSNs, relay nodes and a sink node, are being used in this mechanism. Long distance communication via multi-hop approach consumes less energy compared to single-hop. Furthermore, nodes near the base-station are vulnerable to high energy consumption than farther nodes thereby decreasing network lifetime. In this scheme, the authors have addressed the issue by using relay nodes where the BMSNs cater for sensing purpose of the vital-signs data and forward it to the corresponding relay nodes. Moreover, it is the job of the relay nodes to send forward the received sensory information towards the sink.

6.5 Data-Centric Multi-Objectives QoS-Aware Routing (DMQoS)

DMQoS proposed by Razzaque et al. (2011) is multi objective module based QoS-aware protocol focusing on fulfilling requirements of QoS for the different classes of data being generated. It categorizes data packets into Critical Data Packets (CPs), Delay Driven Data Packets (DPs), Reliability Driven Data Packets (RPs), and Ordinary Data packets (ODs). The body sensor mote that is also known as coordinator, gathers sensed data in raw form from the BMSNs. Body sensor mote, which is a central node behaves like a cluster head and normally contains less restrictions / limitations in comparison to BMSNs in terms of energy and computational resources. After the necessary data is being processed into information and data is being aggregated, the coordinator forwards the data to the destination sink in multi hop approach thereby making use of other BMSNs.

The architecture of routing of DMQoS (Razzaque et al., 2011) contains five modules, i.e. Dynamic Packet Classifier (DPC), Delay Control Module (DCM), Reliability Control Module (RCM), Energy-Aware Geographic Forwarding Module (EAGFM), and Multi-Objectives QoS Aware Queuing Module (MOQoSAQM). The DPC gathers packets of data either from the upper layer or the neighbor node and then categorizes those packets into above four classes discussed above and finally sends them to related modules on a First-In First-Out (FIFO) basis. The EAGFM finally considers that node as a next hop which is having possibly minimum distance and high residual energy with the help of multi-objective Lexicorgraphic Optimization (LO) as given in (Zykina, 2004). The RCM considers the node as a next hop having possibly highest reliability and the DCM chooses the next hop node on using of least possible delay. The responsibility of the MOQoSAQM is to classify and forward the data packets gathered based on four queues using assigned priorities.

To ensure uniform energy consumption among all nodes, a tradeoff is needed between the residual energy and geographic information and the multi-objective LO technique is used for that purpose.

6.6 Energy-Aware Peering Routing (EPR)

EPR (Khan et al., 2012a) focuses on minimizing the consumption of energy and network traffic that is either based on a centralized approach or distributed one. The patient's real time data in a hospital is displayed in this design. In this approach, three kinds of communication devices have been used. Type 1: Body Area Network Coordinator (BANC), Type 2: Nursing Station Coordinator (NSC), and Type 3: Medical Display Coordinator (MDC). The responsibility of BANCs having limited energy is gathering the raw data from BMSNs, aggregate and forwards it to the related MDCs. The responsibility of NCS is to keep the information about peering and communication types of all the BANCs, as it is centrally controlled device and has continuous power supply. Similarly, MDCs are display devices with power supplies that can be replaced. In order to get communication type (point-to-point or point-to-multipoint) and peering information from MDCs, the BANC tries to get its link established during the initial phase. After the needed information have been collected, the BANC discovers the relevant MDCs and will present the data. Energy efficiency in this protocol can be achieved if the broadcasting mechanism of the Hello packets is successfully controlled. Based on aforementioned devices types, neighbor's residual energy along with the geographic information, node with next hop can also be selected at the same time.

6.7 QoS-Aware Peering Routing for Delay-Sensitive Data (QPRD)

QPRD introduced by Khan et al. (2012b) aims to improve EPR (Khan et al., 2012a) by categorizing data packets of patient into two classes, i.e. Delay Sensitive Packets (DSP) and Ordinary Packets (OP). Both QPRD and EPR use same framework and structure discussed in (Khan et al., 2012a). The architecture of QPRD protocol used for routing purpose is comprised of seven different modules, i.e. MAC Transmitter Module (MAC-TM), QoS-Aware Queuing Module (QoS-AQM), Routing Service Module (RSM), Hello Protocol Module (HPM), Packet Classifier (PC), Delay/Reliability Module (D/RM), and MAC Receiver Module (MAC-RM). MAC-TM keeps the hello packets and data packets in a queue using First-in First-out (FIFO) approach and communicates them using CSMA/CA technique while QoS-AQM sends the data packets being gathered to their respective queue. The responsibility of RSM is to gather data packets coming from the PC module and upper layers, classify them as either DSPs or OPs and performs best path selection for each class. Transmission and reception of hello packets is performed by the HPM. The responsibility of the DM is to observe numerous types of delays and send the result to the network layer to perform delay assessment of nodes. Packets sent by other nodes are handled by MAC-RM whereas their classification into data packets as well as hello packets is the responsibility of the PC module.

6.8 QoS-Aware Peering Routing for Reliability-Sensitive Data (QPRR)

Khan et al. (2013) proposed QoS-aware Peering Routing protocol for Reliability-sensitive data (QPRR) aiming to improve the EPR (Khan et al., 2012a) by classifying data of the patient into Reliability Sensitive Packets (RSP) and Ordinary Packets (OP). QPRR makes use of slightly different modular approach as used in QPRD (Khan et al., 2012b). A reliability module replaces the delay module and its responsibility is to assess the link's reliability between any two nodes.

6.9 Reliability Aware Routing (RAR)

In RAR, proposed by Bangash et al. (2014b), data packets are divided into two classes: Normal Data Packets (NDPs) and Reliability-Constraint Data Packets (RCDPs). Identification of RCDPs (highest reliability packets) is important as packet losses may cause a serious condition of the patient, like reporting EEG, ECG etc., whereas NDPs do not require such type of reliability. The proposed Reliability aware scheme belongs to family of modular based routing.

There are five modules in RAR: Packet Classifier, Data Packet Classifier, Reliability-Aware (RA) module, Temperature-Aware (TA) module and Routing Module (RM). The Packet Classifier (PC) module divides the receiving packets from MAC receiver into Hello Packets and Data Packets. Data Packets are further divided into two classes: RCDPs and NDPs by Data Packet Classifier. RCDPs and NDPs are sent to RA module and TA module. The best available route with highest reliability is selected by RA module for RCDPs. TA module facilitates both RCDPs and NDPs by means of providing thermal aware services in accordance with temperature of the neighbor nodes. RM is subdivided into three modules: Routing Table Constructor, Routing Table, and Hello Packet Constructor. The construction and modifications of the routing table is the responsibility of the Routing table Constructor, using the information obtained from received Hello Packets, Path loss Estimator, Reliability Estimator, and Temperature Estimator.

6.10 Zahoor Energy and QoS-aware (ZEQoS)

ZEQoS is another cross-layered modular based peering data dissemination mechanism proposed by Khan et al. (2014). It categories the data packets into non-constrained, reliability-constrained and delay-constrained data packets and uses the same approaches used in EPR (Khan et al., 2012a), QPRD (Khan et al., 2012b) and QPRR (Khan et al., 2013).

6.11 Thermal-aware Multi-constrained QoS Routing (TMQoS)

Another QoS-aware data dissemination mechanism for WBANs is TMQoS introduced by Monowar et al. (2014). TMQoS aims to deliver the required QoS parameters using the heterogeneous natured vital-signs data while maintaining the temperature rise of the implanted BMSNs up to a satisfactory level. In this scheme the sensory data is categorized into four categories: critical, reliability-constrained, delay-constrained and non-constrained data packets.

The MAC receiver of TMQoS (Monowar et al., 2014) receives the packets from the neighbor nodes and categorizes them into Hello and data packets which are transmitted to neighbor nodes by the MAC transmitter. The QoS-aware packet classifier classifies the incoming data packets from the MAC receiver and/or from upper layers into aforementioned four categorize and sends to the multi-constrained QoS-aware route selector. Routing table constructor is responsible to construct and/or updates the routing table while Hello packet construction is the responsibility of the beacon packet constructor. Based on required QoS parameters and least number of hop-counts, appropriate route is selected by the multi-constrained QoS-aware route selector. Once the desired next-hop is selected, the data packet is forwarded to multi-constraint QoS-aware queuing, where two separate queues are maintained for both delay constraint and non-delay constraint packets separately. The delay constraint packets queue has higher priority as compared to non-delay constraint packets queue. The estimation of delay is the job of delay estimator while the reliability is estimated at reliability estimator. Moreover, the duty of the temperature estimator is to estimate the temperature of the BMSNs.

6.12 Critical Data Routing (CDR)

In CDR (Bangash et al., 2015a), the data packets are categorized as critical data packets and non-critical data packets. The classified data packets are kept at QoS aware queues namely critical data queue (CDQ) and non-critical data queue (NCDQ). CDQ is given the highest priority level as compared to NCDQ. The next hop selection is done by taking into consideration the link's quality. Only that path or hop is selected by the proposed algorithm having link quality equivalent to or greater than the threshold level, predefined by the algorithm. The algorithm also checks the path's delay, if found less or equal to already defined threshold level, then data packets with higher priority are forwarded to the next selected hop. Moreover, CDR is a modular based routing scheme.

There are five modules in CDR routing scheme: packet classifier module, data packet classifier module, qos-aware next hop selector module, QoS-aware queues, and routing module. The received packets at MAC receiver are passed to Packet Classifier Module, it discriminates these packets into Hello Packets and data packets. Data packets are further classified into critical data (CD) and non-critical data (NCD) and sent to QoS-aware next hop selector. QoS-aware next hop selector chooses the best available next hop node after looking at the required QoS parameters. In the QoS-aware queue module there are two queues: critical data queue (CDQ) and non-critical data queue (NCDQ). Critical data are queued in CDQ, whereas non-critical data are in NCDQ. CDQ is assigned with higher priority as compare to NCDQ. The routing module is further subdivided into three sub-modules: routing table, hello packet generator and routing table constructor. Routing table constructor constructs and/or updates the Routing table on the basis of received hello packets from neighbors and/or body controller (BC), delay estimator, reliability estimator, temperature estimator, and path loss estimator.

6.13 QoS Aware Inter-Cluster Routing Protocol (QAICR)

A QAICR protocol is proposed in (Saleh et al., 2015) to provide the required reliability and overcome the delay issues in cluster tree network. The incoming packets are separated into hello packets and data packets. The data packets are further categorized in RSP and OP. Delay (sum of both transmission and queuing delay) is used as a routing metric.

The modular base architecture of the QAICR includes: reliability module, packet classifier module, hello protocol module and routing service module. The reliability module monitors messages and acknowledgments being transmitted. The packet classifier categorizes the packets as hello packets and data packets. Hello protocol module builds neighbor tables and keeps information regarding the reliability of the neighbor nodes. The routing service module is responsible to construct the routing table and sort the data packets into RSP and OP. QAICR outperforms QPRR (Khan et al., 2013) in terms of data success ratio, residual energy and throughput.

6.14 Data Centric Routing (DCR)

In Bangash et al. (2015b), the authors proposed data centric routing (DCR), focusing on delay, reliability, temperature rise of BMSNs fixed inside the body and energy consumption metrics. Data packets are categorized as delay-sensitive data (DSD), reliability-sensitive data (RSD) and normal data (ND). DSD packets may tolerate some packet losses but does not allow tolerance on delay. Similarly, RSD may compromise on some sort of delay, but packet losses are not tolerable for RSD packets, whereas ND packets do not have any reliability and/or delay requirements.

DCR scheme is a modular based scheme, having seven modules: Packet Classifier (PC), Data Packet Classifier (DPC), Delay Aware Module (DAM), Reliability Aware Module (RAM), Thermal aware module (TAM), Routing Module (RM) and QoS Aware Module (QoS-AM). MAC receiver captures packets from neighbors and/or Body Controller (BC), Packet discriminates these packets into Hello Packets and Data Packets. DPC categorizes these Data Packets as DSD, RSD and ND Packets and sends them to DAM, RAM and TAM. Delay aware module sends DSD packets upon best possible selected route. Reliability aware module selects best possible route for RSD packets. Thermal aware module routes other data packets such as ND packets to the Desired Next Hop (DNH). Routing module is further sub divided into sub-modules such as Routing Table Constructor, Routing Table (RT) and Hello packet Constructor. Routing module also gets desired information from Delay Estimator, Reliability Estimator, Path loss Estimator and Temperature Estimator. Once the best desired next hops are selected for the data packets, they are queued in two separate QoS aware queues. Delay Constraint Queue (DCQ) is used to queue the DSD packets, while Non-Delay Constraint Queue (NDCQ) is used to queue the RSD and ND packets. Packets in DCQ are given higher priority than the packets in NDCQ.

7. COMPARATIVE STUDY OF QoS-AWARE DATA DISSEMINATION MECHANISMS

The QoS-aware data dissemination mechanisms are modular-based data dissemination mechanism where various modules are used for different tasks. Owing to incorporation of various modules and handling coordination among them is a challenging job in design of such protocols.

QoS-ARSF (Liang & Balasingham, 2007) aims to provide user specific QoS support and it performance is good in terms of reliability and delay. No consideration of energy efficiency is made. Furthermore, due to control packets it incurs more communication and computation overhead. Learning-based Routing RL-QRP proposed by Balasingham (2008) is QoS-aware data dissemination mechanism and is using distributed Q-learning algorithm and geographic information. Performance of RL-QRP is not better in the beginning due to learning process in comparison to QoS-AODV routing protocol (Gerasimov and Simon, 2002), but improves over time. With increase in mobility, packets delivery ratio declines. No energy efficiency is considered in its design. Relay based routing (Ehyaie et al., 2009) performs well by decreasing the power consumption of BMSNs and improving the network lifetime in comparison to single-hop and multi-hop communication. This scheme uses the relay nodes only to improve the energy efficiency; however they can be also used to enhance the reliability and control the temperature effects of the implanted BMSNs.

Distributed QoS-aware routing protocol (Djenouri & Balasingham, 2009) is using separate modules for various task. Moreover, it classifies vital-signs information of human beings into four classes, which are critical, delay-constrained, reliability-constrained and non-constrained data. Against other data dissemination mechanisms, its performance is better in terms of delay-bound data delivery, packets delivery ratio and latency. However, blind dissemination of data packets toward both primary and secondary sinks unnecessarily increases networks traffic thereby potentially giving rise to congestion.

The dual sink issue is addressed in DMQoS routing protocol (Razzaque et al., 2011), where each local base station reports data packets with a single sink. By virtue of various modules, its performance is relatively better than other data dissemination approaches (Djenouri & Balasingham, 2009; Felemban et al., 2006; Razzaque et al., 2008) in terms of energy, reliability and latency. However, with increase in network throughput, its performance deteriorates. Secondly, the Lexicographic Optimization (LO) technique is not the right choice as it considers the parameter with less importance only in case if the parameter with high importance does not give a unique solution.

EPR protocol (Khan et al., 2012a) uses both distributed as well as centralized approaches. Moreover, it is the first data dissemination mechanism that is based the peer-routing approach. It gives better results in term of power consumption and network congestion as compared to DMQoS routing protocol. QPRD (Khan, et al., 2012b) aims to improve EPR by classifying the data packets into non-constrained and delay-constrained data packets. In term of latency, its performance is better than DMQoS at high throughput. QPRR (Khan et al., 2013) is another QoS-aware data dissemination mechanism that aims to improve EPR is. Its performance in terms of packets delivery ratio is better than DMQoS at high throughput. Zahoor Energy-efficient and QoS-aware (ZEQoS) routing protocol (Khan et al., 2014) aims to reduce the energy consumption, delay and packet loss ratio. It is the combination of EPR, QPRR and QPRD.

The aforementioned protocols are limited in scope to be used in a hospital environment. Furthermore, if the nursing station coordinator is not accessible then the body area network coordinator will try to connect with nearest medical display coordinator, compromising the privacy of the patients' data.

TMQoS routing protocol (Monowar et al., 2014) results in better performance in providing the demanded QoS parameter by looking at the structure and nature of data in comparison to Thermal-Aware Routing Algorithm (TARA) (Tang et al., 2005) and Least Total Route Temperature (LTRT) routing protocol (Takahashi et al., 2008), which are temperature-aware data dissemination mechanism whose only aim is to decrease the temperature effects of the BMSNs fixed inside the human body. However, in term of temperature rise, its performance is slightly reduced in comparison to TARA and LTRT. Moreover, it selects next-hop node using the delay, reliability and/or temperature rise information of only those neighbor nodes having least number of hop-counts. However, some of the data packets such as reliability constraint and non-constraint do not impose any such constraints and can tolerate some reasonable delay. Furthermore, it uses redundant transmission for both delay and reliability constraint data packets. This results in more congested network, high energy consumption, more temperature rise and low packet delivery ratio.

RAR (Bangash et al., 2014b), CDR (Bangash et al., 2015a) and DCR (Bangash et al., 2015b) are the only data dissemination mechanisms which take into account the demanded QoS parameters as well as the temperature rise issue of implanted BMSNs. They also consider the high and dynamic path loss due to postural movement and chemistry of human body. RAR, CDR, and DCR outperforms TMQoS routing protocol (Monowar et al., 2014) and LTRT routing protocol (Takahashi et al., 2008) in terms of providing the required QoS parameter(s) using both network models. In terms of temperature increase of the implanted BMSNs, their performance is better as compared to TMQoS but slightly poor as compared LTRT as the later only aims to reduce the temperature rise using network model without relay nodes. Using network model with relay nodes they outperform the LTRT in temperature rise as well.

Table 1 gives a comparison of the aforementioned QoS-aware data dissemination mechanism for WBANs, in terms of temperature rise, mobility, delay, packet delivery ratio (PDR) and energy consumption with other data dissemination mechanisms. The data dissemination mechanisms for intra and inter WBANs discussed above are summarized in Tables 2 and 3 respectively.

8. CONCLUSION

WBANs offer a paradigm change towards proactive organization thereby helping in early detection of and prevention from various diseases. Despite its numerous benefits, designing data dissemination mechanisms for WBANs is a challenging task because of the human body's unique constraints. In this chapter, the WBANs are discussed along with the communication architecture of WBANs. Moreover, the WBANs' general issues and challenges along data dissemination related are identified and discussed. Using the structure and nature of data, the data dissemination mechanisms are being categorized as QoS-aware, thermal-aware, postural-movement-based and cross-layered. Furthermore, it covers a review of existing data dissemination mechanisms specifically designed for WBANs. Each QoS-aware data dissemination mechanism is analyzed in comparison to its relative performance against other data

Table 1. Summary of QoS-Aware data dissemination mechanisms for WBANs

Protocol	Characteristics					
	Intra/Inter	Temperature Rise	Mobility	Delay	Packet Delivery Ratio	Energy Consumption
QoS-ARSF (2007)	Inter	X	√	-	Good	X
RL-QRP (2008)	Inter	X	√	Poor	Very Good	X
LOCALMOR (2009)	Inter	X	√	Good	Very Good	Poor
URIL-WBANs (2009)	Intra	X	√	X	X	Very Good
DMQoS (2011)	Inter	X	√	Good	Very Good	Good
EPR (2012)	Inter	X	√	X	Very Good	Very Good
QPRD (2012)	Inter	X	√	Very Poor	Very Good	Very Good
QPRR (2013)	Inter	X	√	X	Very Good	Good
RAR (2014)	Intra	Very Good	√	X	Very Good	Very Good
TMQos (2014)	Intra	Good	X	Very Good	Very Good	Good
ZEQoS (2014)	Inter	X	√	Very Good	Very Good	Good
CDR (2015)	Intra	Good	√	Very Good	Very Good	Very Good
QAICR (2015)	Inter	X	X	Very Good	Very Good	X
CDR (2015)	Intra	Good	√	Very Good	Very Good	Very Good

(Bangash et al., 2014a)

Table 2. Summary of data dissemination mechanisms for intra-WBANs

Protocols	Characteristics						
	Energy Aware	Delay Aware	Reliability Aware	Data Centric	Thermal Aware	Path Loss Aware	Relay Based
URIL-WBANs (2009)	√	X	X	X	X	X	√
TMQos (2014)	√	√	√	√	√	X	X
RAR (2014)	√	X	√	X	√	√	√
CDR (2015)	√	√	√	X	√	√	√
DCR (2015)	√	√	√	√	√	√	√

Table 3. Summary of data dissemination mechanisms for inter-WBANs

Protocols	Characteristics			
	Energy Aware	Delay Aware	Reliability Aware	Data Centric
QoS-ARSF (2005)	X	X	X	√
RL-QRP (2008)	X	√	√	X
LOCALMOR (2009)	X	√	√	√
DMQoS (2011)	√	√	√	√
EPR (2012)	√	X	X	X
QPRD (2012)	√	√	X	√
QPRR (2013)	√	X	√	√
ZEQoS (2014)	√	√	√	√
QAICR (2015)	X	√	√	X

dissemination schemes along with identification of its strengths and weaknesses. The future data dissemination mechanisms for WBANs should not only provide power efficient but reliable communication along with handling heterogeneous types of BMSNs in real-time applications. Moreover, reliability, latency, mobility, temperature-effects and power consumption should also be taken into consideration while designing any solutions for WBAN.

REFERENCES

Anisi, M. H., Abdullah, A. H., Razak, S. A., & Ngadi, M. (2012). Overview of data routing approaches for wireless sensor networks. *Sensors (Basel)*, *12*(4), 3964–3996. doi:10.3390120403964 PMID:23443040

Arya, V. (2013, August). A quality of service analysis of energy aware routing protocols in mobile ad hoc networks. In *Proceedings of the 2013 Sixth International Conference on Contemporary Computing (IC3)* (pp. 439-444). IEEE.

Bag, A., & Bassiouni, M. A. (2008). Hotspot preventing routing algorithm for delay-sensitive applications of in vivo biomedical sensor networks. *Information Fusion*, *9*(3), 389–398. doi:10.1016/j.inffus.2007.02.001

Bangash, J. I., Abdullah, A. H., Anisi, M. H., & Khan, A. W. (2014a). A survey of routing protocols in wireless body sensor networks. *Sensors, 14*(1), 1322-1357.

Bangash, J. I., Abdullah, A. H., Khan, A. W., Razzaque, M. A., & Yusof, R. (2015). Critical data routing (CDR) for intra wireless body sensor networks. *Telkomnika, 13*(1), 181. doi:10.12928/telkomnika.v13i1.365

Bangash, J. I., Abdullah, A. H., Razzaque, M. A., & Khan, A. W. (2014b). Reliability aware routing for intra-wireless body sensor networks. *International Journal of Distributed Sensor Networks, 10*(10), 786537. doi:10.1155/2014/786537

Bangash, J. I., Khan, A. W., & Abdullah, A. H. (2015). Data-centric routing for intra wireless body sensor networks. *Journal of Medical Systems, 39*(9), 91. doi:10.100710916-015-0268-5 PMID:26242749

Ben-Othman, J., & Yahya, B. (2010). Energy efficient and QoS based routing protocol for wireless sensor networks. *Journal of Parallel and Distributed Computing, 70*(8), 849–857. doi:10.1016/j.jpdc.2010.02.010

Boulis, A., Smith, D., Miniutti, D., Libman, L., & Tselishchev, Y. (2012). Challenges in body area networks for healthcare: The MAC. *IEEE Communications Magazine, 50*(5), 100–106. doi:10.1109/MCOM.2012.6194389

Chipara, O., He, Z., Xing, G., Chen, Q., Wang, X., Lu, C., ... Abdelzaher, T. (2006, June). Real-time power-aware routing in sensor networks. In *Proceedings of the 2006 14th IEEE International Workshop on Quality of Service* (pp. 83-92). IEEE. 10.1109/IWQOS.2006.250454

Coello, C. A. (2000). An updated survey of GA-based multiobjective optimization techniques. *ACM Computing Surveys, 32*(2), 109–143. doi:10.1145/358923.358929

Dagtas, S., Pekhteryev, G., Sahinoglu, Z., Cam, H., & Challa, N. (2008). Real-time and secure wireless health monitoring. *International Journal of Telemedicine and Applications, 2008*, 1–10. doi:10.1155/2008/135808 PMID:18497866

Darwish, A., & Hassanien, A. E. (2011). Wearable and implantable wireless sensor network solutions for healthcare monitoring. *Sensors (Basel), 11*(6), 5561–5595. doi:10.3390110605561 PMID:22163914

Djenouri, D., & Balasingham, I. (2009, September). New QoS and geographical routing in wireless biomedical sensor networks. In *Proceedings of the 2009 Sixth International Conference on Broadband Communications, Networks, and Systems* (pp. 1-8). IEEE. 10.4108/ICST.BROADNETS2009.7188

Ehyaie, A., Hashemi, M., & Khadivi, P. (2009, June). Using relay network to increase life time in wireless body area sensor networks. In *Proceedings of the 2009 IEEE International Symposium on a World of Wireless, Mobile and Multimedia Networks & Workshops* (pp. 1-6). IEEE. 10.1109/WOW-MOM.2009.5282405

Felemban, E., Lee, C. G., & Ekici, E. (2006). MMSPEED: Multipath Multi-SPEED protocol for QoS guarantee of reliability and. Timeliness in wireless sensor networks. *IEEE Transactions on Mobile Computing, 5*(6), 738–754. doi:10.1109/TMC.2006.79

Gerasimov, I., & Simon, R. (2002, April). A bandwidth-reservation mechanism for on-demand ad hoc path finding. In *Proceedings 35th Annual Simulation Symposium. SS 2002* (pp. 27-34). IEEE. 10.1109/SIMSYM.2002.1000079

Honeine, P., Mourad, F., Kallas, M., Snoussi, H., Amoud, H., & Francis, C. (2011, May). Wireless sensor networks in biomedical: Body area networks. In *Proceedings of the International Workshop on Systems, Signal Processing and their Applications, WOSSPA* (pp. 388-391). IEEE. 10.1109/WOSSPA.2011.5931518

Kandris, D., Tsagkaropoulos, M., Politis, I., Tzes, A., & Kotsopoulos, S. (2011). Energy efficient and perceived QoS aware video routing over wireless multimedia sensor networks. *Ad Hoc Networks*, *9*(4), 591–607. doi:10.1016/j.adhoc.2010.09.001

Kandris, D., Tsioumas, P., Tzes, A., Nikolakopoulos, G., & Vergados, D. (2009). Power conservation through energy efficient routing in wireless sensor networks. *Sensors (Basel)*, *9*(9), 7320–7342. doi:10.339090907320 PMID:22399998

Khan, J. Y., Yuce, M. R., Bulger, G., & Harding, B. (2012). Wireless body area network (WBAN) design techniques and performance evaluation. *Journal of Medical Systems*, *36*(3), 1441–1457. doi:10.100710916-010-9605-x PMID:20953680

Khan, Z., Aslam, N., Sivakumar, S., & Phillips, W. (2012). Energy-aware peering routing protocol for indoor hospital body area network communication. *Procedia Computer Science*, *10*, 188–196. doi:10.1016/j.procs.2012.06.027

Khan, Z., Sivakumar, S., Phillips, W., & Robertson, B. (2012, November). QPRD: QoS-aware peering routing protocol for delay sensitive data in hospital body area network communication. In *Proceedings of the 2012 Seventh International Conference on Broadband, Wireless Computing, Communication and Applications* (pp. 178-185). IEEE. 10.1109/BWCCA.2012.37

Khan, Z. A., Sivakumar, S., Phillips, W., & Robertson, B. (2013). A QoS-aware routing protocol for reliability sensitive data in hospital body area networks. *Procedia Computer Science*, *19*, 171–179. doi:10.1016/j.procs.2013.06.027

Khan, Z. A., Sivakumar, S., Phillips, W., & Robertson, B. (2014). ZEQoS: A new energy and QoS-aware routing protocol for communication of sensor devices in healthcare system. *International Journal of Distributed Sensor Networks*, *10*(6), 627689. doi:10.1155/2014/627689

Kumar, P., & Lee, H. J. (2012). Security issues in healthcare applications using wireless medical sensor networks: A survey. *Sensors*, *12*(1), 55-91.

Lee, Y. S., Lee, H. J., & Alasaarela, E. (2013, July). Mutual authentication in wireless body sensor networks (WBSN) based on Physical Unclonable Function (PUF). In *Proceedings of the 2013 9th International Wireless Communications and Mobile Computing Conference (IWCMC)* (pp. 1314-1318). IEEE.

Li, B. Y., & Chuang, P. J. (2013). Geographic energy-aware non-interfering multipath routing for multimedia transmission in wireless sensor networks. *Information Sciences*, *249*, 24–37. doi:10.1016/j.ins.2013.06.014

Liang, X., & Balasingham, I. (2007, October). A QoS-aware routing service framework for biomedical sensor networks. In *Proceedings of the 2007 4th International Symposium on Wireless Communication Systems* (pp. 342-345). IEEE. 10.1109/ISWCS.2007.4392358

Liang, X., Balasingham, I., & Byun, S. S. (2008, October). A reinforcement learning based routing protocol with QoS support for biomedical sensor networks. In *Proceedings of the 2008 First International Symposium on Applied Sciences on Biomedical and Communication Technologies* (pp. 1-5). IEEE.

Lin, L., Yang, C., Wong, K., Yan, H., Shen, J., & Phee, S. (2014). An energy efficient MAC protocol for multi-hop swallowable body sensor networks. *Sensors, 14*(10), 19457-19476.

Monowar, M. M., Mehedi Hassan, M., Bajaber, F., Hamid, M. A., & Alamri, A. (2014). Thermal-aware multiconstrained intrabody QoS routing for wireless body area networks. *International Journal of Distributed Sensor Networks, 10*(3), 676312. doi:10.1155/2014/676312

Movassaghi, S., Abolhasan, M., & Lipman, J. (2013). A review of routing protocols in wireless body area networks. *Journal of Networks, 8*(3), 559–575. doi:10.4304/jnw.8.3.559-575

Movassaghi, S., Abolhasan, M., Lipman, J., Smith, D., & Jamalipour, A. (2014). Wireless body area networks: A survey. *IEEE Communications Surveys and Tutorials, 16*(3), 1658–1686. doi:10.1109/SURV.2013.121313.00064

Nazir, B., & Hasbullah, H. (2013). Energy efficient and QoS aware routing protocol for clustered wireless sensor network. *Computers & Electrical Engineering, 39*(8), 2425–2441. doi:10.1016/j.compeleceng.2013.06.011

Ngai, E., Zhou, Y., Lyu, M. R., & Liu, J. (2010). A delay-aware reliable event reporting framework for wireless sensor–actuator networks. *Ad Hoc Networks, 8*(7), 694–707. doi:10.1016/j.adhoc.2010.01.004

Quwaider, M., & Biswas, S. (2009, October). Probabilistic routing in on-body sensor networks with postural disconnections. In *Proceedings of the 7th ACM international symposium on Mobility management and wireless access* (pp. 149-158). ACM. 10.1145/1641776.1641803

Quwaider, M., Rao, J., & Biswas, S. (2010). Body-posture-based dynamic link power control in wearable sensor networks. *IEEE Communications Magazine, 48*(7), 134–142. doi:10.1109/MCOM.2010.5496890

Rashidi, P., & Mihailidis, A. (2012). A survey on ambient-assisted living tools for older adults. *IEEE Journal of Biomedical and Health Informatics, 17*(3), 579–590. doi:10.1109/JBHI.2012.2234129 PMID:24592460

Razzaque, M., Hong, C. S., & Lee, S. (2011). Data-centric multiobjective QoS-aware routing protocol for body sensor networks. *Sensors (Basel), 11*(1), 917–937. doi:10.3390110100917 PMID:22346611

Razzaque, M. A., Alam, M. M., Mamun-Or-Rashid, M., & Hong, C. S. (2008). Multi-constrained QoS geographic routing for heterogeneous traffic in sensor networks. *IEICE Transactions on Communications, 91*(8), 2589–2601. doi:10.1093/ietcom/e91-b.8.2589

Saleh, A. B., Sibley, M. J., & Mather, P. (2015, March). QoS Aware Inter-Cluster Routing Protocol for IEEE 802.15. 4 Networks. In *Proceedings of the 2015 17th UKSim-AMSS International Conference on Modelling and Simulation (UKSim)* (pp. 538-543). IEEE.

Sayrafian-Pour, K., Yang, W. B., Hagedorn, J., Terrill, J., & Yazdandoost, K. Y. (2009, September). A statistical path loss model for medical implant communication channels. In *Proceedings of the 2009 IEEE 20th International Symposium on Personal, Indoor and Mobile Radio Communications* (pp. 2995-2999). IEEE. 10.1109/PIMRC.2009.5449869

Shen, H., Bai, G., Tang, Z., & Zhao, L. (2014). QMOR: QoS-aware multi-sink opportunistic routing for wireless multimedia sensor networks. *Wireless Personal Communications*, *75*(2), 1307–1330. doi:10.100711277-013-1425-0

Srinivasan, P., & Kamalakkannan, P. (2012, December). REAQ-AODV: Route stability and energy aware QoS routing in mobile Ad Hoc networks. In *Proceedings of the 2012 Fourth International Conference on Advanced Computing (ICoAC)* (pp. 1-5). IEEE. 10.1109/ICoAC.2012.6416845

Su, S., Yu, H., & Wu, Z. (2013). An efficient multi–objective evolutionary algorithm for energy–aware QoS routing in wireless sensor network. *International Journal of Sensor Networks*, *13*(4), 208–218. doi:10.1504/IJSNET.2013.055583

Takahashi, D., Xiao, Y., Hu, F., Chen, J., & Sun, Y. (2008). Temperature-aware routing for telemedicine applications in embedded biomedical sensor networks. *EURASIP Journal on Wireless Communications and Networking*, *2008*, 26.

Tang, Q., Tummala, N., Gupta, S. K., & Schwiebert, L. (2005, June). TARA: thermal-aware routing algorithm for implanted sensor networks. In *Proceedings of the International Conference on Distributed Computing in Sensor Systems* (pp. 206-217). Springer. 10.1007/11502593_17

Ullah, S., Higgins, H., Braem, B., Latre, B., Blondia, C., Moerman, I., ... Kwak, K. S. (2012). A comprehensive survey of wireless body area networks. *Journal of Medical Systems*, *36*(3), 1065–1094. doi:10.100710916-010-9571-3 PMID:20721685

Ullah, S., Shen, B., Riazul Islam, S. M., Khan, P., Saleem, S., & Sup Kwak, K. (2010). A study of MAC protocols for WBANs. *Sensors (Basel)*, *10*(1), 128–145. doi:10.3390100100128 PMID:22315531

World Health Organization (WHO). (2018). Ageing and Health. Rederived from https://www.who.int/news-room/fact-sheets/detail/ageing-and-health

World Health Organization (WHO). (2018). World Health Statistics 2018. Rederived from https://www.who.int/gho/publications/world_health_statistics/2018/en/

World Population Aging. (2017). "Population Division", Department of Economic and Social Affairs, United Nations, 2018. Rederived From https://www.un.org/en/development/desa/population/publications/pdf/ageing/WPA2017_Highlights.pdf

Xiao, Y., Shen, X., Sun, B. O., & Cai, L. (2006). Security and privacy in RFID and applications in telemedicine. *IEEE Communications Magazine*, *44*(4), 64–72. doi:10.1109/MCOM.2006.1632651

Yang, G. Z. (2014). *Body Sensor Networks* (1st ed.). London, UK: Springer Berlin Heidelberg, London. doi:10.1007/978-1-4471-6374-9

Zykina, A. V. (2004). A lexicographic optimization algorithm. *Automation and Remote Control*, *65*(3), 363–368. doi:10.1023/B:AURC.0000019366.84601.8e

ADDITIONAL READING

Bag, A., & Bassiouni, M. A. (2006, October). Energy efficient thermal aware routing algorithms for embedded biomedical sensor networks. In *Proceedings of the 2006 IEEE International Conference on Mobile Ad Hoc and Sensor Systems* (pp. 604-609). IEEE. 10.1109/MOBHOC.2006.278619

Bag, A., & Bassiouni, M. A. (2008). Hotspot preventing routing algorithm for delay-sensitive applications of in vivo biomedical sensor networks. *Information Fusion, 9*(3), 389–398. doi:10.1016/j.inffus.2007.02.001

Bag, A., & Bassiouni, M. A. (2008, February). Routing algorithm for network of homogeneous and id-less biomedical sensor nodes (RAIN). In *Proceedings of the 2008 IEEE Sensors Applications Symposium* (pp. 68-73). IEEE.

Bag, A., & Bassiouni, M. A. (2009). Biocomm– A cross-layer medium access control (MAC) and routing protocol co-design for biomedical sensor networks. *International Journal of Parallel. Emergent and Distributed Systems, 24*(1), 85–103. doi:10.1080/17445760802335345

Bara'a, A. A., & Khalil, E. A. (2012). A new evolutionary based routing protocol for clustered heterogeneous wireless sensor networks. *Applied Soft Computing, 12*(7), 1950–1957. doi:10.1016/j.asoc.2011.04.007

Javaid, N., Abbas, Z., Fareed, M. S., Khan, Z. A., & Alrajeh, N. (2013). M-ATTEMPT: A new energy-efficient routing protocol for wireless body area sensor networks. *Procedia Computer Science, 19*, 224–231. doi:10.1016/j.procs.2013.06.033

Lee, Y. S., Lee, H. J., & Alasaarela, E. (2013, July). Mutual authentication in wireless body sensor networks (WBSN) based on Physical Unclonable Function (PUF). In *Proceedings of the 2013 9th International Wireless Communications and Mobile Computing Conference (IWCMC)* (pp. 1314-1318). IEEE.

Liang, X., Balasingham, I., & Byun, S. S. (2008, October). A reinforcement learning based routing protocol with QoS support for biomedical sensor networks. In *Proceedings of the 2008 First International Symposium on Applied Sciences on Biomedical and Communication Technologies* (pp. 1-5). IEEE.

Lin, L., Yang, C., Wong, K., Yan, H., Shen, J., & Phee, S. (2014). An energy efficient MAC protocol for multi-hop swallowable body sensor networks. *Sensors, 14*(10), 19457-19476.

Maskooki, A., Soh, C. B., Gunawan, E., & Low, K. S. (2011, January). Opportunistic routing for body area network. In Proceedings of the 2011 IEEE Consumer Communications and Networking Conference (CCNC) (pp. 237-241). IEEE. doi:10.1109/CCNC.2011.5766463

Milenkovic, A., Otto, C., & Jovanov, E. (2006). Wireless sensor networks for personal health monitoring: Issues and an implementation. *Computer Communications, 29*(13-14), 2521–2533. doi:10.1016/j.comcom.2006.02.011

Movassaghi, S., Abolhasan, M., & Lipman, J. (2013). A review of routing protocols in wireless body area networks. *Journal of Networks*.

Oey, C., & Moh, S. (2013). A survey on temperature-aware routing protocols in wireless body sensor networks. *Sensors (Basel), 13*(8), 9860–9877. doi:10.3390130809860 PMID:23917259

Quwaider, M., & Biswas, S. (2009, December). On-body packet routing algorithms for body sensor networks. In *Proceedings of the 2009 first international conference on networks & communications* (pp. 171-177). IEEE. 10.1109/NetCoM.2009.54

Quwaider, M., & Biswas, S. (2009, October). Probabilistic routing in on-body sensor networks with postural disconnections. In *Proceedings of the 7th ACM international symposium on Mobility management and wireless access* (pp. 149-158). ACM. 10.1145/1641776.1641803

Quwaider, M., & Biswas, S. (2010). DTN routing in body sensor networks with dynamic postural partitioning. *Ad Hoc Networks*, 8(8), 824–841. doi:10.1016/j.adhoc.2010.03.002 PMID:25530740

KEY TERMS AND DEFINITIONS

BMSNs: Bio-Medical Sensor Nodes (BMSNs) are the sensor nodes, which are fixed either with the body or inside the body.

Data Dissemination: Data dissemination is procedure that how the generated or received data packets can be forwarded towards the destination.

Delay: Delay of a data packet is time calculated by taking the difference between the time once it is generated at the source BMSN and the time it delivered to the BC.

Inter-WBAN: It is the segment of the network where different BCs process, aggregate and forward the received vital-signs information towards the sink(s).

Intra-WBAN: It is the local body area network of various BMSNs where they report the sensory data of patients to the Body Coordinator (BC) which is the base station located locally.

Path Loss: WBANs implies higher and dynamic on and in-body path loss. The reasons behind the dynamic and high path loss in WBANs are the human body's postural movements and the in-body wireless communication (in case of implanted BMSNs).

QoS: Heterogeneous natured sensor nodes generate various kinds of data packets containing the vital-signs information and require different QoS provisions.

Reliability: Reliability is the ratio of the number of data packets delivered to BC to number of data packets transmitted by the source BMSNs.

Routing: Routing refers to the procedure of choosing the next hop node while forwards data from one BMSN to another or sink.

Temperature-Rise: Energy consumption of sensor node's circuitry and absorption of antenna radiation are the two main factors contribute to the temperature rise issue of BMSNs fixed inside the body. This temperature rise will affect the human tissues, which are heat sensitive organs and may cause some damage to the tissues if continued for long period of time.

WBANs: The merger of pervasive computing, wireless sensor technologies and bio-medical engineering has led to the emergence of a promising technology known as Wireless Body Area Networks (WBANs).

Vital Signs: It the measurement of the basic functions through which the status of the human body can be evaluated such as temperature, heartbeat, electromyography (EMG), pH-level, blood pressure, electrocardiogram (ECG), electroencephalogram (EEG), respiration rate.

ENDNOTES

1   Body temperature is the amount heat produced and sustained by human body processes.

2   Heartbeat is the number of times the heart beats in one minute.

3   pH stands for potential hydrogen and is the measure of hydrogen-icon concentration.

4   Electromyography (EMG) is an examination to evaluate the electrical activity of skeletal muscles

5   Blood pressure is the pressure of the blood against the walls of artery.

6   Electrocardiogram (ECG) is an examination that checks the heart problems with electrical activity.

7   Electroencephalogram (EEG) is a test and recording the brain activity.

8   Respiration rate is the number of breaths that a person takes in one minute.

Chapter 6
Effects of Electromagnetic Radiation of Mobile Phones on the Human Brain

Junaid Ahmad Malik
https://orcid.org/0000-0003-4411-2015
Government Degree College, Bijbehara, India

ABSTRACT

With the expanding use of wireless cellular networks, concerns have been communicated about the possible interaction of electromagnetic radiation with the human life, explicitly, the mind and brain. Mobile phones emanate radio frequency waves, a type of non-ionizing radiation, which can be absorbed by tissues nearest to where the telephone is kept. The effects on neuronal electrical activity, energy metabolism, genomic responses, neurotransmitter balance, blood–brain barrier permeability, mental psychological aptitude, sleep, and diverse cerebrum conditions including brain tumors are assessed. Health dangers may likewise develop from use of cellular communication, for instance, car accidents while utilizing the device while driving. These indirect well-being impacts surpass the immediate common troubles and should be looked into in more detail later on. In this chapter, we outline the possible biological impacts of EMF introduction on human brain.

1. INTRODUCTION

New advances are creating regular day to day existence to support individual. Communication through mobile and portable devices is right now the speediest fashioning correspondence system in the media transmission industry. Due to the extended number of customers using the mobile phone, the stress is by and by connected towards electromagnetic radiations transmitted by the mobile phones itself. Electromagnetic radiation can be entreated into ionizing and non-ionizing radiation. Ionizing radiation is the radiation with high essentialness which can clear tight securities among electrons and atoms achieving tissue hurt while non-ionizing radiation is the radiation that has enough imperativeness to vibrate the particles and atoms anyway don't remove the electrons in the atom (Robert et al., 2007). This radiation

DOI: 10.4018/978-1-7998-2521-0.ch006

for the most part occurs at low repeat go. Mobile phone is organized with low power handset to transmit voice and data to base station is arranged at very few kilometers. These radiations cause issues like headaches, genuine anguish in ear, foggy vision, memory adversity, shivering, unbearable sensations, feeling snoozing, excessive touchiness (Tyagi et al., 2011) have been seen while using cell phones. Experts have found that these signs are progressively essential in people with higher introduction to radiation of mobile phone.

While utilizing the cellular communication, electromagnetic wave is moved to the body which messes with the health especially at the spot near ear skull area where they are known to impact the neurones. The radiations intrude with the electromagnetic powers that two neurones interface each other with. This can provoke deafness and migraines. People using telephones are slanted to hypertension and distinctive symptoms, for instance, hot ears, consuming skin, cerebral agonies and weakness. There have been various assessments into the relationship between mobile phones and memory trouble as appears in Table 1. Considering their more diminutive heads, progressively thin skulls and higher tissue conductivity, children may gulp more verve from a given phone than adults. Widespread guidelines on introduction levels to microwave frequency and periodicity limit the power levels of remote devices and it is remarkable for remote contraptions to outperform the standards. In any case, these guidelines simply think about thermal effects, as non-thermal effects have not yet been conclusively delineated (Binhi et al., 2002). This paper shows that the non-thermal radiation impacts the human temperament. Global System for Mobile Communications or GSM is the world's most conspicuous standard for phone frameworks. GSM is a cellular system, which suggests that phones partner with it by means of searching for cells in the prompt province. GSM frameworks work in different particular transporter frequency ranges. GSM frameworks work in the 900 MHz or 1800 MHz bands. Where these groups were by then employed, the 850 MHz and 1900 MHz bands are used somewhat, paying little mind to the frequency and periodicity assigned by an administrator; it is parceled into timeslots for solitary phones to use (Masiliunas et al., 2018).

This grants eight full-rate or sixteen half-rate exchange channels per radio frequency. These eight radio timeslots (or eight burst periods) are accumulated into a Time-Division Multiple Access (TDMA) plot. Half rate redirects utilize substitute diagrams in the comparable timeslot. The transmission control in the handset is obliged to a furthest reaches of 2 watts in GSM 850/900 and 1 watt in GSM 1800/1900 (Tyagi et al., 2011). Code Division Multiple Access (CDMA) is a channel get to methodology used by various radio correspondence headways. One of the key thoughts in data correspondence is the likelihood that it empowers a couple of transmitters to send information at the same time over a solitary correspondence channel. This empowers a couple of customers to share a band of frequencies. This thought is called multiple access. CDMA uses spread-go advancement and an uncommon coding plan where each transmitter is doled out a code to empower various customers to be multiplexed over the identical physical channel. The transmission control in the handset is confined to a furthest reaches of 6 to 7 milli Watts (Robert et al., 2007). Table 2 shows the points of interest of GSM and CDMA wireless progressions and their ability level.

Another speedier fifth Generation (5G) media transmission framework has as of late been affirmed by the Federal Communications Commission (FCC) with new receiving wires which is as of now being introduced and tried. 5G will incorporate the higher millimetre wave frequencies at no other time utilized for web and interchanges innovation. The 5G organization proposes to include frequencies in the microwave range in the low-(0.6 GHz - 3.7 GHz), mid-(3.7GHz - 24 GHz), and high-band frequencies (24 GHz and higher) for faster transactions. This radiation, similar to the 2G, 3G, and 4G broadcast communication frameworks, has not had pre-advertise testing for long haul wellbeing impacts regardless of the way that individuals will be presented persistently to this microwave radiation. 5G high range can drive change of cells and actuates tumors which may later become malignant in growth and nature. Introduction to the 5G radiation expands the creation of ROS. Responsive Oxygen Species (ROS) are a typical piece of cellular procedures and signalling. Overproduction of ROS that isn't offset with either endogenous cancer prevention agents [Superoxide Dismutase (SOD), Catalase (CAT), Glutathione Peroxidase (GPx), Glutathione (GSH), Melatonin (MLT)], or exogenous cell backups (Vitamin C, Vitamin E, carotenoids, polyphenols) permits the development of free radicals that oxidize and harm DNA, proteins, layered lipids and mitochondria (Verma et al., 2019). There is a specific worry for 5G applications as the eyes would likewise get huge radiation particularly for close to handle exposures. Electromagnetic affectability of 5G range has the qualities like cerebral pains, sleep deprivation, discombobulating, sickness, absence of concentration, heart palpitations, and melancholy (Masiliunas et al., 2018; Tocci, 2019).

Electromagnetic radiation is a kind of vitality demonstrating wave-like demeanour as it travels through the space. Electromagnetic radiation has both electric and magnetic fields, which sway in form inverse to each other and inverse to the course of energy blow-out. Electromagnetic radiation can be gathered into ionizing radiation and non-ionizing radiation, in perspective on whether it is prepared for ionizing particles and breaking mixture bonds non-ionizing radiation is connected with two noteworthy potential dangers: electrical and regular (Delgado et al., 1982). The normal effect of electromagnetic fields is to cause dielectric warming. Complex natural effects of progressively delicate non-thermal electromagnetic fields moreover exists, including fragile Extremely Low Frequency appealing fields (Harland & Liburdy, 1997) and adjusted Radio Frequency and microwave fields (Aalto et al., 2006). Magnetic and attractive fields impel hovering streams inside the human body and nature of these alluring fields depends really on the intensity of the impinging magnetic field. These streams cause nerves and muscles to fortify which accordingly impacts natural techniques. The effect of the feeble EM radiations on people can be recognized as course of action of events which fuses prologue to EM radiations which when absorbed alters the organic field organizations, storing up of essentialness and information into the body fluid, change in the valuable exercises of cell which finally results into some disease (Eighteenth Int. Crimean Conference, 2008). The number of wireless customers has extended exponentially starting late and it has become a noteworthy device in human routine life. Evaluations propose there are around 1.6 billion phone customers through the world and the numbers are growing (Wikipedia, Online) and thus the level of establishment of more electromagnetic radiations.

2. MOBILE PHONE SIGNAL

Diverse test settings are utilized, to research the impact RF-EMF introduction on cerebrum action and neurobehavioral execution. The incidences of eagerness for RF-EMF identified with cell phone signals extend from roughly 450 to 2600 MHz. The most generally focused of these frequencies is the 900 MHz Global System for Mobile Communication (GSM), however the quantity of studies including UMTS handset signals (1800-1900 MHz) has expanded in the course of the most recent years. Other than various frequencies utilized, likewise the Pulse Modulation (PM) of the sign can contrast between the studies. The idea of PM is to move a narrowband corresponding signal, similar to a telephone call, over a wideband baseband station or, in a portion of the plans, as a piece stream over another advanced transmission framework. Cell phone signals are pulsated at various frequencies, contingent upon their drive. A cell phone has an essential rhythm at a repetition of 217 Hz. At the point when a receiver is effectively utilized in 'talk mode,' each 26 pulses are gathered under another ELF beat at around 8 Hz. Cell phones utilizing battery sparing (DTX innovation) have an extra pulse at 2 Hz during listening mode. In stand-by a telephone will pulse less regular to keep in touch with the base station (Hung et al., 2007).

Other than a PM signal, likewise a Continuous Wave (CW) signal can be utilized. This is an electromagnetic influx of consistent plentifulness and repetition. Early age telephones utilized such a CW signal, however these were quickly supplanted by advanced GSM, utilizing PM signals.

3. NEURONAL RESPONSES IN VITRO

At high radiation partition (SAR 6.8-100 W/kg) isolated neurons respond to both steady and beat microwaves (2.45 GHz) with a decrease in unconstrained development, an extension in layer conductance, a prolongation of the obstinate period following depolarization and a lessening of the perseverance time (Wachtel et al., 1975; Seaman & Wachtel, 1978; McRee & Wachtel, 1980; Arber & Lin, 1984; Arber & Lin, 1985; McRee & Wachtel, 1986). In Helix aspersa neurons, the electrophysiological impacts are dissolved after Ca^{2+} chelation with EDTA, recommending that changes in calcium homeostasis might be incorporated (Arber & Lin, 1984, 1985).

In one more assessment, in which synaptosomes orchestrated from rat cerebral cortex were introduced to beat 2.8 GHz microwaves, a development in 32P linking with phosphoinositides has been depicted at mean SAR $\geq$ 10 W/kg nonetheless not at lower retention degrees, proposing a thermal impelling of inositol assimilation (Gandhi & Ross, 1989). Meanwhile phosphoinositides are related with the assemblage of calcium from non-mitochondrial limit goals (Berridge & Irvine, 1984), extended calcium enactment could provoke drawn-out calcium efflux degrees, as observed in synaptosomes (Lin-Lui and Adey, 1982). The raised extracellular calcium concentration may, along these lines, settle neuronal layers through surface charge screening, explaining the viewed electrophysiological aggravations.

A few investigations revealed that in vitro microwave effects may be on a very basic level impacted by ELF sufficiency guideline. Exceptional introduction of chick cerebrum tissue toward microwaves (147 MHz) sinusoidally amplitude balanced at frequencies some place in the scope of 6 and 20 Hz, provoked the appearance of calcium particles into the extracellular partition (Bawin et al., 1975; Blackman et al., 1979).

Considering these examinations together, it is recommended that nonthermal microwave introduction impacts cell work in a general sense at ELF guideline incidences in the 6-20 Hz go. These frequencies are in the extent of EEG development and may explain that ELF magnetic and attractive fields can gather hippocampal rhythmical theta activity (Bawin et al., 1984, 1986, 1996). At present, there isn't much of information for whether higher guideline frequencies used in TDMA and CDMA portable correspondence frameworks may in like manner upset neuronal limit. Regardless, as changes of calcium efflux have as of late been represented specifically ELF repetition windows up to 510 Hz (Blackman et al., 1988), further assessments should be done to clarify whether such windows are of congruity also for mobile correspondence.

4. EFFECTS ON DNA DAMAGE

Succeeding intense presentation of rodents to persistent and beat microwaves at entire body arrived at the midpoint of SAR of 0.6 or 1.2 W/kg aimed at 2 hours; a portion subordinate increment in sole and double strand DNA breaks has recently stood accounted for in the mind (Lai and Singh, 1995, 1996). These perceptions excited impressive intrigue on account of the potential ramifications as for carcinogenesis. In light of this information, two different examinations were performed in vitro utilizing an all-around portrayed presentation arrangement through precise temperature settings. During the investigations mouse fibroblasts, human glioblastoma cells, besides rodent synapses remained uncovered for 2 hour to persistent 2.45 GHz microwaves (mean SAR 1.2 W/kg) or for 24 hour to frequency tweaked CDMA 836-848 MHz microwaves (mean SAR 0.6 W/kg) (Malyapa et al., 1997, 1998). In spite of delicate estimation method in the said examination, no expansion of DNA harm can be distinguished both for following introduction or after a 4 hour delay. A potential clarification aimed at this distinction is the way that the tests done by Lai and Singh (1995 and 1996) existed done with driving forces discharged at 1/1000 of the inter-pulse time. The present introduction arrangement varies extensively from TDMA procedures in versatile correspondence, where driving forces equivalent one eighth or 33% of inter-pulse period, contingent upon singular framework outlines. Accordingly, the pinnacle control was a lot greater than the average power, which possibly will have represented the watched DNA harm.

Figure 1. Schematic summary of the possible mechanisms of RF-EMF exposure in central nervous system (Source: Kim et al., 2019)

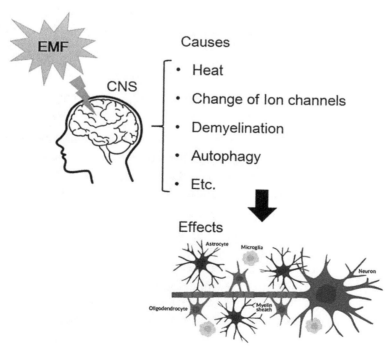

5. RISK OF BRAIN TUMOR

Various apprehensions have been raised with respect to the association between radiofrequency signals radiated from these gadgets and the conceivable danger of creating ceaseless sicknesses. Even though existing rules express that cell phones transmit energy levels very low to cause any injurious health influences, there has been developing discussion concerning whether a relative hazard has not been set up because of the various degrees of introduction when the examination is at first directed. Particularly since early cell phones were created with a simple innovation, and produced radiofrequency torrents of just 800 – 900 megahertz (MHz) (Benson et al., 2017; Linet & Inskip, 2010). All things considered, various endeavors have been made to assess this association dependent on the standard of cell phone utilization today—with a significant part of the exploration concentrating on the impacts of cell phone use and the improvement of tumors, especially in the head and neck locale. Specifically, investigation has concentrated on tumors specific to the temporal region of the brain—a spot proposed to encounter the most presentation to cell phone radiation—including tumors like, meningiomas, gliomas, and acoustic neuromas (Christensen et al., 2004). However, in spite of this developing database of logical investigation, the subject still stays dubious. While some case-control examines, appeared in Table 1, have implied to discover an association between cerebrum tumors and expanded cell phone utilization by means of a tumor "promoter" impact, other case-control inquiry discover no momentary impacts of mobile phone electromagnetic field presentation on the brain pathology (Bernier, 2017; Mandala et al., 2014).

Lahkola et al. (2006) analysed the impact of cell phone use on a danger of building up an assortment of intracranial tumors by leading a meta-investigation including 12 examinations. The Odds Ratio (OR) was seen as unimportant at 0.98 (95% certainty interim; CI = 0.83 - 1.16) for every single intracranial tumor identified with cell phone use. For gliomas, the pooled OR was 0.96 (95% CI 0.78 - 1.18), for meningiomas it was 0.87 (95% CI 0.72 - 1.05), and for acoustic neuromas it was 1.07 (95% CI 0.89 - 1.30). Kan et al. (2007) directed a comparable report inspecting the OR for high-grade gliomas, meningiomas, and acoustic neuromas. The pooled OR was venerated at being lower than 1, and the chances proportion for low-grade glioma was seen as unimportant with an OR = 1.14 (95% confidence interval; CI = 0.91 to 1.43).

6. EFFECTS ON BLOOD-BRAIN BARRIER PERMEABILITY

Effects of microwave introduction on blood-mind obstruction porousness have been analyzed either alone or in blend in with static magnetic fields, as used for Magnetic Resonance Imaging (MRI). Aggravations of the blood-brain barrier penetrability were reviewed by surveying the extravasation of external tracers or of inside serum constituents. Most scientists agree that steady and beat microwave presentation grows blood–mind block in vitro (Schirmacher et al., 2000) and in vivo (Albert & Kerns, 1981; Frey et al., 1975; Lin & Lin, 1982; Merritt et al., 1978; Oscar & Hawkins, 1977; Sutton & Carrol, 1979), yet a few researchers are at fluctuation to these revelations, in every occasion on condition that restriction allied compression reactions were avoided (Preston et al., 1979).

Since different authors portrayed extended vulnerability of the blood-cerebrum obstruction exactly on elevated SAR joined via temperature upsurge (Merritt et al., 1978), blood-mind boundary collapse subsequent to microwave light may be a direct result of thermal impacts. Various investigators, nevertheless, centered around that the disrupting impact may occur under thermally controlled conditions (Frey et al., 1975; Oscar & Hawkins, 1977).

The neuropathological significance of the development of blood-cerebrum limit porousness is probably low in light of the fact that even the most articulated changes impelled by microwave presentation are little diverged from developed models of blood-mind hindrance disrupting impacts (Fritze et al., 1997). Additionally, blood-cerebrum hindrance changes are quickly convoluted. The penetrability addition to Evans blue diminished adequately 10 min after presentation of rodents at cerebrum matter SAR of 240 W/kg, and completely disappeared after 30 min (Lin & Lin, 1982). So additionally, the penetrability augmentation to horseradish peroxidase was completely exchanged inside 1 h following microwave introduction at control densities of 10 µW/cm^2 (Albert & Kerns, 1981).

7. EFFECTS ON HIPPOCAMPUS

The morphological and biochemical adjustments brought about via RF-EMF experiences were examined in bodily research. Now, pre-birth introduction brings about smaller size, lesser birth weight besides future generations critical debilitation of the hippocampus, pyramidal cell and glial cells (Bas et al., 2009; Hosseini-Sharifabad et al., 2012). Neuronal harm in the focal sensory system has been accounted for because of both pre-birth or early grown-up exposures to electromagnetic radiation (Mausset et al., 2001; Salford et al., 2003). Bas et al. (2009) proposed that EMF introduction may influence the original arrangement of cells in the Cornu Ammonis (CA) of the hippocampus throughout the embryonic improvement. And hence could bring about disintegration of social and subjective capacities including wisdom plus transient retention. Albeit numerous in vitro and in vivo trial ponders have been played out, the potential impacts of EMF introduction on the focal sensory system are as yet hazy (Lazzaro et al, 2013; Altunkaynak et al., 2016). X-ray having a place with hippocampus were explored via stereological and spectroscopic examination likewise nervous system tests in therapeutic understudies that announced utilizing cell phones for < 30 min day by day use by the head and for >90 min everyday use by the head. Conflicting proof occurs around the impacts of RF-EMF on psychological capacities besides relationship with hippocampal capacities (Haarala et al., 2003). Deniz et al., (2017) evaluated hippocampal capacities utilizing OsiriX 3.2.1 programming in people using wireless gadgets for < 30 min everyday use by the head and for >90 min day by day use by the head. Be that as it may, no critical distinction was resolved between the groups as far as hippocampal capacities. In the course of such a specific circumstance, there are not much examinations up to now exploring the impacts of mobiles on hippocampal capacities in the human cerebrum utilizing MR pictures. Wang et al. (2016) researched major variations in grey plus white matter related with cellular network usage thru exploring functional Magnetic Resonance Images (fMRI) in undergrads. They recommended that the overemployment of cellular network may become the main root cause for the changes in brainy framework and the said adjustments can comprehend the impacts of EMF on the cerebrum and hidden neuronal components. In this investigation, they executed spectroscopic and neurocognitive examinations in order to assess relationships through volumetrical qualities. Their discoveries indicated a critical contrast among the assemblages in the stroop and digit area (in reverse) exams, including the appraisal of consideration. The examination might be significantly critical to understanding absence of consideration and fixation. Moreover, they additionally watched a diminished capacity to smother boosts in the persons who use the mobile phones for an extended duration. In any case, they decided no critical distinction in additional neurological errands among the assemblages. Schoeni et al. (2015) explored the impacts of night-time mobile usage on the subjective capacities in young people, utilizing neurocognitive examinations to gauge verbal and figural retention. They recommended that night-time utilization of cell phones may prompt an expansion in wellbeing side effects, for example, fast exhaustion and cerebral pain. Notwithstanding, and as opposed to the outcomes, they watched no impact of presentation to EMF discharged via mobile gadgets on attention limit and retention. Notwithstanding these impacts of cell phones on psychological execution, Movvahedi et al. (2014) examined the momentary impacts of RF energy on response period and transient retention in primary institute understudies. The investigators recommended that electromagnetic emission displayed valuable consequences for momentary and temporary retention (Figure 1).

In conclusion, the utilization of cell phones for in excess of 90 min in a day is related with expanded issues of fixation and consideration. In any case, prolonged utilization of cell phones is found to have no effect on memory assignments and hippocampal volume as depicted in Table 1. Further investigation including large quantities of subjects is currently required so as to approve these discoveries and so as to decide to what extent the changes in hippocampus are brought up in exposed people contrasted with controls.

8. EFFECTS ON SLEEP AND COGNITIVE OCCUPATIONS

a. Effects on Sleep

The discussion on whether there are changes in sleep routine in view of microwave introduction relies upon discoveries by Reite et al. (1994), who definite that exceptional presentation of human subjects for only 15 min to adequacy adjusted microwaves (0.1-100 µW/kg as a primary concern tissue) prompts a shortening of the sleep starting inaction and augmentation in the length of stage 2 sleep as appears in Table 1. As per these observations, Pasche et al. (1996) found a reducing in sleep starting inertness and augmentation in the total entirety of the sleep following remarkable (20 minutes) introduction of patients encountering psychophysiological a sleeping disorder to plentifulness controlled microwaves. Regardless, the microwave repeat used in these assessments (27.12 MHz) was not in the extent of compact particular devices. Under conditions even more immovably related to phones night-time introduction to a GSM signal (50 µW/cm²) for 8 hours provoked a limitation of sleep starting idleness and a general decline of Rapid Eye Movement (REM) rest in strong subjects (Mann & Roschke, 1996). The full-scale sleep time and relative proportion of moderate wave rest remained not affected. In advanced trials of a comparable social occasion, polysomnographic changes as a result of mobile phone introduction couldn't be reproduced, neither at low (20 µW/cm²) nor at incredibly high (5 µW/cm²) control densities (Wagner et al., 1998, 2000). In a further especially controlled assessment, healthy males were exhibited to beat 900 MHz fields (spatial apex SAR 1 W/kg), either in subbing 15 min on/15 min off pauses which were unpredictably applied for the length of the night (Borbely et al., 1999) or for 30 min once proximately going before sleep (Huber et al., 2000). In the two assessments an extension of EEG powers during non-REM rest was observed. Presently, the debatable discoveries do not suggest an undeviating opinion on if portable correspondence impacts sleep in humans. Subsequently these variations may impact the overall success; potential associations between wireless devices and sleep require further evaluation.

b. Effects on Cognitive Functions

A couple of researchers accept that electromagnetic fields may similarly connect with intellectual capacities. The central discovering was a restriction of response times after prologue to ELF (Gavalas et al., 1970) or GSM microwave arenas (Preece et al., 1999; Koivisto et al., 2000a, 2000b), particularly throughout assignments which need contemplation or control of information in the occupied commemoration. A connection to consideration is in like manner prescribed by the recognition that evoked or preliminary moderate mind possibilities were balanced distinctly during handling of complex memory or visual observing tasks yet not thru fewer requesting tests (Eulitz et al., 1998; Freude et al., 1998, 2000; Krause et al., 2000).

9. 3G, 4G AND 5G MOBILE NETWORKS

Some time ago 3G portable systems were generally preferred by mobile clients. In any case, that has now offered route to the considerably more progressed, 4G LTE system. Hugely amazing and including quicker transmission capacity, this system gives exceptionally quick support of portable Internet clients. Be that as it may, much the same as everything else, this is likewise not without its drawbacks. The most recent claim is that the fourth-age innovation is a few times to a greater degree a wellbeing peril than any of its ancestors. At the point when cell phones had quite recently entered the market, they were prevalently used to make calls while moving and type out instant messages. Anyhow, this system changed in only a couple of years' time. While 3G made it conceivable to peruse the Internet on cell phones, the following fourth generation—4G—has made it workable for clients to stream rich media content right on their cell phones and tablets.

Analysts uncovered the right ear of 18 members to Long Term Evolution (LTE) radio frequency radiation for 30 minutes. The consumed measure of radiation in the cerebrum was well inside international (ICNIRP) mobile phone lawful points of confinement and the wellspring of the radiation was kept 1 cm from the ear. To take out investigation predispositions the scientists utilized a double visually blind, hybrid, randomized plan, presenting members to genuine and hoax exposures. The outcomes exhibit that RF radiation from LTE 4G innovation influences mind neural movement in both the closer cerebrum site and in the remote region, including the left half of the cerebrum. As indicated by the Global Mobile Suppliers Association "LTE is the quickest producing portable framework innovation ever". The United States is the biggest LTE vitrine on the world. By March 2013 the worldwide cumulative of LTE memberships was by now 91 million subscribers. Over portion of these, 47 million, were American 4G subscribers (Bin Lv et al., 2013).

In 2018, a peer reviewed report presented by the National Toxicology Program (NTP) of the US National Institute of Environmental Health Sciences discovered RF-EMF of 900 MHz, utilized by 3G and 4G systems, encouraged occurrences of detrimental heart schwannomas (disease that assaults nerve tissues) in male and female rats. The report likewise discovered proof that the radiation caused glioma (harmful tumor in the cerebrum) in rats. Malignant growth isn't the main disease that such radiations can reason. Researchers have so far connected 5G to at any rate 20 infirmities, including heart maladies, type-2 diabetes and mental unsettling influences, for example, misery, tension and self-destructive inclinations. To raise the worries, on March 5 2019, 230 safety authorities and researchers from 40 nations requested the Nordic nations to stop 5G till the "potential risks of intense and long-lasting wellbeing

Table 1. Different studies exploring impacts of RF-EMF on brain activity during rest by EEG

Study	Study Subjects	Exposure	Duration	Blinding	Main Outcomes
Croft et al. (2002)	16 M, 8 F	900 MHz, PM 217 Hz	3 x 20 min	Single	Increase alpha, decrease delta power
Curcio et al. (2005)	10 M, 10 F	902.4 MHz, PM 217, 0.25 W/Kg	45 min	Double	Increase EEG power alpha band (effect larger for EMF on during EEG)
D'Costa et al. (2003)	5 M, 5 F	900 MHz, PM 217	5 x 5 min	Single	Decrease alpha and beta power
Hietanen et al. (2000)	10 M, 9 F	900, 1800 MHz	20 min	Single	No effects
Hinrikus et al. (2008b)	30 M, 36 F	450 MHz, PM 7, 14 & 21, 40 & 70, 217, 1000 Hz 0.303 W/kg	20 min	Double	Alteration alpha and beta rhythm
Hinrikus et al. (2008a)	4 M, 9 F	450 MHz PM 7, 14, 21 Hz 0.35 W/kg	40 min	Double	Increase in alpha and beta rhythm (for PM 14 & 21 Hz)
Huber et al. (2002)	16 M	900 MHz CW & PM 2, 8, 217, 1736 Hz 1 W/kg	30 min	Double	Alpha power increase, PM signal
Kleinlogel et al. (2008)	15 M	900, 1950 MHz PM 217 Hz 1 W/kg	30 min	Double	No effects
Kramarenko & Tan (2003)	10 M (adults) 10 M (12 years)	900 MHz PM 217 Hz	Duration of a call	-	Abnormal slow waves in delta range
Reiser et al. (1995)	18 M, 18 F	902.4 MHz PM 217 Hz	15 min	Single	Increase in EEG power in alpha and beta band
Roschke & Mann (1997)	36 M	900 MHz PM 217 Hz	3.5 min	Single	No effects

M – males, F – females. Exposure parameters given are Frequency (MHz), Pulse Modulation (PM) frequency and estimated Specific Absorption Rate W/kg (SAR)

(Source: Maartje Brouwer, 2010)

impacts of introduction to 5G have been completely explored by industry-autonomous researchers". Prior in September 2017, upwards of 180 specialists from 36 nations, including India, asked the EU to set up an autonomous team to survey the effect of 5G on human wellbeing. In 2015, US researchers made an intrigue to the UN secretary general, WHO and all UN member countries to install 5G after the wake of evaluating its wellbeing impacts (Down to Earth, 2019).

As the adjudicators are out on the safekeeping of 5G, a few researchers propose planning systems dependent on less destructive fiber optic cables. These can be multiple times quicker than 5G. We ought to feat wired connotations which can bring rate of 10 Gb every second. Above all, we ought to perceive the truth about cell phones: an emanating gadget. They ought to be overhauled to limit client exposures and use them sparingly (Down to Earth, 2019). 4G and 5G innovations reason numerous damages to human wellbeing. Malignancy is just a single issue, and one that is effectively fathomed. 4G and 5G cause 720! (Factorial) various illnesses in individuals and can destroy everything that lives however a few types of microorganisms (Michrowski, 2018). As per Peter Tocci, known ICMR impacts incorporate endocrine disturbance (host of diseases), breakdown of blood-mind obstruction, DNA strand breaks, hindrance of DNA repair, sperm harm, regenerative issues, chemical imbalance, Alzheimer's - and some more. In spite of the fact that not to be rejected, malignant growth, the 'well known' concern, is really a lesser one in the panoply of impacts – as in, ecocide and possible end of reproduction (Trower, 2013).

10. MOBILE PHONES AND PUBLIC HEALTH

Cellular phones are presently a basic part of current communications. In various countries, over an enormous section of the people use mobile phones and the market is growing rapidly. In specific parts of the world, mobile phones are the most dependable or the principle phones accessible. Given the tremendous number of mobile phone customers, it is basic to explore, appreciate and screen any potential general prosperity influence. Cellular phones transport by transmitting radio waves over an arrangement of fixed receiving wires named base stations. Radiofrequency waves are electromagnetic fields, and not under any condition like ionizing radiation, for instance, X-rays or gamma rays, can neither disrupt chemical bonds nor reason ionization in the human body (Figure 1).

11. EXPOSURE LEVELS

Mobile phones are low-powered radiofrequency transmitters, employed at frequencies some place in the range of 450 and 2700 MHz with top powers in the extent of 0.1 to 2 watts. The handset possibly transmits control once it is turned on. The power (and thusly the radiofrequency prologue to a customer) flips rapidly with extending great ways from the receiver. A person utilizing a mobile phone 30-40 cm far from their body - for example while chatting, getting to the Internet, or using a "hands free" gadget - will hence have a much lower introduction to radiofrequency arenas than someone holding the phone against his head.

Despite using "without hands" devices, which fend off mobile phones from the head and body during phone calls, exposure is in like manner lessened by compelling the number and length of calls. Using the phone in regions of good reception moreover lessens introduction as it empowers the phone to transmit at diminished power. The usage of specialized devices for lessening radiofrequency field introduction has not been exhibited to be convincing. Mobile phones are consistently denied in clinics and on planes, as the radiofrequency sign may interfere with certain electro-therapeutic contraptions and route frameworks or navigation.

12. ARE THERE ANY HEALTH EFFECTS?

Incalculable examinations have been performed over the span of the recent two decades to review whether mobile phones represent to a potential prosperity peril. Until this point in time, no major antagonistic wellbeing impacts have been set up as being realized by mobile phone usage. A few examinations by prominent researchers on the impact of RF-EMF on brain activity have been depicted in Table 1.

a. Short-term Effects

Tissue warming is the principle arrangement of collaboration between radiofrequency energy and the human body. On the frequencies used by phones, most of the energy is devoured by the skin and other recognizable tissues, realizing superfluous temperature climb in the cerebrum or certain different tissues of the body (Masiliunas et al., 2018).

Different contemplates have inquired about the effects of radiofrequency fields on cerebrum electrical activity, mental work, sleep, rest, pulse and circulatory strain in volunteers. Until this point in time, ask about doesn't suggest any dependable confirmation of disagreeable prosperity impacts from prologue to radiofrequency fields at levels underneath those that reason tissue warming. Further, analysis has not had the alternative to offer assistance for a causal association between introduction to electromagnetic fields and self-reported signs, or "electromagnetic sensitivity".

b. Long-term Effects

Epidemiological explore about examining potential long stretch perils from radiofrequency presentation has generally scanned for a connection between mind tumors and wireless use. Regardless, considering the way that various malignancies are not discernable until various years after the affiliations that provoked the tumor, and since mobile phones were not comprehensively used until the mid-1990s, epidemiological assessments at present can simply assess those infections that become clear inside shorter timespans. Nevertheless, significances of animal research dependably show no extended threatening development risk for long stretch prologue to radiofrequency fields (Masiliunas et al., 2018).

A couple of gigantic worldwide epidemiological studies have been done or are consistent, including case-control contemplates about an imminent associate partner studies assessing different prosperity endpoints in adults. The greatest survey case-control focus on adults, Interphone, encouraged by the International Agency for Research on Cancer (IARC), was expected to choose if there are interfaces between usage of mobile phones and head and neck maladies in adults.

The worldwide pooled examination of data collected from 13 partaking countries found no extended risk of glioma or meningioma with wireless usage of more than ten years. There are a couple of indications of an extended risk of glioma for the people who point by point the most raised 10% of total significant stretches of cell phone use, in spite of the way that there was no anticipated example of growing peril with increasingly prominent length of use. The masters contemplated that inclinations and bungles limit the nature of these conclusions and check a causal comprehension. Considering on these data, IARC has orchestrated radiofrequency electromagnetic fields as possibly malignancy causing among the people (2B), a class used when a causal alliance is seen as strong, anyway when probability, inclination or confusion can't be blocked with reasonable assurance.

While an extended peril of cerebrum tumors is not developed, the extending usage of wireless network gadgets and the nonappearance of data for a gadget use after some timespans longer than 15 years warrant further research of mobile phone use and brain malignant development possibility. In particular, with the continuous notoriety of phone use among increasingly young people, and along these lines a perhaps longer lifetime of introduction, WHO has progressed further research on this regard. A couple of studies looking at potential prosperity impacts in children and youngsters are in progress.

13. FACTORS AFFECTING

1. Cell Phone and Human Body Distance

In case cell phone moves even an inch from the body, it can remarkably diminish radiation introduction. Prominence of the sign reduces as the square of the great ways from the source. This suggests if we double the distance from the source, the signal quality would be manifold times less. On the off chance that we increase 10 times the space between the cell phone and our head, the signal quality will be 100 times less, and similarly at 100 times of detachment, signal quality becomes10,000 times a smaller amount (Figure 1).

2. Distance from the Tower

Diverse correspondence aspects release distinctive proportion of radiation. With the help of a sensible meter we can measure how a great deal of radiation is gotten at a particular spot. Around a lone zenith (tower), radiation may not be uniform. The energy from a remote tower receiving wire, like that of other media transmission radio wires, is facilitated toward horizon (corresponding to the earth surface), with some plunging disseminate. Cell phones dialog with adjoining cell tower basically through Radiofrequency (RF) waves, a sort of vitality in the electromagnetic range between FM radio waves and microwaves. Like FM radio waves, microwaves, undeniable light, and warmth, they are sorts of non-ionizing radiation. This suggests they can't cause illness by genuinely hurting DNA. Right when an individual makes a cell phone call, a signal is sent from the phone's radio wire to the nearest base station receiving device. The base station responds to this signal by designating it an open radiofrequency channel. RF waves interchange the voice information to the base station. The voice signals are then sent to a exchange centre, which moves the call to its goal line. Voice signals are then and there given off forward and backward during the call, so impacts human cerebrum.

3. Specific Absorption Rate (SAR)

SAR is the estimation of rate by which a body ingests vitality when the body is exhibited to radio frequency electromagnetic waves (RF-EMWs). We can in like manner state that it is an extent of maintenance of EM wave vitality by tissues. It is portrayed as power held per mass of tissue and has unit's watts/kilogram. Degree of consistency is observed either for whole body or for a little model volume of tissues (Scarella et al., 2006). As showed by ICNIRP rules, for obliging prologue to time moving electric, attractive and electromagnetic fields, the most outrageous SAR regard for mobile phones has been set at 2 Watts/Kg restricted for the head and trunk (of a human) in the frequency scope of 10 MHz to 10 GHz These guidelines have been made as a group with Environment Health Division of the World Health Organization (WHO). In India, FCC bounds for the open introduction is 1.6 W/kg for 1 gram volume found the center estimation of SAR (Tyagi et al., 2010).

4. Age of the Person

When contrasted with grown-ups, youngsters have huge impact on their mind while talking on the cell phone since kids are developing all the more quickly, they have more cell dividing ability, so radiations disturbs all the more no. of cells. Likewise, kids have a slenderer skull compared with grown-ups so they have bigger effect (Riadh et al., 2011). It is additionally demonstrated that embryos are higher touchy to radiations than others.

5. GSM and CDMA

Examinations show that cellular network radiations sway human cerebrum and GSM worked wireless phone has higher effect on brain commotion when stood out from CDMA worked phones, as appears in Table 2.

14. EXPOSURE LIMIT GUIDELINES

Radiofrequency introduction limits for wireless cellular network customers are given the extent as Specific Absorption Rate (SAR) - the pace of radiofrequency strength ingestion per unit mass of the body. As of now, two overall bodies have made introduction rules for workers and for the general populace, except for patients encountering restorative management or treatment. These standards rely upon a nitty gritty assessment of the open coherent verification.

15. WHO RESPONSE

Owing to open and managerial concern, WHO developed the International Electromagnetic Fields (EMF) Project in 1996 to overview the sensible evidence of possible ominous health impacts from electromagnetic fields. WHO is leading an appropriate risk appraisal of all thought about prosperity results from radiofrequency fields introduction by 2016. Likewise, and as noted over, the International Agency for Research on Cancer (IARC), a WHO specific office, has examined the malignancy causing capacity of radiofrequency fields, as from phones in May 2011. WHO moreover recognizes and progresses investigate requirements for radiofrequency fields and prosperity to fill openings in data through its assessment plans. WHO makes open information materials and advances talk among specialists, governments, industry and the overall public to raise the level of perception about potential contrasting health risks of mobile phones.

Table 2. Energy scope of GSM and CDMA networks

GSM	1-2 Watt	Burst
CDMA	6-7 mWatt	Continuous

16. RECOMMENDATIONS AND FUTURE WORK

From the above investigation, it shows the results of electromagnetic radiation on human wellbeing using the available two cell phone developments in the Country viz. GSM 2G and 3G using EEG and Matlab. The effort on the same is being finished in the inspection office with different subjects and using the recently referenced cell phone correspondence advances using assorted kind of change, transmitted power and working frequency. Response of human mind is being examined under three conditions: when no phone is used, when a GSM 2G portable phone is used and utilizing a GSM 3G network. The characteristics of brain signals so gained would make sense of which kind of specialized gadgets is constantly increasingly sensible for person in concern with human wellbeing. Results gained will help organizing a class of specialized gadgets which have insignificant effect on human prosperity.

Future examinations focusing on long haul wireless cellular network presentation (10 years or more) ought to be accompanied so as to uncover understanding into this flawed issue, and ideally tip the scale in an indisputable manner. It is felt that manifestations in view of wireless use particularly those that impact the health of an individual can be constrained or wiped out by spreading awareness on the theme especially on confined use and not getting habituated to the gadgets.

17. CONCLUSION

The intent of this chapter is to show that wireless innovation is the most overwhelming natural and health threats. At present, there is minimal verification that pulsed or consistent microwave presentation at power and frequencies perceived with portable wireless cellular communication could interfere with the utilitarian and essential functioning of the brain. Under exploratory conditions, most of the positive results portrayed so far could be credited to thermal impacts. Such effects are presumably not going to occur during ordinary use of mobile phones. Other natural stresses observed under exploratory conditions could be related to technical responses, for instance, restriction stress, which unanesthetized animals may suffer when they are placed in obliging animal holders. Preliminary game arrangements should, along these lines, be arranged with maintenance to reproduce the authentic presentation situations for human customers of wireless cellular networks.

So additionally, collaborations with human behaviour, conduct or neurological diseases are best inconsequentiality. In particular, no vital relationship can be set up with the rate or the development of brain tumors under either trial or quantifiable situations. The effects of cell phone usage require steady perception, monitoring, observing and an effective reporting framework in such way can go far in helping specialists to figure formulate policies that will check the evil impacts owing to phone usage.

REFERENCES

Aalto, S., Haarala, C., Brück, A., Sipilä, H., Hämäläinen, H., & Rinne, J. O. (2006). Mobile phone affects cerebral blood flow in humans. *Journal of Cerebral Blood Flow and Metabolism*, 26(7), 885–890. doi:10.1038j.jcbfm.9600279 PMID:16495939

Albert, E. N., & Kerns, J. M. (1981). Reversible microwave effects on the blood-brain barrier. *Brain Research, 230*(1-2), 153–164. doi:10.1016/0006-8993(81)90398-X PMID:7317776

Wang, Y., Zou, Z., Song, H., Xu, X., Wang, H., d'Oleire Uquillas, F., & Huang, X. (2016). Altered grey matter volume and white matter integrity in college students with mobile phone dependence. *Frontiers in Psychology, 7*, 597. PMID:27199831

Altunkaynak, B. Z., Altun, G., Yahyazadeh, A., Kaplan, A. A., Deniz, O. G., Turkmen, A. P., ... Kaplan, S. (2016). Different methods for evaluating the effects of microwave radiation exposure on the nervous system. *Journal of Chemical Neuroanatomy, 75*, 62–69. doi:10.1016/j.jchemneu.2015.11.004 PMID:26686295

Arber, S. L., & Lin, J. C. (1984). Microwave enhancement of membrane conductance: Effects of EDTA, caffeine, and tetracaine. *Physiological Chemistry and Physics and Medical NMR, 16*, 469–475. PMID:6443226

Arber, S. L., & Lin, J. C. (1985). Microwave-induced changes in nerve cells: Effects of modulation and temperature. *Bioelectromagnetics, 6*(3), 257–270. doi:10.1002/bem.2250060306 PMID:3836669

Bas, O., Odaci, E., Mollaoglu, H., Ucok, K., & Kaplan, S. (2009). Chronic prenatal exposure to the 900 megahertz electromagnetic field induces pyramidal cell loss in the hippocampus of newborn rats. *Toxicology and Industrial Health, 25*(6), 377–384. doi:10.1177/0748233709106442 PMID:19671630

Bawin, S. M., Kaczmarek, L. K., & Adey, W. R. (1975). Effects of modulated VHF fields on the central nervous system. *Annals of the New York Academy of Sciences, 247*(1), 74–81. doi:10.1111/j.1749-6632.1975.tb35984.x PMID:1054258

Bawin, S. M., Satmary, W. M., Jones, R. A., Adey, W. R., & Zimmerman, G. (1996). Extremely-low-frequency magnetic fields disrupt rhythmic slow activity in rat hippocampal slices. *Bioelectromagnetics, 17*(5), 388–395. doi:10.1002/(SICI)1521-186X(1996)17:5<388::AID-BEM6>3.0.CO;2-#PMID:8915548

Bawin, S. M., Sheppard, A. R., Mahoney, M. D., Abu-Assal, M., & Adey, W. R. (1986). Comparison between the effects of extracellular direct and sinusoidal currents on excitability in hippocampal slices. *Brain Research, 362*(2), 350–354. doi:10.1016/0006-8993(86)90461-0 PMID:3942883

Bawin, S. M., Sheppard, A. R., Mahoney, M. D., & Adey, W. R. (1984). Influences of sinusoidal electric fields on excitability in the rat hippocampal slice. *Brain Research, 323*(2), 227–237. doi:10.1016/0006-8993(84)90293-2 PMID:6098340

Benson, V. S., Pirie, K., Schüz, J., Reeves, G. K., Beral, V., & Green, J. (2017). Mobile phone use and risk of brain neoplasms and other cancers: Prospective study. *International Journal of Epidemiology, 42*(3), 792–802. doi:10.1093/ije/dyt072 PMID:23657200

Bernier, R. H. (2017). What constitutes a public health problem? Epimonitor. Retrieved from http://epimonitor.net/List_of_Public_H ealth_Issues.htm

Berridge, M. J., & Irvine, R. F. (1984). Inositol triphosphate, a novel second messenger in cellular signal transduction. *Nature, 312*(5992), 315–321. doi:10.1038/312315a0 PMID:6095092

Bin, Lv., Zhiye, C., Tongning, W., Qing, S., Duo, Y., Lin, M., ... Yi, X. (2013). The alteration of spontaneous low frequency oscillations caused by acute electromagnetic fields exposure. *Clinical Neurophysiology*. PMID:24012322

Binhi, V. N., Repiev, A. & Edelev. (2002). *Magnetobiology: underlying physical problems*. San Diego, CA: Academic Press.

Blackman, C. F., Benane, S. G., Elliott, D. J., House, D. E., & Pollock, M. M. (1988). Influence of electromagnetic fields on the efflux of calcium ions from brain tissue in vitro: A three-model analysis consistent with the frequency response up to 510 Hz. *Bioelectromagnetics*, *9*(3), 215–227. doi:10.1002/bem.2250090303 PMID:3178897

Blackman, C. F., Elder, J. A., Weil, C. M., Benane, S. G., Eichinger, D. C., & House, D. E. (1979). Induction of calcium-ion efflux from brain tissue by radio-frequency radiation: Effects of modulation frequency and field strength. *Radiation Research*, *14*, 93–98.

Borbely, A. A., Huber, R., Graf, T., Fuchs, B., Gallmann, E., & Achermann, P. (1999). Pulsed high-frequency electromagnetic field affects human sleep and sleep electroencephalogram. *Neuroscience Letters*, *275*(3), 207–210. doi:10.1016/S0304-3940(99)00770-3 PMID:10580711

Christensen, H. C., Schüz, J., Kosteljanetz, M., Skovgaard, P. H., Boice, J. D., McLaughlin, J. K., & Johansen, C. (2004). Cellular Telephones and Risk for Acoustic Neuroma. *American Journal of Epidemiology*, *159*(3), 277–283. doi:10.1093/aje/kwh032 PMID:14742288

Croft, R. J., Chandler, J. S., Burgess, A. P., Barry, R. J., Williams, J. D., & Clarke, A. R. (2002). Acute mobile phone operation affects neural function in humans. *Clinical Neurophysiology*, *113*(10), 1623–1632. doi:10.1016/S1388-2457(02)00215-8 PMID:12350439

Curcio, G., Ferrara, M., Moroni, F., D'Inzeo, G., Bertini, M., & De Gennaro, L. (2005). Is the brain influenced by a phone call? An EEG study of resting wakefulness. *Neuroscience Research*, *53*(3), 265–270. doi:10.1016/j.neures.2005.07.003 PMID:16102863

D'Costa, H., Trueman, G., Tang, L., & ... . (2003). Human brain wave activity during exposure to radiofrequency field emissions from mobile phones. *Australasian Physical & Engineering Sciences in Medicine*, *26*, 162–167. doi:10.1007/BF03179176 PMID:14995060

Delgado, J. M., Leal, J., Monteagudo, J. L., & Gracia, M. G. (1982). Embryological changes induced by weak, extremely low frequency electromagnetic fields. *Journal of Anatomy*, *134*(3), 533–551. PMID:7107514

Deniz, O. G., Kaplan, S., Selçuk, M. B., Terzi, M., Altun, G., Yurt, K. K., ... Davis, D. (2017). Effects of short and long term electromagnetic fields exposure on the human hippocampus. *Journal of microscopy and ultrastructure, 5*(4), 191-197.

Down to Earth. (2019). 5G: A dangerous generation.

Eulitz, C., Ullsperger, P., Freude, G., & Elbert, T. (1998). Mobile phones modulate response patterns of human brain activity. *Neuroreport*, *9*(14), 3229–3232. doi:10.1097/00001756-199810050-00018 PMID:9831456

Freude, G., Ullsperger, P., Eggert, S., & Ruppe, I. (1998). Effects of microwaves emitted by cellular phones on human slow brain potentials. *Bioelectromagnetics, 19*(6), 384–387. doi:10.1002/(SICI)1521-186X(1998)19:6<384::AID-BEM6>3.0.CO;2-Y PMID:9738529

Frey, A. H., Feld, S. R., & Frey, B. (1975). Neural function and behaviour: Defining the relationship. *Annals of the New York Academy of Sciences, 247*(1), 433–439. doi:10.1111/j.1749-6632.1975.tb36019.x PMID:46734

Fritze, K., Sommer, C., Schmitz, B., Mies, G., Hossmann, K. A., Kiessling, M., & Wiessner, C. (1997). Effect of GSM microwave exposure on blood-brain barrier. *Acta Neuropathologica, 94*, 465–470. doi:10.1007004010050734 PMID:9386779

Gandhi, C. R., & Ross, D. H. (1989). Microwave induced stimulation of ^{32}Pi-incorporation into phosphoinositides of rat brain synaptosomes. *Radiation and Environmental Biophysics, 28*(3), 223–234. doi:10.1007/BF01211259 PMID:2552495

Gavalas, R. J., Walter, D. O., Hamer, J., & Rossadey, W. (1970). Effect of lowlevel, low-frequency electric fields on EEG and behavior in Macaca nemestrina. *Brain Research, 18*(3), 491–501. doi:10.1016/0006-8993(70)90132-0 PMID:4995199

Haarala, C., Bjornberg, L., Ek, M., Laine, M., Revonsuo, A., Koivisto, M., & Hämäläinen, H. (2003). Effect of a 902 MHz electromagnetic field emitted by mobile phones on human cognitive function: A replication study. *Bioelectromagnetics, 24*(4), 283–288. doi:10.1002/bem.10105 PMID:12696088

Harland, J. D., & Liburdy, R. P. (1997). Environmental magnetic fields inhibit the antiproliferative action of tamoxifen and melatonin in a human breast cancer cell line. *Bioelectromagnetics, 18*(8), 555–562. doi:10.1002/(SICI)1521-186X(1997)18:8<555::AID-BEM4>3.0.CO;2-1 PMID:9383244

Hietanen, M., Kovala, T., & Hamalainen, H. (2000). Human brain activity during exposure to radiofrequency fields emitted by cellular phones. *Scandinavian Journal of Work, Environment & Health, 26*(2), 87–92. doi:10.5271jweh.516 PMID:10817372

Hinrikus, H., Bachmann, M., Lass, J., Karai, D., & Tuulik, V. (2008a). Effect of low frequency modulated microwave exposure on human EEG: Individual sensitivity. *Bioelectromagnetics, 29*(7), 527–538. doi:10.1002/bem.20415 PMID:18452168

Hinrikus, H., Bachmann, M., Lass, J., Tomson, R., & Tuulik, V. (2008b). Effect of 7, 14 and 21 Hz modulated 450 MHz microwave radiation on human electroencephalographic rhythms. *International Journal of Radiation Biology, 84*(1), 69–79. doi:10.1080/09553000701691679 PMID:18058332

Hosseini-Sharifabad, M., Esfandiari, E., & Hosseini-Sharifabad, A. (2012). The effect of prenatal exposure to restraint stress on hippocampal granule neurons of adult rat offspring. *Iranian Journal of Basic Medical Sciences., 15*, 106–107. PMID:23493456

Huber, R., Graf, T., Cote, K. A., Wittmann, L., Gallmann, E., Matter, D., ... Achermann, P. (2000). Exposure to pulsed high-frequency electromagnetic field during waking affects human sleep EEG. *Neuroreport, 11*(15), 3321–3325. doi:10.1097/00001756-200010200-00012 PMID:11059895

Huber, R., Treyer, V., Borbely, A. A., Schuderer, J., Gottselig, J. M., Landolt, H.-P., ... Achermann, P. (2002). Electromagnetic fields, such as those from mobile phones, alter regional cerebral blood flow and sleep and waking EEG. *Journal of Sleep Research*, *11*(4), 289–295. doi:10.1046/j.1365-2869.2002.00314.x PMID:12464096

Hung, C. S., Anderson, C., Horne, J. A., & McEvoy, P. (2007). Mobile phone 'talk-mode' signal delays EEG-determined sleep onset. *Neuroscience Letters*, *421*(1), 82–86. doi:10.1016/j.neulet.2007.05.027 PMID:17548154

Kan, P., Simonsen, S. E., Lyon, J. L., & Kestle, J. R. W. (2007). Cellular Phone Use and Brain Tumor: A Meta-Analysis. *Journal of Neuro-Oncology*, *86*(1), 71–78. doi:10.100711060-007-9432-1 PMID:17619826

Kleinlogel, H., Dierks, T., Koenig, T., Lehmann, H., Minder, A., & Berz, R. (2008). Effects of weak mobile phone - Electromagnetic fields (GSM, UMTS) on well-being and resting EEG. *Bioelectromagnetics*, *29*(6), 479–487. doi:10.1002/bem.20419 PMID:18431738

Koivisto, M., Krause, C. M., Revonsuo, A., Laine, M., & Hamalainen, H. (2000b). The effects of electromagnetic field emitted by GSM phones on working memory. *Neuroreport*, *11*(8), 1641–1643. doi:10.1097/00001756-200006050-00009 PMID:10852216

Koivisto, M., Revonsuo, A., Krause, C., Haarala, C., Sillanmaki, L., Laine, M., & Hamalainen, H. (2000a). Effects of 902 MHz electromagnetic field emitted by cellular telephones on response times in humans. *Neuroreport*, *11*(2), 413–415. doi:10.1097/00001756-200002070-00038 PMID:10674497

Kramarenko, A. V., & Tan, U. (2003). Effects of high-frequency electromagnetic fields on human EEG: A brain mapping study. *The International Journal of Neuroscience*, *113*(7), 1007–1019. doi:10.1080/00207450390220330 PMID:12881192

Krause, C. M., Sillanmaki, L., Koivisto, M., Haggqvist, A., Saarela, C., Revonsuo, A., ... Hamalainen, H. (2000). Effects of electromagnetic field emitted by cellular phones on the EEG during a memory task. *Neuroreport*, *11*(4), 761–764. doi:10.1097/00001756-200003200-00021 PMID:10757515

Lahkola, A., Tokola, K., & Auvinen, A. (2006). Meta-Analysis of Mobile Phone Use and Intracranial Tumors. *Scandinavian Journal of Work, Environment & Health*, *32*(3), 171–177. doi:10.5271jweh.995 PMID:16804618

Lai, H. (1996). Single- and double-strand DNA breaks in rat brain cells after acute exposure to radiofrequency electromagnetic radiation. *International Journal of Radiation Biology*, *69*(4), 513–521. doi:10.1080/095530096145814 PMID:8627134

Lai, H., & Singh, N. P. (1995). Acute low-intensity microwave exposure increases DNA single-strand breaks in rat brain cells. *Bioelectromagnetics*, *16*(3), 207–210. doi:10.1002/bem.2250160309 PMID:7677797

Lazzaro, V., Capone, F., Apollonio, F., Borea, P. A., & Cadossi, R. (2013). A consensus panel review of central nervous system effects of the exposure to low-intensity extremely low-frequency magnetic fields. *Brain Stimulation*, *6*(4), 469–476. doi:10.1016/j.brs.2013.01.004 PMID:23428499

Lin, J. C., & Lin, M. F. (1982). Microwave hyperthermia-induced blood-brain barrier alterations. *Radiation Research*, *89*(1), 77–87. doi:10.2307/3575686 PMID:7063606

Lin-Lui, S., & Adey, W. R. (1982). Low frequency amplitude modulated microwave fields change calcium efflux rates from synaptosomes. *Biolectromagnetics, 3*(3), 309–322. doi:10.1002/bem.2250030303 PMID:7126280

Linet, M., & Inskip, P. (2010). Cellular Telephone Use and Cancer Risk. *Reviews on Environmental Health, 25*(1), 51–55. doi:10.1515/REVEH.2010.25.1.51 PMID:20429159

Malyapa, R. S., Ahern, E. W., Bi, C., Straube, W. L., La Regina, M., Pickard, W. F., & Roti, J. L. (1998). DNA damage in rat brain cells after in vivo exposure to 2450MHz electromagnetic radiation and various methods of euthanasia. *Radiation Research, 149*(6), 637–645. doi:10.2307/3579911 PMID:9611103

Malyapa, R. S., Ahern, E. W., Straube, W. L., Moros, E. G., Pickard, W. F., & Roti, J. L. (1997). Measurement of DNA damage after exposure to electromagnetic radiation in the cellular phone communication frequency band (835.62 and 847.74 MHz). *Radiation Research, 148*(6), 618–627. doi:10.2307/3579738 PMID:9399708

Mandala, M., Colletti, V., Sacchetto, L., Manganotti, P., Ramat, S., Marcocci, A., & Colletti, L. (2014). Effect of Bluetooth Headset and Mobile Phone Electromagnetic Fields on the Human Auditory Nerve. *Laryngoscope, 124*(1), 255–259. doi:10.1002/lary.24103 PMID:23619813

Mann, K., & Roschke, J. (1996). Effects of pulsed high-frequency electromagnetic fields on human sleep. *Neuropsychobiol, 33*(1), 41–47. doi:10.1159/000119247 PMID:8821374

Masiliunas, R., & Vitkute, D. Stankevi˘cius, E., Matijo˘saitis, V. & Petrikonis, K. (2018). Response inhibition set shifting and complex executive function in patients with chronic lower back pain. Medicina, 53, 26-33.

Mausset, A. L., de Seze, R., Montpeyroux, F., & Privat, A. (2001). Effects of radiofrequency exposure on the GABAergic system in the rat cerebellum: Clues from semiquantitative immunohistochemistry. *Brain Research, 912*(1), 33–46. doi:10.1016/S0006-8993(01)02599-9 PMID:11520491

McRee, D. I., & Wachtel, H. (1980). The effects of microwave radiation on the vitality of isolated frog sciatic nerves. *Radiation Research, 82*(3), 536–546. doi:10.2307/3575320 PMID:7384419

McRee, D. I., & Wachtel, H. (1986). Elimination of microwave effects on the vitality of nerves after blockage of active transport. *Radiation Research, 108*(3), 260–268. doi:10.2307/3576914 PMID:3492008

Merritt, J. H., Chamness, A. P., & Allen, S. J. (1978). Studies on blood-brain barrier permeability after microwave radiation. *Radiation and Environmental Biophysics, 15*(4), 367–377. doi:10.1007/BF01323461 PMID:756056

Michrowski, A. (2018). What you should know about the coming 5G – and what to do about it. Whole Life Expo 2019.

Movvahedi, M. M., Tavakkoli-Golpayegani, A., Mortazavi, S. A., Haghani, M., Razi, Z., & Shojaie-Fard, M. B. (2014). Does exposure to GSM 900 MHz mobile phone radiation affect short-term memory of elementary school students. *Journal of Pediatric Neurosciences, 9*(2), 121–124. doi:10.4103/1817-1745.139300 PMID:25250064

Oscar, K. J., & Hawkins, T. D. (1977). Microwave alteration of the blood– brain barrier system of rats. *Brain Research, 126*(2), 281–293. doi:10.1016/0006-8993(77)90726-0 PMID:861720

Pasche, B., Erman, M., Hayduk, R., Mitler, M. M., Reite, M., Higgs, L., ... Lebet, J. P. (1996). Effects of low energy emission therapy in chronic psychophysiological insomnia. *Sleep, 19*(4), 327–336. doi:10.1093leep/19.4.327 PMID:8776791

Preece, A. W., Iwi, G., Davies-Smith, A., Wesnes, K., Butler, S., Lim, E., & Varey, A. (1999). Effect of a 915-MHz simulated mobile phone signal on cognitive function in man. *International Journal of Radiation Biology, 75*(4), 447–456. doi:10.1080/095530099140375 PMID:10331850

Preston, E., Vavasour, E. J., & Assenheim, H. M. (1979). Permeability of the blood-brain barrier to mannitol in the rat following 2,450 MHz microwave irradiation. *Brain Research, 174*(1), 109–117. doi:10.1016/0006-8993(79)90807-2 PMID:487114

Habash, R.W. (2011). *Non-Invasive microwave hyperthermia* [PhD Thesis]. ECE Deptt, IISc, Bangalore, India.

Reiser, H., Dimpfel, W., & Schober, F. (1995). The influence of electromagnetic fields on human brain activity. *European Journal of Medical Research, 1*, 27–32. PMID:9392690

Reite, M., Higgs, L., Lebet, J. P., Barbault, A., Rossel, C., Kuster, N., ... Amato, D. B. P. (1994). Sleep inducing effect of low energy emission therapy. *Bioelectromagnetics, 15*(1), 67–75. doi:10.1002/bem.2250150110 PMID:8155071

Robert, L., Lee, F., Keinrath, C., Scherer, R., & Bisch, H. (2007). Brain-Compute Communication: Motivation, Aim, and Impact of Exploring a Virtual Apartment. *IEEE Transactions on Neural Systems and Rehabilitation Engineering, 15*(4), 473–482. doi:10.1109/TNSRE.2007.906956 PMID:18198704

Roschke, J., & Mann, K. (1997). No Short-Term Effects of Digital Mobile Radio Telephone on the Awake Human Electroencephalogram. *Bioelectromagnetics, 18*(2), 172–176. doi:10.1002/(SICI)1521-186X(1997)18:2<172::AID-BEM10>3.0.CO;2-T PMID:9084868

Salford, L. G., Brun, A. E., Eberhardt, J. L., Malmgren, L., & Persson, B. R. (2003). Nerve cell damage in mammalian brain after exposure to microwaves from GSM mobile phones. *Environmental Health Perspectives, 111*(7), 881–883. doi:10.1289/ehp.6039 PMID:12782486

Scarella, O. C., Lanteri, S., Beaume, G., Oudot, S., & Piperno, S. (2006). Realistic numerical modeling of human head tissue exposure to electromagnetic waves from cellular phones. *Comptes Rendus Physique, 7*(5), 501–508. doi:10.1016/j.crhy.2006.03.002

Schirmacher, A., Winters, S., Fischer, S., Goeke, J., Galla, H. J., Kullnick, U., ... Stogbauer, F. (2000). Electromagnetic fields (1.8 GHz) increase the permeability to sucrose of the blood-brain barrier in vitro. *Bioelectromagnetics, 21*, 338–345. doi:10.1002/1521-186X(200007)21:5<338::AID-BEM2>3.0.CO;2-Q PMID:10899769

Schoeni, A., Roser, K., & Roosli, M. (2015). Symptoms and cognitive functions in adolescents in relation to mobile phone use during night. *PLoS One, 10*(7), 0133528. doi:10.1371/journal.pone.0133528 PMID:26222312

Seaman, R. L., & Wachtel, H. (1978). Slow and rapid responses to CW and pulsed microwave radiation by individual Aplysia pacemakers. *The Journal of Microwave Power, 13*(1), 77–86. doi:10.1080/1607 0658.1978.11689079 PMID:213605

Sutton, C. H., & Carrol, F. B. (1979). Effects of microwave-induced hyperthermia on the blood-brain barrier of the rat. *Radiat Sci, 14*(6S), 329–334. doi:10.1029/RS014i06Sp00329

Tocci, P. G. (2019). *Wireless Technology: Ultra Convenient. Endlessly Entertaining. Criminally Instigated.* Terminally Pathological.

Trower, B. (2013). Wi-Fi- A thalidomide in the making. Who cares?

Tyagi, A., Duhan, M., & Bhatia, D. (2011). *Effect of Mobile Phone Radiation on Brain Activity GSM Vs CDMA.* IJSTM.

Tyagi, A., Jain, V., Bhatia, D., & Duhan, M. (2010). Review of Effect of Electromagnetic Radiations of Mobile Phone on Human Health. In *Proceeding of Control Instrumentation System Conference.* Academic Press.

Verma, S. C., Tejaswini, T. M., & Pradhan, D. (2019). Harmful effects of 5G radiations: review. In *Proceedings of IRAJ International Conference* (pp. 71-75). Academic Press.

Wachtel, H., Seaman, R., & Joines, W. (1975). Effects of low-intensity microwaves on isolated neurons. *Annals of the New York Academy of Sciences, 247*(1), 46–62. doi:10.1111/j.1749-6632.1975.tb35982.x PMID:1054247

Wagner, P., Roschke, J., Mann, K., Fell, J., Hiller, W., Frank, C., & Grozinger, M. (2000). Human sleep EEG under the influence of pulsed radiofrequency electromagnetic fields. Results from polysomnographies using submaximal high power flux densities. *Neuropsychobiol, 42*, 207–212. doi:10.1159/000026695 PMID:11096337

Wagner, P., Roschke, J., Mann, K., Hiller, W., & Frank, C. (1998). Human sleep under the influence of pulsed radiofrequency electromagnetic fields: A polysomnographic study using standardized conditions. *Bioelectromagnetics, 19*(3), 199–202. doi:10.1002/(SICI)1521-186X(1998)19:3<199::AID-BEM8>3.0.CO;2-X PMID:9554698

Wikipedia. (n.d.). Mobile Phone. Retrieved From http://en.wikipedia.org/wiki/Mobile_phone

ADDITIONAL READING

Hardell, L. (2017). Effects of Mobile Phones on Children's and Adolescents' Health: A Commentary. *Child Development, 89*(1), 137–140. doi:10.1111/cdev.12831 PMID:28504422

Kim, J. H., Yu, D. H., Kim, H. J., Huh, Y. H., Cho, S. W., Lee, J. K., ... Kim, H. R. (2017). Exposure to 835 MHz radiofrequency electromagnetic field induces autophagy in hippocampus but not in brain stem of mice. *Toxicology and Industrial Health, 34*(1), 23–35. doi:10.1177/0748233717740066 PMID:29166827

Lingvay, D., Borş, A. G. & Borş, A. M. (2018). Electromagnetic pollution and its effects on living matter. *Electrotehnica, Electronica, Automatica (EEA), 66*(2), 5-11.

Vila, J., Turner, M. C., Gracia-Lavedan, E., Figuerola, J., Bowman, J. D., Kincl, L., ... Cardis, E. (2018). Occupational exposure to high-frequency electromagnetic fields and brain tumor risk in the INTEROCC study: An individualized assessment approach. *Environment International, 119*, 353–365. doi:10.1016/j.envint.2018.06.038 PMID:29996112

Xu, Y., Jia, Y., Kirunda, J. B., Shen, J., Ge, M., Lu, L., & Pei, Q. (2018). Dynamic Behaviors in Coupled Neuron System with the Excitatory and Inhibitory Autapse under Electromagnetic Induction. *Complexity, 2018*, 1–13. doi:10.1155/2018/3012743

KEY TERMS AND DEFINITIONS

4G: 4G is the fourth generation of broadband cell cellular network innovation and is succeeding third generation network (3G). In other words, it tends to be characterized as a portable correspondence standard sought to supplant 3G, permitting remote internet access at a lot higher speed.

Brain: A brain is an organ which fills serves as the center point of the sensory system in all vertebrate and most invertebrate creatures. It is situated in the skull, by and large near the tangible organs for faculties like vision. It is the most multifarious organ in a vertebrate's body. In man, the cerebral cortex involves around 14-16 billion neurons.

Carcinogen: A carcinogen is any stuff, radionuclide, or radiation that encourages, the formation of cancer cells. A carcinogen has a tendency to damage or disrupt the genome or the cellular metabolic pathways.

CDMA: Code-division multiple access (CDMA) is a channel access technique utilized by different radio correspondence developments. In contrast to the GSM and TDMA technologies, CDMA communicates over the whole frequency range accessible. CDMA does not appoint a particular frequency to its clients on the communication system.

Cerebrum: Cerebrum is the biggest section of the vertebrate brain which fills the major space of the skull area and comprising of two cerebral halves partitioned by a profound furrow and joined by the corpus callosum, a transverse band of nerve filaments.

Electromagnetic: An electromagnet is a magnet that runs on electricity. In contrast to a perpetual magnet, the quality of an electromagnet can without much of a stretch be changed by changing the measure of electric flow which passes through it. Electromagnetic power is a principal physical power that is liable for communications between excited particles which materialise on account of their charge and for the discharge and retention of photons.

EMF: An electromagnetic field (EMF) is an attractive field created by moving electrically excited entities. It is brought about by the movement of an electric charge. A fixed charge will create just an electric field in the encompassing space. In the event that the charge is moving, an magnetic field is likewise brought.

GSM: GSM (Global System for Mobile Communication) is a wireless computerized cellular system that is broadly utilized by cell phone clients. GSM utilizes a variety of Time Division Multiple Access (TDMA) and is the most commonly utilized among the three computerized remote communication advancements: TDMA, GSM and CDMA. GSM digitizes and packs information, then sends it down a channel with two different streams of client information, each in its own time slot. It works at either the 900 MHz or 1800 MHz frequency band.

Hippocampus: Hippocampus is an multifaceted brain fragment interleaved intensely into temporal lobe. It has a principal job in learning, wisdom, retention and memory. It is a delicate and susceptible structure that gets persuaded by an assortment of inducements.

Magnetic Field: The magnetic field is the zone around a magnet where there is attractive power. It is a vector field that portrays the attractive impact of electric charges in relative movement and polarized materials.

Mobile: It is characterized as a phone with an entrance to a cell radio framework and consequently can be utilized over a wide zone, without a physical association with a system. A mobile is a remote handheld gadget that enables clients to make and get calls and to send instant messages. The initial age of mobiles could just make and get calls. The present mobiles, nevertheless, are stuffed with numerous extra highlights, for example, internet browsers, games, cameras, video players and even navigational frameworks.

Network: A network is characterized as an assemblage of at least two PC frameworks connected together. A network comprising of a group of broadcasting stations that entirely transmit similar missions.

Phone: A phone is equipment that we use when dialling somebody's telephone number and chat with them. In other words, the telephone can be characterized an electrical framework that we use to converse with another person at somewhere else, by dialing a number on a bit of equipment and talking into it.

Radiation: Radiation is the emanation or transmission of vivacity as waves or particles through space or through a substantial medium. This incorporates electromagnetic energy, for example, radio waves, visible light, and x- rays. particle radiation, for example, α, β, and neutron radiation.

SAR: Specific Absorption Rate (SAR) is a proportion of the rate at which the energy is consumed by the human body when presented to a radio frequency (RF) electromagnetic field. It is characterized as the power engrossed per mass of tissue and has units of watts per kilogram (W/kg).

Chapter 7
Mobile Apps for Human Nutrition:
A Review

Muzamil Ahmad

ⓘ https://orcid.org/0000-0003-3173-6814
The University of Agriculture, Peshawar, Pakistan

Muhammad Abbas Khan
The University of Agriculture, Peshawar, Pakistan

Mairaj Bibi
Bolan University of Medical and Health Sciences, Pakistan

Zia Ullah
The University of Agriculture, Peshawar, Pakistan

Syed Tanveer Shah
The University of Agriculture, Peshawar, Pakistan

ABSTRACT

Lack of proper diet causes many diseases like night blindness, gum death, rickets, osteomalacia, etc. Similarly, undernutrition will cause a low intelligence quotient (IQ), osteoporosis, anemia, scurvy, pellagra, etc. Over-nutrition will result in obesity, Type II diabetes mellitus, and ischemic heart diseases. Also, the unhygienic intake of food, intake of food on no fixed time, intake of fast food intake of other unhealthy stuff can lead to irregularities in the human body. Adopting healthy habits, physical activity, exercise, sports, and walking can lead to a healthy lifestyle of an individual. In addition, today's busy schedule and less time availability restricts individuals to visit the doctors or nutritionists. Many mobile applications were developed for monitoring and calculating an energy level as well as healthy nutrition. This review chapter has assessed the use and features of various mobile phone health applications, which helps individuals to overcome and monitor the above-mentioned health-related issues.

DOI: 10.4018/978-1-7998-2521-0.ch007

1. INTRODUCTION

The main purpose of this review paper is to educate those who are facing hurdles in visiting physicians for their regular health checkups and ask for their regular nutritional balance, due to any reason such as belonging to remote areas, having a busy schedule, having no knowledge about varieties of apps used in assessment of Human Nutrition. They always need a reliable and efficient source that is time saving, costless and provide them an easy way for nutritional assessment on their doorsteps to maintain a balance nutrition and healthy life, therefore, keeping in view the above, the use of smart gadgets and mobile apps and their progression in innovation plays a vigorous role in maintaining a balance nutrition and equip one to have enough knowledge about the usage and function of variety of collected nutritional apps on a single click (Boushey, Spoden, Zhu, Delp, & Kerr, 2017). This review includes a variety of nutritional apps along with their workflow regarding diet coach, food diary, weight loss, calories counter and pregnancy applications.

Along with this, it is mandatory to know the basic knowledge of human nutrition. Human Nutrition id the area of Medical Sciences which deals with nutrients and their influences on human routine eating, health and exercises. Nutrition or nutrients provide growth and development to human beings as well as to plants. In Nutrition mostly appropriate diet is that which contains the micro and macronutrients. Furthermore, in nutrition we study about nutrients which give energy, e.g., when an individual takes some food, it separates in smaller molecules which discharges energy in the form of Adenosine Tri Phosphate (ATP) as shown in the reaction below.

$$C_6H_{12}O_6 \rightarrow 6H_2O + 6CO_2 + Energy (ATP)$$

The reaction above shows that nutrients undergo catabolism process to give us energy. Similarly, nutrients are essential in human life for example, a fetus is totally reliant on her mom for nutrition. Insufficient nutrition causes diseases, influences growth and nourishment of a child. A poor diet with a smaller amount of iron causes iron deficiency which results in tiredness and retard in attention in studies. The absence of vitamin A causes night blindness, the absence of vitamin C causes gum bleeding, the absence of vitamin D causes rickets in kids and osteomalacia in adults, and the absence of meats causes macrocytic anemia and so on (Organization, 2000).

Furthermore, both abundance and insufficiency of nutrients causes diseases like low IQ, osteoporosis, anemia, scurvy, pellagra, night blindness and so forth and over nutrition brings about obesity, Type II diabetes mellitus (Because of Intake of Abundance Glucose), ischemic (heart sicknesses) (Because of Intake of Overabundance Cholesterol) (Alamgir, Sami, & Salahuddin).

2. BACKGROUND

Even many papers published on nutritional mobile phone applications, no studies yet have been analyzed that covers the functions of various nourishing applications, altogether. Before, individuals utilize conventional dietary evaluation strategies (Pen or Paper), which required day by day recording of every food consumed and its vitality content (Jospe, Fairbairn, Green, & Perry, 2015).

This strategy for recording was challenging especially to get precise outcomes for revealing relationship between diet and health. Besides, record keeping trouble (Either because of lapse of memory or wrong estimation of food size), tediousness, perpetual storage absence, non-simple access to printed record for worldwide analysts, laboriousness for resource inadequate nations, insufficient dietary content knowledge etc. brought about poor checking of individual's nutrition (Boushey et al., 2017).

Furthermore, the conducted surveys demonstrated that individuals are eager to spend cost on effective nutritional assessment systems (for example paid mobile phone applications), also, adjustment to mobile phones applications, which are used for digitalizing nutritional evaluations, has given a chance to assess intake of nutrients and giving feedback (Carter, Burley, Nykjaer, & Cade, 2013).

3. OBJECTIVE

The study conducted aims to review the primary functions of nutrition related prominent mobile phone applications accessible in Google Play Store, and so forth and to divert and redirect the frame of mind of individuals (who are eager to get advantages of mobile phone applications used to upgrade human health for example professional health students, market and the scholarly world and so on.) towards the use of mobile phone applications.

4. HUMAN NUTRITION APPS

In this section the functions of numerous human nutrition mobile applications are discussed. Some of the best apps that help in monitoring human health will be scrutinized for better results.

4.1 Calorie Counter by Fatsecret

The least demanding to utilize calorie counter and best weight reduction and eating less junk food applications available. The best part is that Fat Secret is freely available. This application monitor one's food, weight and exercise, using the world's most elevated quality nutrition and food database and make connect with a worldwide network of individuals hoping to roll out an improvement to remain fit and healthy to accomplish one's objectives.

The application synchronizes with Fat Secret Professional, the most advantageous approach to share one's food, exercise, and weight with his/her favored health expert. An individual's health expert will get free access to straightforward and useful assets to screen his performance and furnish one with input, guidance, and backing. The Calorie Counter application is shown in the Figure 1.

Fat Secret is quick, easy to utilize and includes coordination with outside services and instruments to enable one to prevail with his eating routine:

- A standardized tag scanner and auto-complete capacities.
- An eating routine schedule to see one's calories expended and consumed.
- An awesome network that is prepared to offer help and turbo charge one's weight reduction.
- Image acknowledgment of foods, dinners, and items so one can take photographs with the camera and monitor nutrition with pictures.
- A weight tracker.
- Detailed announcing and objectives for every one of one's calories and macros.

Figure 1. Calorie counter by Fatsecret
(*FatSecret, 2019*)

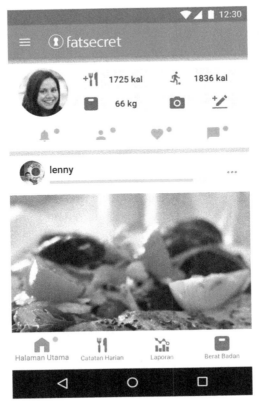

- A simple to utilize a food diary to plan and monitor what an individual is eating.
- Photo collection. (Photo diet, Food snap, Instant calorie)
- A diary to record one's progress.
- Reminders for suppers, weigh-ins, and diaries.
- Notifications for help, remarks, and followers.
- Fantastic plans and dinner thoughts.
- Sharing and communicating with one's expert on the choice.
- Samsung Health, Google Fit and Fit bit exercise monitoring integration.
- An activity diary to record every one of the calories they consume.

4.2 Calorie Counter Pro by Mynetdiary

One of the most worthwhile restorative applications is MyNetDairy. This Application is tied in with searching for caloric worth, eating fewer carbs, and exercise. This application, truth be told, has helped individuals in getting thinner. A large number of clients have lost 0.6kg weight week by week and 12.27kg in the initial a half year. Individuals using this application stay fit and sound by knowing how much calories they are getting from sugars, proteins, and fats and afterward as indicated by the caloric estimations of these macronutrients, individuals choose the low fitting caloric eating regimen. In the event that somebody has the information that Carbohydrates give 4.1kcal, proteins give 4.1kcal, fats give 9kcal, they will like to accept sugars and proteins more when contrasted with fats. Getting warnings from this application in an individual's mobile phone. An individual will set its different times of eating, exercise, rest and rest. The Figure 2 shows the Calorie Counter PRO application.

4.3 My Diet Diary Calorie Counter by MedHelp

Arrive at one's weight objective quicker with My Diet Diary, one's eating routine, and wellness partner. The most effortless approach to get in shape, keep up the weight or put on weight. The exquisite and least complex weight reduction application to follow one's food, calories, work out, weight, cholesterol, carbs, calories consumed, other nutrition information. Demonstrated accomplishment as a large number of individuals worldwide has use this application to arrive at their weight objective. The Figure 3 shows My Diet Diary Calories Counter.

My Diet Diary Calorie Counter provides the following features:

• Daily eating fewer carbs tips.

Figure 2. Calorie counter PRO by MyNetDiary (Inc, 2019)

Figure 3. My diet diary calorie counter by MedHelp (StayWell, 2019)

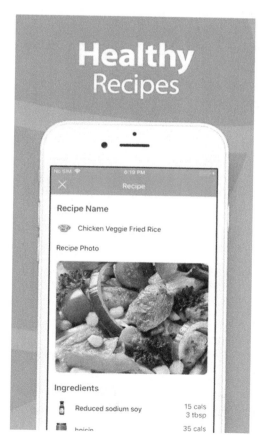

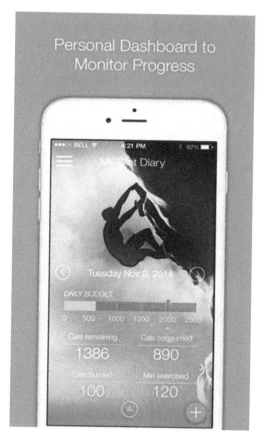

- Add food from our database of 150,000+ foods and solid plans for regardless of what diet you are on: Atkins, sans gluten, Paleo, Jenny Craig, Weight watchers, and so on.
- Automatically give insights regarding each and every food: protein, gluten, carbs, calories, nutrients, cholesterol, and minerals.
- Easy to peruse reports and charts to view patterns.
- A day by day calorie counter and track other food information (protein, carbs, cholesterol, sugar, fiber, and so on).
- The most straightforward approach to follow what an individual eat and see a full wholesome outline.
- Journal to follow one's everyday work out, calories consumed, and minutes worked out.
- Detailed everyday journal synopsis to see one's general improvement and how to improve.
- Set weight reduction objective and utilize individual's calorie tracker to begin following their calorie spending plan and diet.
- Daily diet and wellness tips.
- Reminders to enable one to remain on track.
- Connect and see one's average improvement from your Fit bit, Jawbone Up, or other action Global Positioning System (GPS) beacons or step tallying.
- View weight diagrams, calories expended graphs, diet rundown, and reports following one's weight reduction.
- Calculate all out micro and macronutrients.
- Connect one's fit bit, Jawbone Up and more for a far-reaching perspective on the entirety of his wellness and nourishing data.
- Not on eating routine? Have diabetes? Utilize a sustenance log, diary, and tracker to see a breakdown of calories from carbs and fats.
- Log more than 65 activities to see calories consumed and calories lost.
- See calories and fat one ignited with our progression counter.
- Track cardio, strolling, biking, running, advance counter, and the sky is the limit from there.
- Daily wellness tips.
- Basal Metabolic Rate (BMR) calculator and Body Mass Index (BMI) mini-computer.

4.4 Ultimate Food Value Diary - Diet & Weight Tracker

Everybody is extraordinary and all one's weight reduction adventures are similarly unique so this application gives an individual the decision to pick the arrangement that suits them and it is illustrated in the Figure 4.

Settle up with stunning highlights:

- Food, Alcohol, Exercise, and Daily objective adding calculator.
- Standardized barcode scanner greater than three million standardized identifications.
- Boundless nourishment and exercise top choices.
- Configurable in metric and majestic.
- Worth estimator - Calculate nourishment esteems dependent on simply the calorific worth.
- Cloud information reinforcement and reestablish with programmed reinforcements and the capacity to duplicate information between Android gadgets.

Figure 4. Ultimate food value diary - diet & weight tracker
(Ltd, 2019)

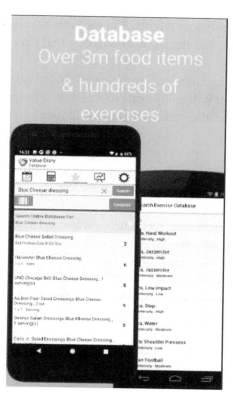

Figure 5. Noom weight loss coach
(Noom, 2017)

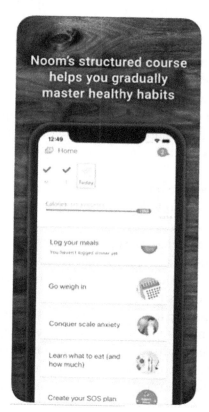

- Online Food and Restaurant with a huge number of food and cafe things, loaded with everyday nutrition, tidbits and liquor things.
- Capacity to track body estimations
- Dinner Maker enabling one to amass things as a supper with programmed divide computation.
- Track sound decisions, in addition, to record one's everyday notes.
- Weight reduction following diagrams, target and achievements.
- Worked in food and exercise databases.
- Pedometer support - Record one's means on his wellness band or smart watch and have the application consequently convert them to exercise earned inside the application for all plans - matches up with Fit bit and Google Fit.

4.5. Noom Weight Loss Coach

Noom's demonstrated brain research-based methodology distinguishes one's profound established considerations and triggers and constructs a custom course of action to enable one to shape sound propensities, quicker.

Included in the New York Times, Women's Health, Shape, Forbes, ABC and then some, the Figure 5 shows the application having just helped more than 45 million individuals overall form health propensities and accomplish their health objectives.

Individuals who use Noom lose a normal of 18 pounds in only four months. Figure out how to explore one's condition, challenge one's considerations, ace triggers, and defeat any boundary that may come to one's direction.

Regardless of whether it's passionate eating, yearnings at late morning, trouble with social eating, or a sweet tooth. Noom's experimentally supported arrangement will enable one to make an arrangement to beat any hindrance and practice more advantageous propensities until one have aced them.

This Application gives the accompanying element:

- Flexible training intended to enable one to set and accomplish his short-and long term objectives.
- Tools to follow one's weight, nourishment, work out, circulatory strain, and glucose across the board place.
- An interactive substance with over 250+ new articles, including pick one's-own-experience style advisers to apply Psych Tricks of this application into one's everyday life, flawlessly.
- Scientifically-demonstrated brain science way to deal with "stunt" one's body into structure solid propensities, quicker.
- Custom feast + exercise Plans accessible to take one's advancement to the following level.
- Smarter innovation to distinguish one's difficulties progressively and keep him on track.
- Personalized criticism from one's mentor dependent on him.
- This application has most complete food database, with over a large portion of a million new and refreshed nutrition logging choices and scanner tags to make one's experience far and away superior.

4.6. Nutrition Lookup

This application get quick, solid wholesome data in a hurry. Spark People's Nutrition Lookup application is an advantageous and simple approach to settle on the most advantageous decision inevitably. Fueled by Spark People's broad nutrition database, this little however compelling application enables one to look into wholesome data for many food at the dash of a catch.

What one Get with Nutrition Lookup:

- Detailed healthful data for more than 3 million foods.
- Easy-to-comprehend charts that show the breakdown of calories, starches, fats, and proteins for any accessible food.
- Bar code filtering for a straightforward query of bundled foods. One can open camera from inside this application, examine the Universal Product Code (UPC) name and discover the food right away. Nutrition Lookup application are shown in Figure 6.

Figure 6. Nutrition lookup
(SparkPeople, 2016)

Figure 7. Easy diet diary
(Ltd, 2012-2019)

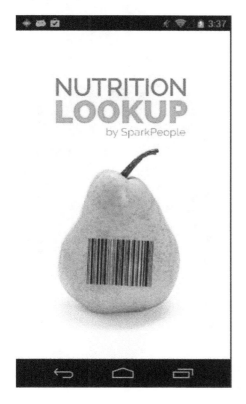

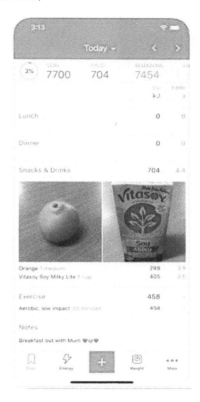

4.7. Easy Diet Diary

Simple eating routine dairy is another restorative application shown in the Figure 7 gets more fit of individual, its works like a connecter, here individual records his dietary eating routine record just as exercise and weight and afterward subsequent to doing this they counsel their dietary dairy to a dietician, nutritionist and to a health experts, so by doing this, individuals get sound life tips and stay solid forever.

4.8. Nutritionist-Dieting Made Easy

The most thorough and restoratively significant application to control weight and exercise. Nutritionist recommends the correct food and tells the amount that one ought to eat. So this nutritionist application that is mentioned in the Figure 8 has changed the way of life of individuals particularly the manner in which they eat.

4.9. Map My + App (Walk, Run, Ride, Fitness)

Among the most effective applications, this is a walk, run, ride, and wellness significant application. Here individuals are propelled that they can get more fit from multiple points of view like strolling, running,

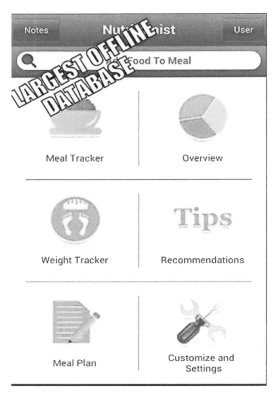

Figure 8. Nutritionist-Dieting made easy
(Outlier, 2015)

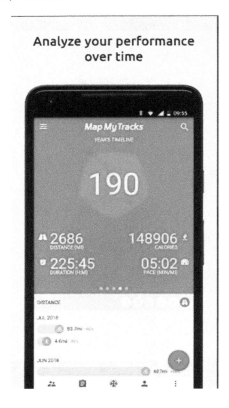

Figure 9. Map my + app (walk, run, ride, fitness)
(MapMyFitness, 2019)

riding and cycling after each supper or whenever of the day. So by doing this they will be fit and will have a solid life until the end of time. The Figure 9 shows Map My plus App.

4.10. Body Tracker - Body Fat Tracker

With regards to rapidly and effectively computing one's muscle versus fat ratio, nothing beats Body Tracker. Clients are guided bit by bit through the whole procedure. Muscle versus fat computations can be taken in record time - with no preparation.

Body Tracker is astoundingly simple to use, regardless of whether one have no related knowledge computing his muscle to fat ratio. All one need is a measuring tape, fat caliper, or muscle versus fat scale, and Body Tracker will tell one precisely the best way to take his estimations. Simply enter estimations, and Body Tracker will do every one of the counts for an individual - and spare his outcomes. On the off chance that one don't have a clue how to take caliper or tape estimations, simply see the pictures or video included inside Body Tracker.

Body Tracker gives one a decision of a few techniques to compute one's muscle to fat ratio and clearly shows in the Figure 10.

Figure 10. Body tracker - body fat tracker
(LLC, 2012)

Figure 11. Perfect produce
(SparkPeople, Perfect Produce, 2013)

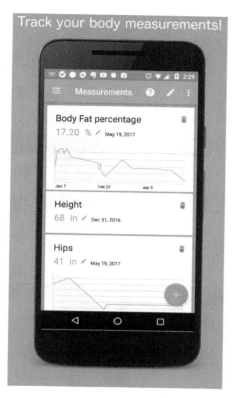

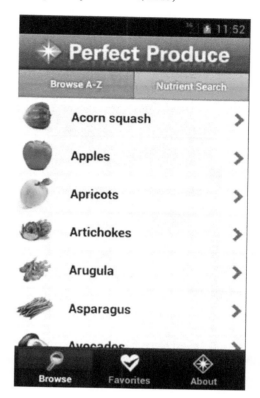

4.11. Perfect Produce

One need to eat more foods grown from the ground, yet wind up now and again confounded in the producing path or the kitchen? How would one pick the best grapefruit? How would one shield avocados from turning darker so rapidly? How would one appropriately store apples? Also, what precisely does fennel resemble? (Furthermore, how would one set it up?) So much produce such a large number of inquiries. That is the reason Spark People made Perfect Produce, a speedy and simple instrument that demystifies the produce area of the general store. Haul out this application at the grocery store or in the kitchen. Sound supper arranging and shopping for food recently turned into that a lot simpler.

Made by Spark People, the web's greatest eating regimen webpage, Perfect Produce is shown in the Figure 11.

Thousands of solid plans with foods grown from the ground as the fundamental fixing.

Information on purchasing, putting away and setting up every one of the foods grown from the ground found in many grocery stores.

The capacity to scan for items dependent on dietary substance discover nutrition high in fiber, calcium, or vitamin C, and that's just the beginning.

Eating at any rate 5 servings of foods grown from the ground day by day is probably the most ideal approaches to get in shape and eat healthy, as indicated by the individuals and specialists at Spark People.

Figure 12. WW (Formerly Weight Watchers)
(Weight Watchers,International, Inc., 2019)

Figure 13. MyFitnessPal
(LLc, 2009-2019)

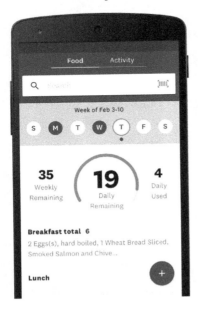

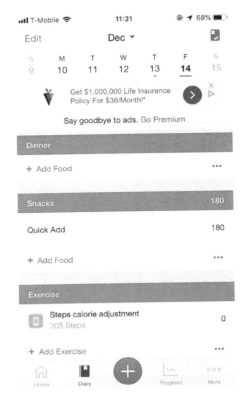

This application makes getting your "five per day" simpler, and, with plans of this application, makes them considerably more delicious and fascinating to eat.

4.12. WW (Formerly Weight Watchers)

With this latest WW (Formerly Weight Watchers) application depicts in the Figure 12. one would have access to this user friendly fitness and food tracker, a huge number of delectable recipes, and the help one have to get more fit and build healthy addiction for the life.

- Recipes.
- With 4K plus WW recipes, deciding what to eat is easy. Choosing what to eat is simple. Browse by choosing classifications, for example, "Fast and easy" to find out delectable meals to fulfill any taste. Construct and store dishes one like to make remaining on track easier.
- Fitness & Food Tracker.

Effectively track what one eat by using the Scanning of Barcode or searching of this application database about two lac twenty five thousands of foods. Supported by science of human nutrition, Smart Points system will guide one to a healthy dieting which can contains a lot of fruits, protein and vegetables.

Review an individual's fitness objectives with the activity tracker. It will tell one the best way to synchronize his fitness mobile and covert his day by day moves into Fit Points, the application measurement for activity.

4.13. MyFitnessPal

Here is another application about weight reduction and a healthy life. In this application, clients change diet with interims that how many staples will be taken in breakfast lunch and in supper. Before the day's over, he/she will ascertain the entire day's calories and check whether he/she has accomplished the everyday objectives or not. This application which is shown in the Figure 13 helped many individuals to stay fit and solid.

4.14. Pregnancy Health & Fitness

Pregnancy Health and Fitness step by step including all the data hopeful mother requirements for a solid pregnancy from origination until birth. Just enter one's infant's expected date in this application to get to week by week refreshes about one's body, her child's development and master tips for a fit and solid pregnancy.

This application gives an all-encompassing interpretation of pregnancy health and could be seen by an individual in the Figure 14. Including Fetal Development Images.

See what one's infant resembles as one's pregnancy advances, alongside insights concerning one's infant's weight, size, and improvement. Additionally, get nourishment rules to enable one to eat the best supplements infant needs at explicit occasions.

A Week-by-Week Countdown realize what side effects and changes to expect, including normal solutions for basic pre-birth protests as one's body prepare to carry one's infant into the world.

- *Pre-birth Articles and Tips*

There is such a long way to go regarding pregnancy, labor, and conveyance (regardless of whether one will have a homebirth or clinic birth) that it can appear to be overpowering. That is the reason that the team of this application has taken their best articles and consolidated them into simple to-peruse, straightforward tips so one can learn on their timetable.

SparkPeople.com is a main sound living site that has helped a large number of individuals get in shape, get fit and improve their health since 2001. The enlisted dietitians of this application affirmed fitness coaches and pre-birth health and wellness specialists built up this proof-based Pregnancy Health application to enable ladies to proceed with their smart dieting and exercise propensities during pregnancy and past - on the grounds that solid children start with sound mothers.

- *Exercise Demonstrations for Expectant Moms*

The affirmed maternity wellness specialists of this application made a progression of safe activities and exercise advisers for assistance the mom-to-be remain fit, put on the appropriate measure of weight, and advance generally speaking maternal health.

Figure 14. Pregnancy health & fitness
(SparkPeople, Pregnancy Health & Fitness, 2016)

Figure 15. Healthy recipes & calculator
(SparkPeople, Healthy Recipes & Calculator, 2017)

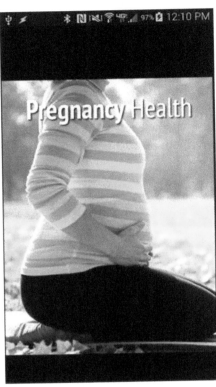

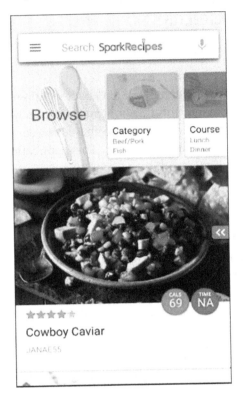

4.15. Healthy Recipes & Calculator

An individual is a single tick away from more than 500,000 plans from the world's biggest solid plans site, SparkRecipes.com. These plans have been attempted and tried by home cooks simply like you, and this application is intended to make it simple for an individual to prepare top choices in any place he go as show in the Figure 15. Make eating tasty, nutritious suppers a snap - all without burning up all available resources.

This Application Gives to Clients:

- Discover plans that fit individual's dietary needs: Whether an individual's eating routine is without gluten, low carb or veggie-lover, this application have the plans for individuals. Channel for one's dietary needs and find delectable plans, quick.
- Search application formula database one's own way: Looking for a sound breakfast dish? Need a low-fat pasta dish the children will eat? With Healthy Recipes, it's anything but difficult to locate another formula that possesses all the necessary qualities. Search by dinner, cooking, event, course, or planning time.
- Coordinate with one's wellness following application: all plans one spare to his "Top picks" rundown will naturally be synchronized to wellness following this application in the event that one

use it also. Show signs of improvement thought of what one eat and how solid it is. Furthermore, track the plans one find in this application is a free diet following application with a tap.

- Spare one's top choices: Found a formula that one adore? Spare it to one "Top picks" list so one can return to it. Need to see these plans from anyplace on the web? Make a free Spark Recipes account and match up one's preferred plans over the entirety of one's gadgets.
- See calories, carbs, and 10 other key supplements for every formula - SparkRecipes.com is a sister webpage to SparkPeople.com, the #1 solid living site in the US. Recognizing what an individual eat is the initial move towards watching what one eat, so all application plans highlight itemized healthful data. We make it simple to figure precisely what's in what one is eating. Searching for low fat, low carb suppers? This application have secured one. Simply searching for simple plans that rush to make? This application have those as well.

4.16. Weight My Diet Weight Tracker

The application is illustrated in the Figure 16 which Provides Weigh My Diet. Weight Tracking, Measurements tracking and Diet Weight Loss Tracking.

Its Features are mentioned below:

Record an individual's weight. (Optionally, individual's weights with cloths and without cloths wearing can be separately recorded.)

It record the weight in Pounds, Kilograms or Stones, and change all figures instantly. One can see a Chart/Graph of the amendments to one's weight time to time with a best fit graph line and so on.

4.17. Best Boiled Egg Diet Plan

In the Figure 17 shown the Best Boiled Egg Diet Plan application which provides a summarized list of egg (ingredient) consumption's benefits and claims that its use will lose 24pounds weight in two weeks. This application provides a 7-days easy and simple Meal plan with new features where an individual can select healthier snacks during the diet to eat them in-between two regular meals.

4.18. Track-Calorie Counter

Nutritionix Track is a tracking application for fitness created and maintained by a group of registered dietitians. Making habit of a day by day fitness tracking is a viable method to progress towards an individual's health objectives, so the mission of the Track application is to remove the truly difficult work from keeping up of individual's food log. The following application of Track-Calorie Counter is shown in Figure 18.

4.19. Simple Diet Diary

Like different applications, the following shown Figure 19 is one of the most simple applications for weight reduction, as the name shown here an individual simply needs to record everyday dietary arrangement in his dairy and as indicated by the determined calories they do practice and along these lines, they get more fit by keeping up the day by day record.

Figure 16. Weight my diet weight tracker
(zeronica.com, 2015)

Figure 17. Best boiled egg diet plan
(Apps, 2019)

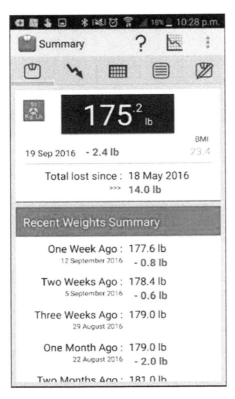

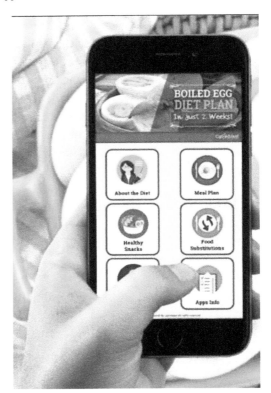

4.20. Healthy Slow Cooker Recipes

Healthy Slow Cooker Recipes from Spark People together the least demanding, most delicious moderate cooker plans from SparkRecipes.com across the board application. It's never been simpler to locate such a straightforward, healthy among unique applications.

In this application which is below illustrated in the Figure 20, You'll find top of the easy plans for soups, bean stews, stews, primary dishes, treats, and that's only the tip of the iceberg, all made right in your moderate cooker. Besides, the plans call for simple, bravo fixings so you can eat well without going through the greater part of your day in the kitchen. This is what else you can anticipate from our application:

Detailed, simple to-adhere to formula guidelines for each formula.

A total food breakdown of each formula, including calories, fat, cholesterol, sodium, protein, carbs and the sky is the limit from there.

Honest formula appraisals from this application enormous network of home cooks.

Simple social coordination with Facebook and Interest, so you can impart your preferred plans to your companions.

A formula box to spare your preferred plans across the board place.

Figure 18. Track-Calorie counter
(Nutritionix, 2019)

Figure 19. Simple diet diary
(Stone, 2019)

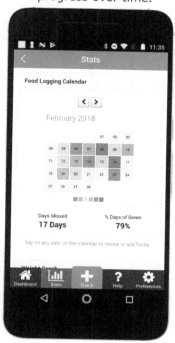

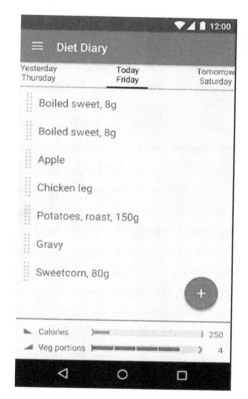

4.21. Dining Note: Simple Food Diary

The Figure 21 shows the pictorial demonstration of another significant application from a medical perspective. Here an individual is instructed to make diet, practice and other day by day exercises (breakfast, lunch, supper, espresso, water consumption, snakes and so on) of day by day schedule. In light of these exercises an individual watches that they have arrived at their objectives of weight reduction or not.

4.22. Health Diet Foods Fitness Help

Health Diet Foods Fitness Help is demonstrated in the Figure 22, which advises individuals to get in chart. Dietician gives health tips with the goal that individuals for magnificence tips will receive these tips of health all-around quickly and will have a solid life. These health tips helps in fixing all the health related issues like stomach issues and many more. Along these tips, managing this will keep up the strong life of individuals.

4.23. Health, Nutrition and Diet Guide

The Figure 23 shows the approaching picture of this application of Health, Nutrition and Diet Guide, the dietician backing to keep up the health of individuals by giving tips for the counteractive action of

Figure 20. Healthy slow cooker recipes
(SparkPeople, Healthy Slow Cooker Recipes, 2016)

Figure 21. Dining note: simple food diary
(In, 2018)

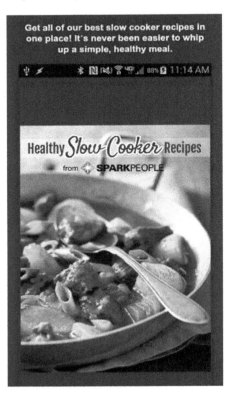

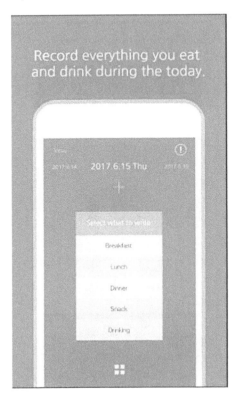

infections like hypertension, diabetes mellitus, tension, hypersensitivities, and sleep deprivation, and so forth, so, an individual after these tips will have a solid way of life. These tips keep up a sound life as well as lessen weight.

4.24. Smoothie Recipes: 500+ Healthy Smoothies

This application, illustrated in Figure 24, contains extraordinary determinations of smoothie plans that will most likely fulfill your sense of taste with flavorful ingredients. It gives simple ingredients and headings to solid organic product plans which is ideal for the conscious health users. This application has a tremendous accumulation of 500+ smoothie plans from around the world. It's possible but difficult to explore and locate your enticing smoothie formula and start setting it up right away.

Sound Smoothie Recipes has the majority of your answers a basic fingertip away. Look at it to discover which smoothie you like the most.

4.25. BodyFast Intermittent Fasting: Coach, Diet Tracker

Intermittent fasting is another method for weight reduction. Here individuals are educated in an instructing focus on intermittent fasting or you can say that fasting on exchange days. Fasting is useful and causes weight reduction to many degrees and it misfortune weight as well as keep from numerous different

Figure 22. Health diet foods fitness help
(*RecoveryBull.com, 2019*)

Figure 23. Health, nutrition and diet guide
(*Facts, 2018*)

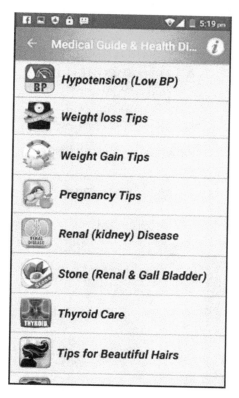

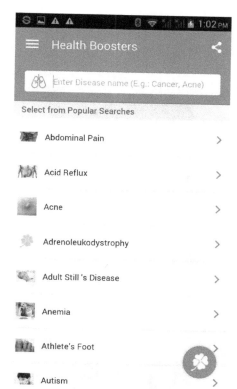

sicknesses like diZero Calories - fasting tracker for weight reduction and diabetes mellitus. The Figure 25 helps in easy access to this application.

4.26. Zero Calories - Fasting Tracker for Weight Loss

Zero Calories - fasting tracker, describe in the Figure 26, is additionally similar to the previously mentioned applications which aids in weight reduction yet the distinction here is that here the individual is educated to expand the fasting time and length of the fast.

4.27. YAZIO Calorie Counter, Nutrition Diary & Diet Plan

Calorie Counter application by YAZIO that is shown in Figure 27, is another restorative application for weight reduction. Here individuals are educated to note every day food intake like proteins, fats, water consumption and espresso just as exercise and afterward calculate the full day by day calories that the individual has consumed by doing every one of these exercises thus the most ideal method for getting more fit.

Figure 24. Smoothie recipes: 500+ healthy smoothies
(chavan, 2019)

Figure 25. BodyFast intermittent fasting: coach, diet tracker
(UG, 2019)

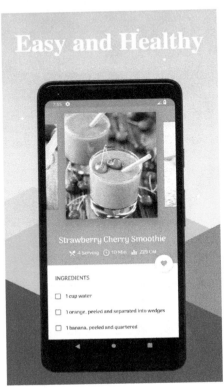

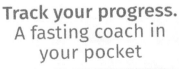

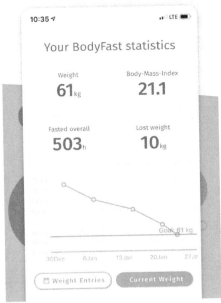

4.28. Total Keto Diet: Low Carb Recipes & Keto Meals

This is a comparative sort of application as referenced previously. Here people are educated to utilize low carbs plans so that if there will be low glucose level in blood, an ever-increasing number of fats will be catabolized and will create increasingly more ketone bodies so the principle advantage to individual utilizing this application, mentioned in the Figure 28, is that all fats in body will be catabolized and fit weight will be diminished and individual can get in shape through this component all-around effectively.

4.29. Cronometer

This is the most exact, far-reaching nutrition tracker available in the market. This application, illustrated in the Figure 29, has helped over 25 lac individuals find their nutrition and meet weight reduction objectives.
    A Highlight of this Application:

- Track more than 60 micronutrients – the most comprehensive information available in the market.
- It is the sole nutrition tracker that gives precise information curated from checked sources.
- All food presented by the clients to the database is checked for exactness by the staff.

Mobile Apps for Human Nutrition

Figure 26. Zero calories - fasting tracker for weight loss
(development, 2019)

Figure 27. YAZIO calorie counter, nutrition diary & diet plan
(GmbH, 2018)

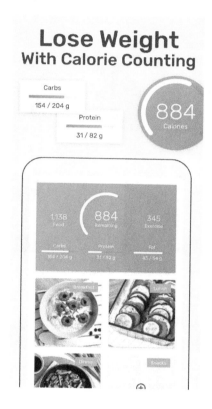

- This application ensures privacy and protection of the whole data of individuals and don't share or sell the data to outsiders.
- Compare custom biometrics as well as nutrients in graphs and view trends after some time.
- The Free form of this application gives more nutritional data than some other application.

4.30. Diet Diary

It is one of the easiest application to use for weight reduction. This application records the day by day diet and exercise, water uptake and game and so forth of an individual and also check every day calories that the individual has consumed in doing these exercises. So along these lines an individual can get in shape all things considered. The pictorial demonstration of this application is in the Figure 30.

5. CONCLUSION

Nowadays mobile devices and smart gadgets are assumed as playing crucial role in keeping up healthy life of the individuals in a sense to alert, aware and persuade the individuals towards the use of mobile applications especially nutrition related mobile applications to make balance nutrition and a healthy

Figure 28. Total keto diet: low carb recipes & keto meals
(Tasteaholics, 2019)

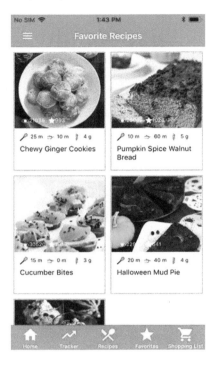

Figure 29. Cronometer
(Inc. C. S., 2019)

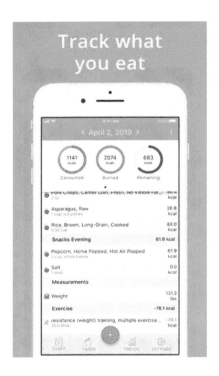

Figure 30. Diet diary
(Yapan, 2017)

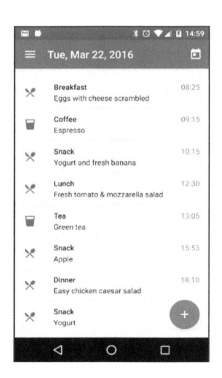

life style. Similarly, if individuals wants to remain healthy, they ought to eat according to the need and activities they performing and keep themselves from overabundance eating. The paper review deciphers the very vital role of these health apps available to a lay man to monitor and sustain good health. These apps help users to have a vigilant eye on their routine diet. Furthermore one should make propensity for daily exercise all through the use of above mentioned mobile phone applications which would definitely improve health and overcome health related issues.

REFERENCES

Alamgir, K., Sami, U., & Salahuddin, K. (2018). Nutritional complications and its effects on human health. *J. Food Sci. Nutr.*, *1*(1), 17–20.

BodyFast UG. (2019, August 5). *BodyFast Intermittent Fasting: Coach, Diet Tracker*. Retrieved from https://play.google.com/store/apps/details?id=com.bodyfast&hl=en

Borisoft - Software development. (2019). *Zero Calories - fasting tracker for weight loss*. Retrieved from https://zerocaloriesfasting.com/index.html

Boushey, C., Spoden, M., Zhu, F., Delp, E., & Kerr, D. (2017). New mobile methods for dietary assessment: Review of image-assisted and image-based dietary assessment methods. *The Proceedings of the Nutrition Society*, *76*(3), 283–294. doi:10.1017/S0029665116002913 PMID:27938425

Boushey, C. J., Spoden, M., Zhu, F. M., Delp, E. J., & Kerr, D. A. (2016). New mobile methods for dietary assessment: review of image-assisted and. *New technology in nutrition research and practice* (p. 12). Dublin: *Proceedings of the Nutrition Society*.

Carter, M. C., Burley, V. J., Nykjaer, C., & Cade, J. E. (2013). Adherence to a smartphone application for weight loss compared to website and paper diary: Pilot randomized controlled trial. *Journal of Medical Internet Research*, *15*(4), e32. doi:10.2196/jmir.2283 PMID:23587561

Carter, M. C., Burley, V. J., Nykjaer, C., & Cade, J. E. (2013). Adherence to a Smartphone Application for Weight Loss. *Journal of Medical Internet Research*, *15*(4). PMID:23587561

Cronometer Software Inc. (2019, August 28). *Cronometer*. Retrieved from https://play.google.com/store/apps/details?id=com.cronometer.android.gold&hl=en

Cylonblast Mobile Apps. (2019, August 31). *Best Boiled Egg Diet Plan*. Retrieved from https://play.google.com/store/apps/details?id=com.cylonblastmobileapps.bestboiledeggdiet&hl=en

Organic Facts. (2018, January 16). *Health, Nutrition & Diet Guide*. Retrieved from https://play.google.com/store/apps/details?id=com.organicfacts.app&hl=en

FatSecret. (2019). *Play Store: Calorie Counter by FatSecret*. Retrieved from https://play.google.com/store/apps/details?id=com.fatsecret.android

Fenlander Software Solutions Ltd. (2019, August 30). *Ultimate Food Value Diary - Diet & Weight Tracker*. Retrieved from https://play.google.com/store/apps/details?id=com.fenlander.ultimatevaluediary&hl=en

Ja Kaun In. (2018). *Dining Note: Simple food diary*. Retrieved from https://apps.apple.com/us/app/dining-note-simple-food-diary/id1194971321

Jospe, M. R., Fairbairn, K. A., Green, P., & Perry, T. L. (2015). Diet app use by sports dietitians: A survey in five countries. *JMIR mHealth and uHealth*, *3*(1), e7. doi:10.2196/mhealth.3345 PMID:25616274

Kiran Chavan. (2019, September 8). *Smoothie Recipes: 500+ Healthy Smoothies*. Retrieved from https://play.google.com/store/apps/details?id=com.kiransmoothie.kiranchavan.juicerecipe&hl=en_US

Linear Software LLC. (2012). *Body Tracker - body fat calc*. Retrieved from https://apps.apple.com/us/app/body-tracker-body-fat-calc/id581557588

MapMyFitness. (2019, September 7). *Map My Fitness Workout Trainer*. Retrieved from https://play.google.com/store/apps/details?id=com.mapmyfitness.android2&hl=en

MyNetDiary Inc. (2019). *Calorie Counter PRO MyNetDiary*. Retrieved from https://apps.apple.com/us/app/calorie-counter-pro-mynetdiary/id352247139

NoomInc. (2017). *Noom*. Retrieved from https://apps.apple.com/us/app/noom/id634598719

Nutritionix. (2019, June 7). *Track - Calorie Counter*. Retrieved from https://play.google.com/store/apps/details?id=com.nutritionix.nixtrack&hl=en

World Health Organization. (2000). Nutrition for health and development: a global agenda for combating malnutrition.

Outlier. (2015, July 22). *Nutritionist-Dieting made easy*. Retrieved from https://play.google.com/store/apps/details?id=com.nutritionist.development&hl=en

RecoveryBull.com. (2019, May 4). *Health Diet Foods Fitness Help*. Retrieved from https://play.google.com/store/apps/details?id=com.medical.guide_health.diet.tips&hl=en

SparkPeople. (2013, January 30). *Perfect Produce*. Retrieved from https://play.google.com/store/apps/details?id=com.sparkpeople.android.produce&hl=en

SparkPeople. (2016, August 26). *Healthy Slow Cooker Recipes*. Retrieved from https://play.google.com/store/apps/details?id=com.sparkpeople.SlowCookerRecipes&hl=en_US

SparkPeople. (2016, August 24). *Nutrition Lookup - SparkPeople*. Retrieved from https://play.google.com/store/apps/details?id=com.sparkpeople.foodLookup&hl=en

SparkPeople. (2016, November 8). *Pregnancy Health & Fitness*. Retrieved from https://play.google.com/store/apps/details?id=com.SparkPeople.pregnancyHealth&hl=en_US

SparkPeople. (2017, August 13). *Healthy Recipes & Calculator*. Retrieved from https://play.google.com/store/apps/details?id=com.sparkpeople.android.cookbook&hl=en

StayWell. (2019). *My Diet Diary Calorie Counter*. Retrieved from https://play.google.com/store/apps/details?id=org.medhelp.mydiet&hl=en

Stone, M. (2019, February 8). *Simple Diet Diary*. Retrieved from https://play.google.com/store/apps/details?id=com.rarepebble.dietdiary&hl=en

Tasteaholics. (2019, August 4). *Total Keto Diet: Low Carb Recipes & Keto Meals*. Retrieved from https://play.google.com/store/apps/details?id=com.totalketodiet.ketodiet&hl=en

Under Armour, Inc. (2019). *MyFitnessPal*. Retrieved from https://apps.apple.com/us/app/myfitnesspal/id341232718

Watchers, W. International, Inc. (2019, September 9). *WW (formerly Weight Watchers)*. Retrieved from https://play.google.com/store/apps/details?id=com.weightwatchers.mobile&hl=en

Xyris Software (Australia) Pty Ltd. (2019). *Easy Diet Diary*. Retrieved from https://apps.apple.com/au/app/easy-diet-diary/id436104108

Can Yapan. (2017, November 25). *Diet Diary*. Retrieved from https://play.google.com/store/apps/details?id=com.canyapan.dietdiaryapp&hl=en

YAZIO GmbH. (2018). *YAZIO — Diet & Food Tracker*. Retrieved from https://apps.apple.com/us/app/yazio-diet-food-tracker/id946099227

zeronica.com. (2015, May 16). *Weight Tracker "Weigh My Diet"*. Retrieved from https://play.google.com/store/apps/details?id=com.zeronica.weighmydiet&hl=en_GB

ADDITIONAL READING

Balapour, A., Reychav, I., Sabherwal, R., & Azuri, J. (2019). Mobile technology identity and self-efficacy: Implications for the adoption of clinically supported mobile health apps. *International Journal of Information Management*, *49*, 58–68. doi:10.1016/j.ijinfomgt.2019.03.005

Braz, V. N., & de Moraes Lopes, M. H. B. (2019). Evaluation of mobile applications related to nutrition. *Public Health Nutrition*, *22*(7), 1209–1214. PMID:29734965

Dallinga, J., Janssen, M., Van Der Werf, J., Walravens, R., Vos, S., & Deutekom, M. (2018). Analysis of the features important for the effectiveness of physical activity–related apps for recreational sports: Expert panel approach. *JMIR mHealth and uHealth*, *6*(6), e143. doi:10.2196/mhealth.9459 PMID:29914863

Elavsky, S., Knapova, L., Klocek, A., & Smahel, D. (2019). Mobile Health Interventions for Physical Activity, Sedentary Behavior, and Sleep in Adults Aged 50 Years and Older: A Systematic Literature Review. *Journal of Aging and Physical Activity*, 1–29. PMID:30507266

Fallaize, R., Franco, R. Z., Pasang, J., Hwang, F., & Lovegrove, J. A. (2019). Popular Nutrition-Related Mobile Apps: An Agreement Assessment Against a UK Reference Method. *JMIR mHealth and uHealth*, *7*(2), e9838. doi:10.2196/mhealth.9838 PMID:30785409

Ferrara, G., Kim, J., Lin, S., Hua, J., & Seto, E. (2019). A Focused Review of Smartphone Diet-Tracking Apps: Usability, Functionality, Coherence With Behavior Change Theory, and Comparative Validity of Nutrient Intake and Energy Estimates. *JMIR mHealth and uHealth*, *7*(5), e9232. doi:10.2196/mhealth.9232 PMID:31102369

Harvey, J., Smith, A., Goulding, J., & Illodo, I. B. (2019). Food sharing, redistribution, and waste reduction via mobile applications: A social network analysis. *Industrial Marketing Management*. doi:10.1016/j.indmarman.2019.02.019

Neriah, D. B., & Geliebter, A. (2019). Weight Loss Following Use of a Smartphone Food Photo Feature: Retrospective Cohort Study. *JMIR mHealth and uHealth, 7*(6), e11917. doi:10.2196/11917 PMID:31199300

Villinger, K., Wahl, D. R., Boeing, H., Schupp, H. T., & Renner, B. (2019). The effectiveness of app-based mobile interventions on nutrition behaviours and nutrition-related health outcomes: A systematic review and meta-analysis. *Obesity Reviews, 20*(10), 1465–1484. doi:10.1111/obr.12903 PMID:31353783

KEY TERMS AND DEFINITIONS

Adenosine Tri Phosphate (ATP): Adenosine triphosphate is an intricate natural-synthetic that gives vitality to drive numerous procedures in living cells, for example, muscle compression, nerve drive spread, and substance union.

Anemia: Disease that occurs due to low Red Cell Count (RCC), characterized by tiredness, confusion, lake of concentration, pallor.

Dementia: Dementia is definitely not a specific infirmity. It's a general term that delineates a social event of symptoms related with a reduction in memory or other thinking aptitudes outrageous enough to lessen a person's ability to perform customary activities.

Diabetes Mellitus (DM): Diabetes mellitus is disabled insulin discharge and variable degrees of fringe insulin obstruction prompting hyperglycemia. Early manifestations are identified with hyperglycemia and incorporate polydipsia, polyphagia, polyuria, and obscured vision.

Diarrhea Dementia Death (DDD): Determination of pellagra is troublesome without the skin sores and is regularly encouraged by the nearness of trademark ones.

Hemolytic Anemia: Hemolytic frailty is a confusion where red platelets are crushed quicker than they can be made. The annihilation of red platelets is called hemolysis. Red platelets convey oxygen to all pieces of your body. On the off chance that you have a lower than typical measure of red platelets, you have sickliness.

Hypertension: Hypertension (HTN or HT), generally called as high blood pressure (HBP), is a long haul ailment where the circulatory strain in the courses is diligently raised. Hypertension normally does not cause side effects.

Insomnia: Lack of sleep because of neurological disorders.

Lipolysis: Breakdown of lipids into fatty acids and glycerol.

Night Blindness: Night blindness is one of the feature of vitamin A deficiency in which the person can see properly at night because of deficiency of Rhodopsin (the main product of vitamin A) that play a vital role in visual cycle.

Osteomalacia: A disease occurs in adults because of deficiency of Vitamin D.

Pellagra: A disease characterized by DDD i.e. diarrhea, dementia and death, caused by deficiency of Niacin (vitamin B3).

Rickets: A disease occurs in children because of deficiency of Vitamin D Causes bowing of legs.

Scurvy: disease characterized by bleeding gums, bleeding from mucosal surfaces because of deficiency of vitamin C, this can be cured by taking citrus fruits and vitamin C supplements.

Wernicke-Korsakoff Syndrome: (WKS): it is a neurological issue. Wernicke's encephalopathy and Korsakoff's psychosis are the intense and incessant stages, separately, of a similar ailment. WKS is brought about by an insufficiency in the B nutrient thiamine. Thiamine assumes a job in using glucose to create vitality for the cerebrum.

Chapter 8
Analysis of Different Image Processing Techniques for Classification and Detection of Cancer Cells

Bukhtawar Elahi

National University of Sciences and Technology, Pakistan

Maria Kanwal

National University of Sciences and Technology, Pakistan

Sana Elahi

Dr. A. Q. Khan Institute of Computer Sciences and Information Technology, Pakistan

ABSTRACT

This chapter gives an analysis of various methodologies for detecting cancer cells through image processing techniques. The challenges during such detections are over-segmentation and computational complexities. Therefore, the algorithms dealing with such problems are analyzed in this chapter. In these algorithms, a watershed and setting up threshold are helpful to overcome segmentation issues. A support vector machine is discussed to detect subtypes of pneumoconiosis for disjointing segments of lungs. For finding lung cancer cells, a segmentation weighted fuzzy probabilistic-based clustering has been used. Multiple variants of thresholding along with classifiers are proposed to detect lungs and liver cancer. Other than that, noise-removal, feature extraction and watershed are used to detect breast cancer. For leukemia, a bimodal thresholding over enhanced images of cytoplasm and nuclei regions has been discussed. kNN classifier, k-mean clustering, and feed-forward neural networks have also been discussed. Results from these techniques vary from 60%-100% depending on the proposed methodology.

DOI: 10.4018/978-1-7998-2521-0.ch008

1. INTRODUCTION

Cancer cells have the power to affect the other healthy cells and the blood vessels surrounding these cancerous cells. This area forms an environment known as microenvironment. The cancerous cells may invade the other cells and spread to influence the other faraway body parts. These cancerous cells form a mass that increases in size to form tumors, lumps or masses. The detection of masses of cancer cells can be detected by using different techniques. Depending on the nature of their invasion, cancer is categorized as malignant or benign as shown in Figure 1.

Benign tumor does not invade or spread to other body parts though its size can be increased. After the removal of this type of tumor it does not affect again but malignant tumor can come back to affect the other body parts. Benign tumor is not life threatening, however, malignant tumor is fatal if it reaches to brain. Malignant tumor invades other surrounding parts but small part of the originally located tumor dislodge and enters into the circulatory system or lymphatic system where it goes to the distant body parts to make them cancerous. Cancer cells use the immune system for their growth and can mask themselves from immune cell and hence immune system becomes unable to remove cancer cells from the body.

There are different types of cancer and their categorization depends on the organ or tissue where it is present and types of cells. Leukemia is the cancer of blood or blood forming cells. Lymphoma is the cancer of lymphatic system. Carcinoma is the cancer of lining that surrounds the skin, digestive tract and lungs. Sarcoma is the cancer of mesodermal cells such as bone, vessels and blood. Melanoma is the cancer of melanocytes containing melanin pigment. Some other cancers include breast cancer, brain and spinal cord cancer etc (Geetha & Selvi, 2015). Lung cancer involves the cancer of trachea, bronchi and lung tissue involving alveoli. Smoking, exposure to radon gas, silica and asbestos, air pollution, lung diseases such as tuberculosis and family history are the main causes of the lung cancer. Lung cancer

Figure 1. Benign VS malignant tumor

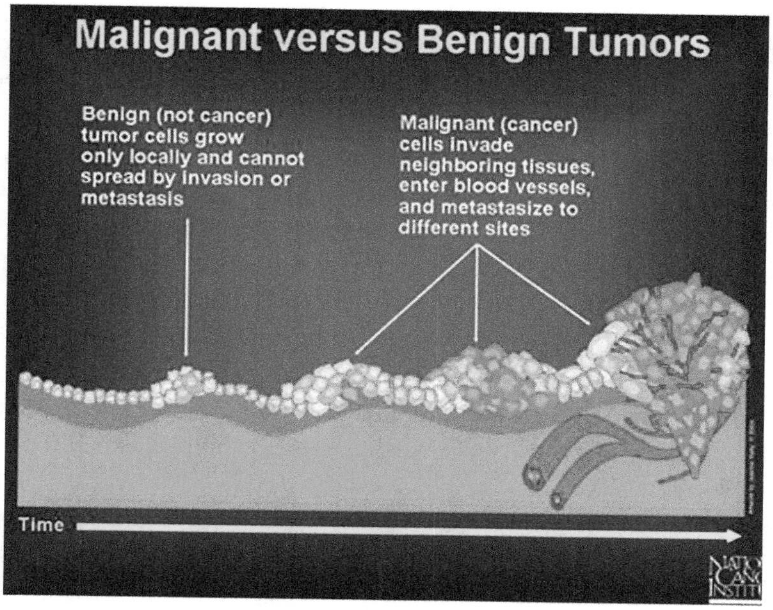

stages are different depending upon the cancer size and its severity. The stage of cancer can be diagnosed with highly precise screening tests.

Skin cancer is the mostly widespread cancer. It starts from the cells that line the superficial layer of the skin. It is localized type of cancer but most destructive in terms of damaging the skin tissues. Basically, there are various kinds of skin cancer that includes squamous cell carcinoma (first kind of skin cancer), basal cell carcinoma (second kind of skin cancer) and melanoma (the third type). Exposure to ultraviolet rays, immunologically suppressed body, family history and exposure to ionizing rays are the main causes of skin cancer. Blood cancer affecting the blood cells number and their function, bone marrow and lymphatic system. Mainly it affects the bone marrow (tissues) where the blood cells are developed. Leukemia, lymphoma and melanoma are the main types of blood cancer. Chemotherapy and radiotherapy could be used as the treatment of his cancer.

Brain tumor originates in the brain and it is a localized tumor known as benign tumor. If not diagnosed early, it can be life threatening. There are some common types of brain tumor that includes gliomas and astrocytic tumors and meningeal tumor. Seizures, vision problem, memory loss problem, speaking, hearing, balancing difficulties are some symptoms of this cancer. Chemotherapy and surgically removal of this tumor are treatments for brain tumors.

2. BACKGROUND

Cancerous cells exhibit a large variety of attributes due to which radiologists have been misinterpreted the results obtained through screening programs. Computer aided classification and detection algorithms are being developed for better interpretation of the results. Reduction of false results, effective and authentic results could now obtain by using detection system (Geetha al., 2015).

Authors (Nilkamal et al, 2014) have proposed the technique of segmentation for detection of skin cancer. In this technique the image is first divided into small segments known as set of pixels. Each pixel is assigned a label that shares same visual behaviors. In segmentation thresholding technique is used in which a value is selected as a threshold value, let say T, and all the values that are below then the threshold are considered as zero and all the values that are above the threshold are considered as one. Zero represent black and one represent white. After thresholding technique, watershed technique is applied and then features are extracted from the image. In feature extraction masking approach has been used.

In another paper by M.Chaithanya Krishna and S.Ranganayakulu skin cancer cells are detected using image processing technique. The technique used in this paper is clustering. Firstly, skin lesion image is acquired. In segmentation step, thresholding-based segmentation, clustering technique and edge detections are used for the detection of skin Melanoma cancer. After that, features extraction techniques are used for the various melanoma parameters like asymmetry, diameter, Border, color by shape analysis and texture size. Miltiades et al. has also proposed a computer aided diagnosis (CAD) system for liver tumor detection. The whole paper is based on two modules classifier module and feature extraction. Liver tumors has been identified through CT liver image and then feature extraction technique has been applied to the CT liver image. The results produced by these techniques are 100 percent for testing set and 97 for validation set (Seo, 2005).

B. Monica Jenefer and V. Cyrilraj has proposed another technique for detecting breast cancer. Firstly, MRI image of the breast cancer is acquired and then noise form image is reduced for enhancement and better quality of image and after this modified watershed segmentation technique is used. Gray level co-occurrence matrix (GLCM) feature extraction technique has been used for feature extraction. In order to get performance metrics Support Vector Machine (SVM) classification is used. The results are 98 accurate in classification and sensitivity was 97.5. (Jenefer et al., 2014). Sundararajan et al. (2010) has proposed vector machine for detection of lungs cancer by using disjoint segments of lungs. Le (2011) has proposed image processing techniques in order to enhance the image of lungs for detection of lungs nodules. Chaudhary et al. 2012) compared the various image processing techniques in order to produce better quality image. Researcher has used threshold and watershed in segmentation technique and monitored which technique produces best accurate result. In image enhancement Gabor filter and Fourier transform techniques are compared.

Hashemi et al. (2013) proposed segmentation for the detection of lungs cancer. First CT scan image of lungs is acquired, then the noise in image is monitored. The noise is reduced by using linear filtering techniques and for pre-processing contrast enhancement technique are used. After that the image is ready for segmentation. Now, the CT scan image is segmented by converting grey scale image into binary image and is differentiates the lungs nodules, malignant and benign by using fuzzy technique.

Anand (2010) gave the idea of neural network technique for detection of lungs tumor. In this technique first CT scan image of lung is acquired then the lungs tumor is detected by coupling the image processing techniques with artificial neural networks in order to differentiate between benign and malignant. Zadeh, Janianpour and Haddadnia (2013) proposed another image analysis approach. In this approach segmentation and automated detection was used to distinguish between cancer cells and normal cells. For detection and segmentation Gaussian smoothing is used and for extraction of image fast Fourier transform has been used.

Naresh (2014) proposed various image processing and data mining techniques to detect lungs cancer. In image processing part image acquisition, removal of noise and segmentation techniques was used. Kaur (2013) used the principal component analysis technique and feature extraction for detection of lungs cancer. Sudha et al. (2012) proposed image processing technique for detection of lungs cancer cell using CT scan image. The whole research is divided into two parts the first one is to use segmentation in which threshold technique is used and in the second part applied the morphological and threshold operations.

This (Aimi Salihah, 2009) research has proposed various image processing techniques for detection of blood cancer. According to this, most of the techniques used thresholding to detect blood cancer cell by counting number of blood cells. First, the image is acquired, and that image is converted into grey scale image which in turn converted into binary image after the whole processing of thresholding where a value of threshold is set which differentiate between white blood cell and red blood cell. If the Red blood cells ratio is zero and white blood cell is 1 then the image is normal image whereas if the ratio of red blood cell is 0.2 and white blood cell is 2.5 then it is abnormal image and person is suffering from blood cancer. If the results produced are not accurate then another threshold value is set, and the experiment is repeated again. The main disadvantage of this technique is it is time consuming by setting threshold value again and again. This research (Patil, 2014) uses the technique of segmentation which consists of two parts thresholding and watershed transformation and the result produced by these two techniques are 81.24% and 85.27% respectively. This proves that the result produced by watershed is better in quality.

Another researcher (Khashman, 2010) proposed a model for detection of blood cancer. This research provides the enhanced image of cytoplasm and nuclei. According to this research, infected cell is detected by bimodal thresholding technique in which two threshold values are used, where the first one is for cytoplasm and the other one is for nuclei. Edges of effected cells are traced, and undesired objects are eliminated by using filtering technique. Result produced by this bimodal threshold technique is 98.33%.

This (Sadeghian et al., 2009) research has introduced zack algorithm for detection of blood cancer. This research provides enhanced image of both parts' cytoplasm and nuclei. The accuracy results produced by this algorithm are 92% for nucleus segmentation and 78% of cytoplasm segmentation.

This research (Joshi, 2013) uses automatic Ostu's technology to detect infected blood cells. *K*-Nearest-Neighbour concept is used here which distinguish between blast cells from lymphocyte cells. This technique is applied on 180 images that are understudy of leukemia. The result produced by this technique is 93% accurate.

These authors (Saikumar, Anoop, & Meghanathan, 2012) used adaptive threshold technique. Instead of setting one value for threshold the adaptive threshold is used where the value of threshold changes according to need. Adaptive threshold is used with Kernel Fuzzy Clustering Method (KFCM). In KFCM the images produced by this technique is fuzzy and the results produced by this technique are better in accuracy and quality of image.

This author (Chandhok, 2012) has proposed another technique of image processing. Two algorithms are used in this research first one is k which is known as clustering and another one technique is neural networks. The output of both techniques is compared according to the time complexity of both algorithms. Image segmentation is used for enhancement of image using neural network which produce less noisy image and artificial neural network (ANN) is used to obtain the better quality of image. Both are compared and check which one is good algorithm for image segmentation.

This research (Ng et al., 2006) has proposed the technique of watershed segmentation and k-means. The advantage of using watershed is that it completely segments the image, on the other hand it provides over-segmentation which is not good for image processing. So, in order to overcome this problem enhanced watershed technique is introduced, in which automated threshold is used. By using automated threshold in watershed technique, the problem of over segment can be reduced.

3. MAIN FOCUS OF THE CHAPTER

The purpose of this chapter is to discover and analyze various methodologies for detecting cancer cells through image processing techniques. Some of the challenges that are usually faced while devising a technique for such task are over-segmentation of image components along with computational complexities. There are multiple proposed algorithms to detect the presence of abnormal cells growth-rate in human body. Among the illness, 39 percent of patients are diagnosed with some form of cancer, while many of them die due late or misdiagnosis of cancer. To aid the cancer-detection process, various techniques are proposed that can detect the growth of abnormal cells in various parts of human body.

4. METHODS AND TECHNIQUES

Fuzzy System

The visualization of the human blood cells that are infected can be done by using a special microscope. Affected cells are analyzed and identified by the doctors through these digital images that are generated by the microscope. The quantity, shape and size of effected cells got changed that is affected by the virus. In Figure 2 affected cells are shown. A digital imaging process can also be applied to these images. Two variables are generated by this process, *Px*, which is linked to the pixels (quantity), and *Sh* (the other variable) which is linked to the cells shape. Either these cells are elliptic, or they are circular in Figure 2, often it's difficult to find the total quantity and number, and also identify the shape of pixels clusters; so these variables (*Px* and *Sh*) estimation must be done in linguistic way.

In Figure 2 normal cells and effected cells are shown by help of microscope with different size and shapes

The proposed method has two sets (fuzzy sets); number of effected cells represented by *Px* (c_2 few infected pixels, c_1 = few infected pixels, c_3. a lot of pixels that are infected) and variable *Sh* represents the shapes of clusters of pixels that are infected (sh_1 for ellipse shape and sh_2 circular shape.

$$Px = \frac{0.1}{c_1} + \frac{0.5}{c_2} + \frac{0.9}{c_3}$$

and

Figure 2. Normal cells and effected cells are shown in microscope with different size and shapes (Talukdar, Deb, & Roy, 2014)

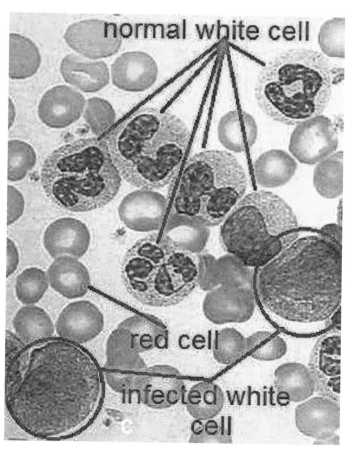

$$Sh = \frac{0.3}{sh_1} + \frac{0.7}{sh_2}$$

The relation among quantity and the shape of infected pixels. Using Cartesian product fuzzy method between variable "*Px*" and variable "*Sh*" gives the resultant relational matrix as

$$Res = Px \times Sh = \begin{pmatrix} 0.1 & 0.1 \\ 0.3 & 0.5 \\ 0.3 & 0.7 \end{pmatrix}$$

In another image when the number of infected pixels found are slightly different;

$$Px' = \frac{0.3}{c_1} + \frac{0.7}{c2} + \frac{9.0}{c3}$$

A new value for fuzzy set (clustered pixels shape) will be produced by using the composition (max-min) with relation R that are associated with new infected pixels quantities.

$$Sh' = Px'\text{o } Res' = \begin{pmatrix} 0.3 & 0.7 & 0.9 \end{pmatrix} \text{o} \begin{pmatrix} 0.1 & 0.1 \\ 0.3 & 0.5 \\ 0.3 & 0.7 \end{pmatrix} = \begin{pmatrix} 0.3 & 0.7 \end{pmatrix}$$

The infection present in the cells can easily be detected by the medical doctor from the above generated result as it is based on the effected cells and the shapes of the effected cells.

Steps

This fuzzy method (proposed by (Talukdar, Deb, & Roy, 2014)) has four different modules (steps):

- First step is the Pre-processing of image.
- Second step in this method is Segmentation of image.
- Third step is extraction of features from the segmented image.
- Fourth step is a decision system which takes decision on the basis of the fuzzy rule.

Image Pre-processing: The data sets of images for blood cells are collected from different sources in JPEG or the Bitmap format. A sample image is made suitable for the particular application through pre-processing of image. The pre-processing of the image includes the enhancement, which implies resizing, sharpening, contrast enhancement, noise removal and highlighting the edges of the image. This procedure enhances the image and remove the unwanted parts of the image.

Image Segmentation: In Image segmentation, the proposed technique selects only that area of image that is of their interest. In this process the image is divided into multiple sections or structures of the interest, so that each section has characteristics similarity. This process is used for extracting useful information from grouped pixels together with region/segment of similarity. The main aim of the segmentation procedure is to modify the image into a meaningful form for the analyzing purpose.

In segmentation a label is assigned to each of the pixel, in such a way that the pixels with the same labels have the common chromatic features. This makes the image analysis task easier. For object recognition, locating boundaries and objects segmentation is used. Segmentation results in a set of outlines extracted from image or in regions that collectively cover the whole image. By taking into consideration the properties of the particular classes, segmentation method is designed. In (Talukdar, Deb, & Roy, 2014), the proposed technique selected the blood cells because they contain the areas of interest. In this proposed technique the thresholding method is applied for the image segmentation.

Feature Extraction: This procedure is also named as description deals. It is taken as sub-dissection of the enhanced image into the principal parts, or separation of some features of an image for the purpose of identification or interpretation of meaningful forms of object, which includes, finding circles or lines or particular shapes.

Fuzzy Set: This set is a comprehensive of traditional set theory. These sets (Fuzzy sets) try to seizure the means human being symbolizes and reason with real world knowledge. In fuzzy set, the degree of membership allowed are between 0 and 1. A Fuzzy logic is a procedure of numerous logic; which works with the reasoning that is not fixed and exact but is approximate. To define the fuzziness of the images and to define the information contained in the images membership function is used. To handle the concepts of the partial truth fuzzy logic had been extended, the truth value may range between completely false and completely true. Fuzzy rules are linguistic rules, the statements that contains the linguistic variables. The use of these linguistic or semantic variables and fuzzy rules uses the acceptance for fuzziness and improbability. In this case, the fuzzy logic simulates the critical capability of human mind to concentrate on the information related to the decision and to summarize the data. For the classification of the desired objects feature extraction is an essential process (Athira Krishnan et al., 2014). It is a vital step in the creation of any of the pattern classification that anticipates in the extraction of the related material that differentiates each (Kasmin et al., 2006).

Complete steps of Fuzzy based system are shown in Figure 3.

Categorization of the Cancer Cells Using Labview

This method has been proposed by (Hossein Ghayoumi Zadeh, 2013). In this technique the image data needs to be transferred into this computer software using a Data acquisition (DAQ) card. After this step, the image is processed by using MATLAB and LABVIEW software. The further steps of this technique image segmentation, image enhancement and others are also carried out with the help of these software. These software has a good quality to connect with the other equipment and it can also control them. LabVIEW is also used as a controlling and processing unit in this technique. By employing the LABVIEW an automatic system can be designed. The algorithm for this proposed technique is given in Figure 4.

In Figure 5, part (a) is the original image of cells that is used for processing. Beside normal cells particular cells are shown in this image. In Figure 5 part (b), authors observed some marked cells which are defected. These defected cells are marked during the image processing step.

Figure 3. Overall steps involved for fuzzy rule-based system

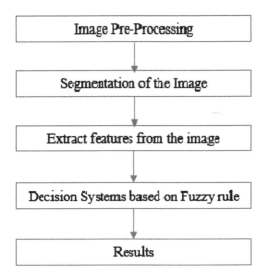

Figure 4. Algorithm of the LABVIEW process

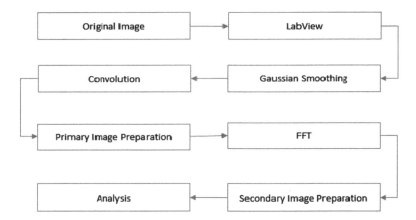

Figure 5. Original image of cells used in image processing
(Hossein Ghayoumi Zadeh, 2013)

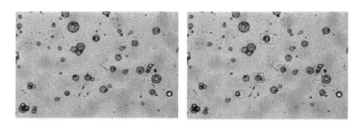

Gaussian Smoothing: The Gaussian smoothing of an image is similar to the mean filtering. These smoothing results are achieved by determining the standard deviation (SD) of the Gaussian filter. The higher the SD of the Gaussian, the larger are the convolution kernels which are needed to represent precisely. The Gaussian method results in a "weighted average" of each of the pixel's neighborhood. Gaussian filter is similar to the mean filter where output is calculated using uniformly weighted average. Therefore, this filter gives a tender smoothing and also preserves the edges of the image better than the mean filter with the same size. Using the equation for the Gaussian filter the mass will be computed as:

$$G\left(a,b\right) = \frac{1}{2\pi\sigma^2} + e^{-\left(\frac{a^2 + b^2}{2\sigma^2}\right)}$$

The mask used in the Gaussian filter is given in Table 1. The output of Gaussian smoothing stage is shown in Figure 6.

Convolution: The Convolution operation is a local operation, in this operation each of the resultant pixel is the weighted summation of the neighboring input pixels. The discrete convolution of T with S, denoted by T * S, is computed as

Table 1. Mask used in the Gaussian filter

1	2	4	2	2
2	4	8	4	2
4	8	16	8	4
2	4	8	4	2
1	2	4	2	1

Figure 6. Cells image after the stage 3 (after applying the Gaussian filter)
(Hossein Ghayoumi Zadeh, 2013)

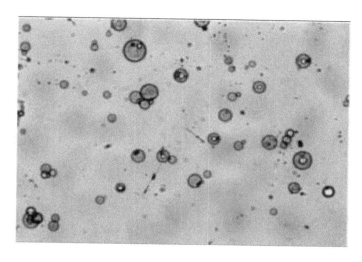

$$\left(T*S\right)\left[x,y\right]\sum\alpha\sum bT\left[a,b\right].S\left[x-a,y-b\right]$$

It is best choice to insert T and S within the image to avoid the effects of wraparound. The mask used in this stage is given in Table 2. The output of this convolution stage is shown in Figure 7.

Image Preparation: In this image preparation step, the thresholded image of the data is drawn and then the image parameters are converted into the metric as shown in Figure 8. After these steps they have done the "proper close" step. The resultant image of this step is presented in Figure 9.

Fast Fourier Transform (FFT): The Fast Fourier transform (FFT) spatial frequency resolution is linked to the dimension of image and also related to equivalent pixel dimension of the image. To examine the output from the various data images this parameter can be acquired easily if the same imaging method is used. The resolution of the image depends upon the distance if the same imaging system is used. After extracting the required parameters for the transformation (i.e. hue, brightness and etc.), The images are convolved by using the double raised cosine kernel:

where M is the image dimension. The objected cells are marked by changing the frequency percentage (truncation) value. The resultant image has the truncation frequency 8% of 6% and the FFT mode of "Low Pass" filter as shown in Figure 10.

Final Step: The final step of this method consists of these stages: Filling of the holes, removing the objects from the border and the Particle Filtering. At the end of procedure, the positions of the targeted cells are extracted out. After the final stage the position of a particular cancer cell is labeled. The signifi-

Table 2. Mask used in the convolution stage

-1	-1	-1
-1	9	-1
-1	-1	-1

Figure 7. Resultant image after applying the convolution mask/filter
(Hossein Ghayoumi Zadeh, 2013)

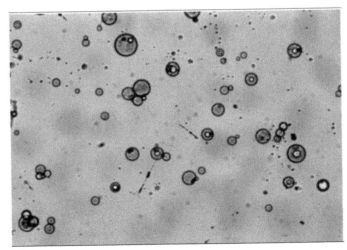

Figure 8. Image quantity changed into metric quantity
(Hossein Ghayoumi Zadeh, 2013)

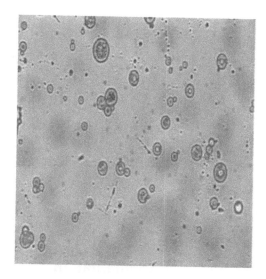

cant point in synthesizing these results is that users can use LabVIEW analysis because of the difference between the results. This LabVIEW analysis can be used to design network that is a neural network for the cancer tissue recognition in the medical images.

By using this technique, the infected cells are highlighted and extracted between other tissues very well. So, this method has been used for cells examination at a large scale. It can also increase the accuracy, accelerate the examination process and the calculating procedure of the effected cells. The effect

Figure 9. Resultant image after convolution stage
(Hossein Ghayoumi Zadeh, 2013)

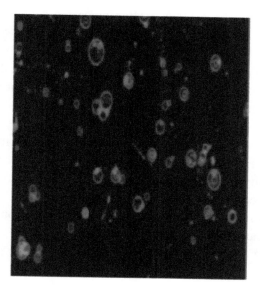

Figure 10. Image after FFT stage
(Hossein Ghayoumi Zadeh, 2013)

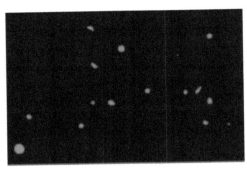

of the medical treatment on the growth of the cancer tissues can easily be observed by counting the number of defected cells.

Cancer Cells Detection Using Color Segmentation

In this method the writer (Shekhar, 2012) presented color segmentation and watershed-based technique for the classification and detection of cancer cells in biopsy images. In the experiment for this technique, various breast cancer cells and various non-cancerous breast cells from various patient and normal females were taken. Each one of these images are of size 24-bit having 447×600 pixels. This techniques has following steps.

Step 1: Classification and detection of the cancer cells nuclei in H and E marked histopathology image. The algorithm for process 1 is given in Table 3.

Step 2: Convert that 24-bit colored jpeg image to an one byte gray scale image afterward changing the contrast of that biopsy image. The pseudo code for this procedure is given in Table 4.

Step 3: Convert the resultant image from process 2(one byte grey scaled image) to a bicolor monochrome and an inverse bicolor monochrome image, after increasing the contrast of the biopsy image. The pseudo code for this procedure is given in Table 5.

In this cancer detection (object level) algorithm the approaches of equalization of adaptive histogram and also the multi-segmentation is used. The main stages of these presented object level cancer classification and detection algorithms are summed up as follows:

- The transformation of this selected biopsy image to the grey scale image.
- Contrast Limited A and H equalization of the biopsy image.
- Adjust the Image intensity of the biopsy image.
- Apply segmentation based on the adaptive thresholding.
- In the segmented biopsy image perform the morphological operation and watershed segmentation.
- Binary large object (Cancer effected object) marking.
- Characteristic extraction of the cancer effected object.

Table 3. Algorithm for Step 1

Input is: a 24-bit colored jpeg image
c_r = Red component significance in 24-bit colored image (c_r: component red)
c_g = The green component significance in colored image
c_b = The blue component significance in colored image
Output: 24-bit color jpeg image
Process
Load the RGB Image to read
Load the colored thresholding image that is to be written
[A B C] = RGB Image size
J from = 0, A
K from = 0, B
condition true($50 < c_r < 160$)
$c_r = 0$
otherwise $c_r = 255$
condition true($0 < c_g < 120$)
$c_g = 0$
otherwise $c_g = 255$
condition true ($120 < c_b < 180$)
$c_b = 0$
otherwise
$c_b = 255$
Ending the K from=0 to B
Ending J from=0 to A
Add c_r, c_g, and c_b components of the image
End

(Shekhar, 2012)

5. RESULTS AND DISCUSSIONS

Cancer Cell Detection Using Fuzzy Systems

From the outputs obtained by threshold output sample (Figure 11, 12, 13) the authors (Talukdar, Deb, & Roy, 2014) counted the defected cells and then made some relationship among cells by applying the fuzzy rules. By using the connections, one medical doctor or physician can easily decide the infection percentages, one is suffering from. Results using Fuzzy systems are shown are Table 6.

The principal aim of this method was to construct an automatic system which can detect the blood cancer cells using the method of soft computing. Major reason of the death around the world is blood cancer and the early detection of blood cancer disease is very key job. The automatic cancer determining system (computer aided) helps the medical doctors as a tool for the cancer cell diagnosis. Fuzzy rule-based methods plays a vital role in cancer classification and detection. The proposed method of fuzzy

Table 4. Algorithm for Step 2

Input is a 24-bit colored jpeg image
RGB Image = a 24-bit colored jpeg image
Grey Image = an 8-bit gray image
[A B C] = a 24-bit colored jpeg image
c_r = Red component significance in 24-bit colored image (c_r: component red)
c_g = The green part significance in colored image
c_b = The blue part significance in colored image
Grey: is image intensity value
Output: is a 8-bit color jpeg image
Start:
Load the RGB Image that is to be read
Load the Gray Image to be written.
[A B C] = size of RGB Image
j from = 0, A
k from = 0, B
Load c_r, c_g, c_b from the RGB Image
condition true (c_r > 160)
$c_r = c_r * 1.5$
condition true (c_r > 255)
$c_r = 255$
otherwise if condition not true
$c_r = c_r / 1.5$
condition (c_r < 0)
$c_r = 0$
condition (c_g > 150)
$c_g = c_g * 1.5$
condition (c_g > 255)
$c_g = 255$
condition not true
$c_g = c_g / 1.5$
condition (c_g < 0)
$c_g = 0$
condition (c_b > 160)
$c_b = c_b * 1.5$
condition (c_b >255)
$c_b = 255$
otherwise
$c_b = c_b / 1.5$
condition (c_b < 0)
$c_b = 0$
Gray = (0.4) * c_r + (0.8) * c_b + (0.48) * c_g
Write the Gray value to Gray Image value
Ending of k from = 0 to B
Ending of j from=0 to A
Close the RGB image and Gray image
End

(Shekhar, 2012)

Table 5. Algorithm for Step 3

Input: a 8-bit gray scaled image
Gray image = a 8-bit gray scaled image image
Mono image = is an image which is Bi-colored monochrome
[*MN*] = size of an an 8-bit grayed image
Intnse = image intensity value
Output is an image i.e. bi-color monochrome
Start
Load the Grey image that is to be read
Load the Mono image that is to be written.
Find the threshold value
[*MN*] = size of Gray Image
J from = 0, M
k from = 0, N
Read the 'Intnse' from the Grey image
check condition (Intnse >160)
true:Intnse = c_r * 1.5
condition true (Intnse >255)
Intnse = 255
condition not true
Intnse = Intnse /1.5
condition true (Intnse < 0)
Intnse = 0
Write down 'Intnse' value to the 'Mono image'
Ending k from = 0, N
Ending J from = 0, M
Close the 'Gray image' and the 'Mono image'
End

(Shekhar, 2012)

techniques and fuzzy rules helped physician and doctors for cancer detection by decreasing their time and effort as they play important role in the cancer detection and cancer classification.

Results Using Color Segmentation Method

In this paper (Singh, 2012) the authors proposed this technique to remove large amount of the connected tissue, fat and the gland tissues from cancer effected tissues within the biopsy image. The cancer cell intensity, the stage of cancer, cancer type and the treatment for that cancer type, they observed all this

Figure 11. (a)Original blood cells image of sample 1, (b) Thresholded output image of sample 1
(Talukdar, Deb, & Roy, 2014)

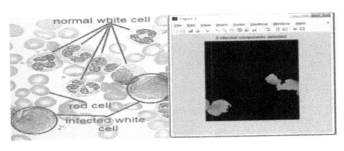

Figure 12. (a) Original blood cells image of sample 2, (b) Thresholded output image of sample 2
(Talukdar, Deb, & Roy, 2014)

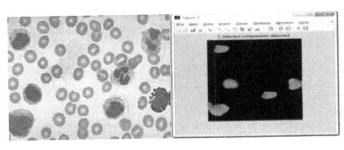

on the basis of the comparison of the pattern of the malignant cancer tissue with the normal tissues. The results from these algorithms are shown in the figures of cancer cells. Figure 14, 15, 16 shows the cancer infected tissue. Figure 14 illustrates a sample high resolution biopsy image. Figure 15 and 16 show the colored image detected cancer tissues.

The accuracy of this classifier has been specified as the ratio of no. of biopsy samples that are accurately categorized to total number of the samples that are examined. This trained classifier then has been examined in the retrieval mode. In retrieval mode the testing vectors has not been taking part in the

Figure 13. (a) Original blood cells image of sample 3, (b) Thresholded output image of sample 3 (showing infected region)
(Talukdar, Deb, & Roy, 2014)

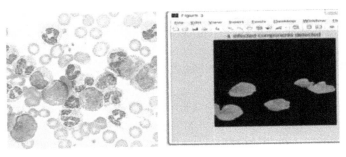

Table 6. Results using Fuzzy systems

Px (No. of Effected Cells)		Sh (Shape of the Cells)		R = Px X Sh (Cartesian Relation)		Px' (The New Image and the No. of Effected Cells)			Sh'= Px'oR (max-min)
C_1(few)	C_2(a few)	C_3(lots)	Sh_1(ellipse)	Sh_2(circle)	R	C_1(few)	C_2(a few)	C_3(lots)	—
1	0.5	0.9	0.3	0.7	[0.1,0.1; 0.3, 0.5;0.3,0.7]	0.3	0.7	0.9	[0.3 0.7]
.2	0.5	0.6	0.2	0.8	[0.2, 0.2; 0.2, 0.5; 0.2, 0.6]	0.2	0.6	0.8	[0.2 0.6]

(Talukdar, Deb, & Roy, 2014)

training procedure. They use the conventional multilayered neural network that has been trained with the gradient descent with the momentum and Levenberg Marquardt and resilient back propagation algorithms.

Table 7 shows the result of the model (Singh,2012) used in categorization of the breast cancer tumor data using the neural network. The general correctness of this categorization in the experimental mode is 98.80%. It shows the results of the methods employed in categorization of the breast cancer tumor samples in malignant, benign and other type malignant.

In the paper (Singh, 2012), for automatic detection of breast cancer and for the classification of the histopathological images the authors presented the approaches of adaptive thresholding, color thresholding and cell level segmentation method based on the watershed approach. FNN had been implemented for the classification of the breast cancer tumor. The general accurateness of this categorization in training mode and validation mode and testing mode are 99.64%, 98.54% and 98.80%. For breast tumor this system provides a fast and more precise cancer cells detection and classification.

Results Using Gabor Filter, FFT Filter and Auto Enhancement

In Image enhancement techniques the best results are obtained by using the Gabor filter. Two other filters the Auto enhancement and FFT filter gave the poor results so for enhancement of image for cancer cells detection Gabor should be preferred (Al-Tarawneh, 2012).

For image segmentation the techniques that are applied are thresholding techniques and Marker Controlled Watershed Segmentation (MCWS)approach. Segmentation of the image using the MCWSA works good if users can distinguish the foreground objects and the background locations.

According to the various experimental particular assessment during the segmentation step the MCWS approach has more quality and precision of 85.165% than the thresholding approach which has accuracy

Table 7. Result using color segmentation process

Case Study	Training Data Correctness %	Validation Data Correctness %	Testing Data Correctness %
Benign	99.32	98.56	98.80
Type 1 (malignant)	99.20	98.58	98.82
Type 2 (malignant)	99.60	98.32	98.76
Type 3 (malignant)	99.20	98.50	98.82

(Singh, 2012)

Figure 14. Biopsy image
(Singh, 2012)

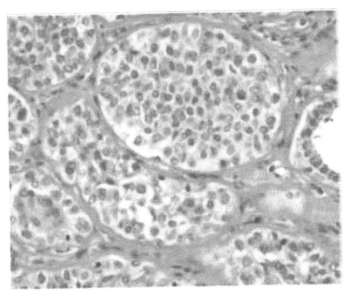

Figure 15. (a) Cancer cell detected color image, (b) Cancer cell detected grey image
(Singh, 2012)

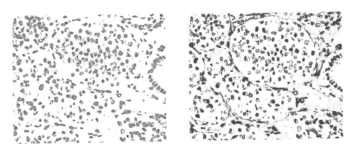

Figure 16. (a) Cancer cell detected Bi-color image, (b) Cancer cell detected color image (c) Cancer cell detected classified image
(Singh, 2012)

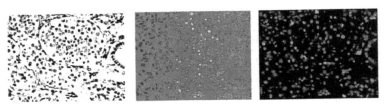

of 81.835%. Sub and final averages for these three techniques are shown in Table 8. The results/output of Gabor filter and FFT filter are shown in Figure 17 and Figure 18, respectively.

6. CONCLUSION

The major cause of death in the world is cancer which is increasing gradually day by day. In his chapter, the different techniques used for detection and classification of various type of cancer are discussed. In this field of medicine, the images are the vital constituents especially in the process of diagnosis of cancer tumors. These digital image processing-based technologies and approaches help the physicians

Table 8. Result using color segmentation process

Subject	Auto Enhancement	Gabor Filter	FFT Filter
Subject 1	37.95	80.975	27.075
Subject 2	47.725	80	36.825
Subject 3	36.825	79.5	25.625
Subject 4	34.775	81.8	25.175
Subject 5	32.85	81.4	22.85
Final Average	38.025	80.735	27.51

(Al-Tarawneh, 2012)

Figure 17. (a) Original Image, (b) Output image after applying Gabor filter (Al-Tarawneh, 2012)

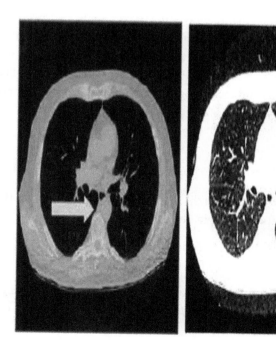

Figure 18. (a) Original Image, (b) Output image after applying FFT filter
(Al-Tarawneh, 2012)

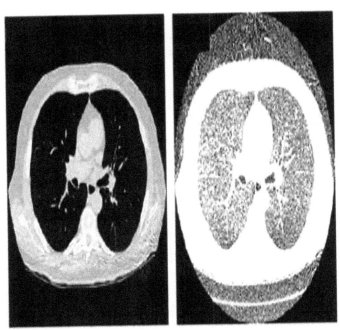

and the medical doctors to have a better clarification, quicker detection and thus increases precision and accuracy of diagnosis for the process of diagnosis of tumors and cancer cells. The aim of the image processing techniques used are to locate, identify and to extract the useful information from the data and then categorize the type of cancer and stage of the cancer. By observing at the results obtained have helped the medical doctors and physicians to choose the most suitable techniques for the optimization of the cancer cells Identifying through the medical imaging. In this chapter an impression of the different type of cancer cell detection techniques and a literature survey on detection and classification of cancer cells by previous researchers is presented. From the literature review and analysis, it shows that the developments of the new methods and technologies are to be required to observe and classify cancer cells more effectively and efficiently.

REFERENCES

Aimi Salihah, A. N., Mustafa, N., & Nashrul Fazli, M. N. (2009). Application of thresholding technique in determining ratio of blood cells for Leukemia detection.

Al-Tarawneh, M. S. (2012). Lung Cancer Detection Using Image Processing Techniques. *Leonardo Electronic Journal of Practices and Technologies*, (20).

Anand, S. V. (2010). Segmentation coupled textural feature classification for lung tumor prediction. In *Proceedings of the 2010 IEEE International Conference on Communication Control and Computing Technologies (ICCCCT)* (pp. 518-524). IEEE.

Athira Krishnan, S. K. (2014). A Survey on Image Segmentation and Feature Extraction Methods for Acute Myelogenous Leukemia Detection in Blood Microscopic Images. *International Journal of Computer Science and Information Technologies, 5*(6), 7877-7879.

Talukdar, N. A., Deb, D., & Roy, S. (2014, August). Automated Blood Cancer Detection Using Image Processing Based on Fuzzy System. *International Journal of Advanced Research in Computer Science and Software Engineering, 4*(8), 1–6.

Chandhok, C. (2012). A novel approach to image segmentation using artificial neural networks and k-means clustering. *International Journal of Engineering Research and Applications, 2*(3), 274–279.

Chaudhary, A., & Singh, S. S. (2012). Lung cancer detection on CT images by using image processing. In *Proceedings of the 2012 International Conference on Computing Sciences (ICCS),* (pp. 142-146). IEEE. 10.1109/ICCS.2012.43

Elgamal, M. (2013). Automatic skin cancer images classification. *(IJACSA). International Journal of Advanced Computer Science and Applications, 4*(3), 287–294. doi:10.14569/IJACSA.2013.040342

Geetha, M. P., & Selvi, D. V. (2015). An impression of cancers and survey of techniques in image processing for detecting various cancers: A review. *International Research Journal of Engineering and Technology, 2.*

Hashemi, A., Pilevar, A. H., & Rafeh, R. (2013). Mass detection in lung CT images using region growing segmentation and decision making based on fuzzy inference system and artificial neural network. *International Journal of Image. Graphics and Signal Processing, 5*(6), 16–24. doi:10.5815/ijigsp.2013.06.03

Jenefer, B. M., & Cyrilraj, V. (2014). An efficient image processing methods for mammogram breast cancer detection. *Journal of Theoretical & Applied Information Technology, 69*(1).

Joshi, M. D., Karode, A. H., & Suralkar, S. R. (2013). White blood cells segmentation and classification to detect acute leukemia. *International Journal of Emerging Trends and Technology in Computer Science, 2*(3).

Kale, S. D., Punwatkar, K. M., & Pusad, Y. (2013). Texture Analysis of Thyroid Ultrasound Images for Diagnosis of Benign and Malignant Nodule using Scaled Conjugate Gradient Backpropagation Training Neural Network. *IJCEM International Journal of Computational Engineering & Management, 16*(6).

Kanakatte, A., Mani, N., Srinivasan, B., & Gubbi, J. (2008, May). Pulmonary tumor volume detection from positron emission tomography images. In *Proceedings of the International Conference on BioMedical Engineering and Informatics BMEI 2008* (Vol. 2, pp. 213-217). IEEE. 10.1109/BMEI.2008.354

Kasmin, F., Prabuwono, A. S., & Abdullah, A. (2012). Detection of leukemia in human blood sample based on microscopic images: A study. *Journal of Theoretical & Applied Information Technology, 46*(2).

Kaur, A. R. (2013). Feature extraction and principal component analysis for lung cancer detection in CT scan images. *International Journal of Advanced Research in Computer Science and Software Engineering, 3*(3).

Khashman, A., & Al-Zgoul, E. (2010). Image segmentation of blood cells in leukemia patients. *Recent advances in computer engineering and applications, 2*(1), 104-109.

Le, K. (2011, January). Chest X-ray analysis for computer-aided diagnostic. In *Proceedings of the International Conference on Computer Science and Information Technology* (pp. 300-309). Springer Berlin Heidelberg.

Naresh, P., & Shettar, R. (2014). Image Processing and Classification Techniques for Early Detection of Lung Cancer for Preventive Health Care: A Survey. *Int. J. of Recent Trends in Engineering & Technology, 11*.

Ng, H. P., Ong, S. H., Foong, K. W. C., Goh, P. S., & Nowinski, W. L. (2006, March). Medical image segmentation using k-means clustering and improved watershed algorithm. In *Proceedings of the 2006 IEEE Southwest Symposium on Image Analysis and Interpretation* (pp. 61-65). IEEE. 10.1109/SSIAI.2006.1633722

Patil, B. G., & Jain, S. N. (2014). Cancer cells detection using digital image processing methods. *International Journal of Latest Trends in Engineering and Technology*.

Sadeghian, F., Seman, Z., Ramli, A. R., Kahar, B. H. A., & Saripan, M. I. (2009). A framework for white blood cell segmentation in microscopic blood images using digital image processing. *Biological Procedures Online, 11*(1), 196–206. doi:10.100712575-009-9011-2 PMID:19517206

Saikumar, T., Anoop, B. K., Murthy, P. S., & Meghanathan, N. (2012). Robust adaptive threshold algorithm based on kernel fuzzy clustering on image segmentation. *Computer Science & Information Technology (CS & IT)*, 99-103.

Seo, K. S. (2005, May). Improved fully automatic liver segmentation using histogram tail threshold algorithms. In *Proceedings of the International Conference on Computational Science* (pp. 822-825). Springer Berlin Heidelberg. 10.1007/11428862_115

Singh, S. (2012). Cancer cells detection and classification in biopsy image. *International Journal of Engineering Science and Technology*.

Sudha, V., & Jayashree, P. (2012). Lung nodule detection in CT images using thresholding and morphological operations. *International Journal of Emerging Science and Engineering, 1*(2), 17–21.

Sundararajan, R., Xu, H., Annangi, P., Tao, X., Sun, X., & Mao, L. (2010, April). A multiresolution support vector machine based algorithm for pneumoconiosis detection from chest radiographs. In *Proceedings of the 2010 IEEE International Symposium on Biomedical Imaging: From Nano to Macro* (pp. 1317-1320). IEEE. 10.1109/ISBI.2010.5490239

Zadeh, H. G., Janianpour, S., & Haddadnia, J. (2013). Recognition and Classification of the Cancer Cells by Using Image Processing and LabVIEW. *International Journal of computer theory and engineering, 5*(1).

Zadeh, H. G., Janianpour, S., & Haddadnia, J. (2013). Recognition and Classification of the Cancer Cells by using Image Processing and Lab VIEW. *International Journal of Computer Theory and Engineering, 5*(1), 104–107. doi:10.7763/IJCTE.2013.V5.656

ADDITIONAL READING

Bhalerao, R. Y., Jani, H. P., Gaitonde, R. K., & Raut, V. (2019, March). A novel approach for detection of Lung Cancer using Digital Image Processing and Convolution Neural Networks. In *Proceedings of the 2019 5th International Conference on Advanced Computing & Communication Systems (ICACCS)* (pp. 577-583). IEEE. 10.1109/ICACCS.2019.8728348

Dutta, A., & Dubey, A. (2019, April). Detection of Liver Cancer using Image Processing Techniques. In *Proceedings of the 2019 International Conference on Communication and Signal Processing (ICCSP)* (pp. 0315-0318). IEEE. 10.1109/ICCSP.2019.8698033

Khan, S., Islam, N., Jan, Z., Din, I. U., & Rodrigues, J. J. C. (2019). A novel deep learning based framework for the detection and classification of breast cancer using transfer learning. *Pattern Recognition Letters*, *125*, 1–6. doi:10.1016/j.patrec.2019.03.022

Pauly, P. S., Rajan, B. K., & Rajan, S. K. (2019, April). Efficient Enhancement of Hepatic and Splenic Carcinoma in Canine using Image Processing. In *Proceedings of the 2019 International Conference on Communication and Signal Processing (ICCSP)* (pp. 0063-0067). IEEE. 10.1109/ICCSP.2019.8698026

Rohith, V., & Ramya, N. (2019). Kidney tumor detection and classification using image processing. *International Journal of Research in Pharmaceutical Sciences*, *10*(3), 2017–2024. doi:10.26452/ijrps.v10i3.1412

KEY TERMS AND DEFINITIONS

ANN: Artificial neural networks are computing systems consisting interconnected group of neurons.

Cancer Identification: Different approaches are used for diagnosis and identification of cancer. Different test and procedures are used to diagnose different cancers.

CT Scan: Computed tomography (CT) scan uses data from several X-rays and combine them to get the image of particular part of that object.

Fuzzy Control System: Fuzzy logic-based control system that takes on continuous values (between 0 to 1) as input.

Image Processing: To extract useful information from images different algorithms and actions are performed on an image.

KNN: K nearest neighbors is a classification algorithm that classifies the object based on k nearest neighbors.

Leukemia: Cancer that effect blood cells.

Lymphoma: Cancer that starts in the lymphocytes.

MRI: Magnetic resonance imaging (MRI) uses radio waves and magnetic fields to get images of the tissues and organs of the body.

Segmentation: In image segmentation, the users select only that area of image that is of their interest. In this process the image is divided into multiple sections or structures of the interest, so that each section has characteristic similarity.

Tumor: A tumor is a mass of tissue that is framed by an aggregation of anomalous cells.

Melanoma: Type of skin cancer.

Chapter 9

Crow–ENN:
An Optimized Elman Neural Network with Crow Search Algorithm for Leukemia DNA Sequence Classification

Rehan Ullah

iD https://orcid.org/0000-0003-0738-9269

The University of Agriculture, Peshawar, Pakistan

Abdullah Khan

iD https://orcid.org/0000-0003-1718-7038

The University of Agriculture, Peshawar, Pakistan

Syed Bakhtawar Shah Abid

The University of Agriculture, Peshawar, Pakistan

Siyab Khan

iD https://orcid.org/0000-0003-4455-9466

The University of Agriculture, Peshawar, Pakistan

Said Khalid Shah

Department of Computer Science, University of Science and Technology, Bannu, Pakistan

Maria Ali

The University of Agriculture, Peshawar, Pakistan

ABSTRACT

DNA sequence classification is one of the main research activities in bioinformatics on which, many researchers have worked and are working on it. In bioinformatics, machine learning can be applied for the analysis of genomic sequences like the classification of DNA sequences, comparison of DNA sequences. This article proposes a new hybrid meta-heuristic model called Crow-ENN for leukemia DNA sequences classification. The proposed algorithm is the combination of the Crow Search Algorithm (CSA) and

DOI: 10.4018/978-1-7998-2521-0.ch009

the Elman Neural Network (ENN). DNA sequences of Leukemia are used to train and test the proposed hybrid model. Five other comparable models i.e. Crow-ANN, Crow-BPNN, ANN, BPNN and ENN are also trained and tested on these DNA sequences. The performance of models is evaluated in terms of accuracy and MSE. The overall simulation results show that the proposed model has outperformed all the other five comparable models by attaining the highest accuracy of over 99%. This model may also be used for other classification problems in different fields because it can achieve promising results.

1. INTRODUCTION

In the past, the speed of producing and sharing scientific knowledge was never been so fast as compared to the present era. New disciplines are being raised by combining different fields of science. One such newly arisen field is bioinformatics, which uses statistics, mathematics and computer science in molecular biology to store, analyze and retrieve biological data. Bioinformatics is growing very fast and it has made itself a basic part of any biological research work. Bioinformatics can serve a biologist to excerpt meaningful information from biological data using different kind of web or computer-based tools, most of which are available freely (Mehmood et al., 2014). Among all these computational techniques machine learning is the most common procedure for analyzing data in the form of protein and DNA sequences. Machine learning is a subfield of AI, which is concerned with designing and development of computer algorithms which get improved with experience. The field of machine learning makes computers capable to aid humans in analyzing complex and large problems. In bioinformatics, machine learning can have applied for the analysis of genomic sequences like the classification of DNA sequences, comparison of DNA sequences, Identification of Unknown DNA sequences etc. Supervised and Unsupervised learning are two broad methodologies which are used commonly in machine learning. (Librecht et al., 2015). Classification is kind of supervised machine learning which is used to classify every element in a dataset into one of the predefined set of groups or classes. Classification is a function of data mining which assigns elements/items in a collection/dataset to some target classes or categories based on some similarities. Classification is aimed to accurately predict a target group or class for every item in a dataset. There are many techniques used for classification like Support Vector Machine (SVM), Decision Trees, Naive Bayes Classification, Artificial Neural Networks (ANN), Bayesian Networks, etc. (Kesavaraj et al., 2013).

This research has combined two machine learning algorithms namely Crow Search Algorithm (CSA) and Elman Neural Network (ENN). The simple ENN has the problem of being stuck in the local minima. It was not able to reach to a global optimum. So, by merging CSA with ENN, this problem is solved.

This research aims to construct a hybrid technique by combining Crow Search Optimization Algorithm (CSA) with Elman neural network (ENN) for leukemia DNA sequences classification. The proposed model is called Crow-ENN. The objective of the proposed hybrid model to construct the proposed optimized machine learning classification model for Leukemia DNA sequences classification and the performance evaluation of the proposed hybrid algorithm by comparing its Mean Square Error (MSE) and accuracy with the existing models.

This study is aimed to classify Leukemia DNA sequences using the proposed hybrid Crow-ENN model. Datasets of Leukemia DNA sequences are taken from NCBI (National Center for Biotechnology Information) database. Two measures are used for the performance evaluation of the proposed model, which are; MSE and Accuracy.

2. RELEVANT LITERATURE

Sarhan, (2009) developed a stomach cancer identification model that is based on ANN and DCT. The proposed methodology extracts feature from stomach microarrays for classification through Discrete Cosine Transform (DCT). The features which are extracted by DCT coefficients are then used by Artificial Neural Network (ANN) to classify whether it is tumor or non-tumor. Next in 2015, (Adetiba et al., 2015) reported a tentative comparison of Support SVM) and ANN combined and their non-combined variants for the prediction of lung cancer. The Voss DNA encoding was applied for mapping the nucleotide sequences of altered genomes and non-altered genomes for gaining the same numerical genomic sequences to train the selected models/classifiers. (Giang et al., 2016) proposed a new model called the convolutional neural network for DNA sequences classification. The study used DNA sequences as simple text data. One-hot vectors are used for representing DNA sequences to the model. (Dakhli et al., 2016) presented a model of the Wavelet Neural Networks which are applied for the DNA sequences classification. (Patel et al., 2016) proposed a model based on the back-propagation algorithm for the classification of breakable genome sequences. (Kumar, 2016) developed an ANN approach to classify Acute Myelogenous Leukemia (AML) and Acute Lymphocytic Leukemia (ALL). Kassim et al. (2017) proposed a Convolutional Neural Network (CNN) based deep learning model for classification of whole genomic sequences of an organism. Zaman et al. (2017) proposed a model for gene sequences classification using Back Propagation Neural Network (BPNN). In the bioinformatics field, different machine learning approaches i.e. ANN or (SVM) are applied for analyzing and classifying gene sequences. BPNN is very efficient and effective for the classification of sequences of hypertension gene and it identifies the illness. Bzhalava et al. (2018) trained Artificial Neural Network (ANN) and Random Forest (RF) by the use of metagenomic sequences that were classified taxonomically into the virus and non-virus classes. Zheng et al. (2019) introduced a nucleotide-level Convolutional Neural Networks (CNNs) for classification of pre-miRNAs. "one-hot" encoding and padding are used for the conversion of pre-miRNAs into matrixes of the same shape. By simulating the proposed models on the test dataset and comparing them with some traditional machine learning models, it is showed that the proposed model gave better results. The prediction accuracies of all the proposed models were about 90%. Tan et al. (2019) proposed a deep recurrent neural network-based ensemble model for identifying enhancers. The features of deep ensemble networks were made from 6 kinds of dinucleotide physicochemical properties, which performed better as compared to other features. The proposed ensemble method can classify enhancers with an accuracy of 75.5%. While in classifying enhancers as strong and weak sequences, the proposed model attained an accuracy of 68.49%. Wen et al. (2019) established a convolutional neural network and k-mers based classification approach for mRNA and lncRNA. First, lncRNA and mRNA sequences are converted into k-mer frequency matrix, then the convolutional neural network is trained by inputting the k-mer frequency matrix. The classification model has the highest accuracy with 1-mers, 2-mers, and 3-mers that is 98.72% in humans, 87.97% in mice and 99.63% in chickens, which is the better accuracy as compared to the accuracies of random forest, decision tree, logistic regression, and SVM.

3. ARTIFICIAL NEURAL NETWORKS (ANN)

In simple words, artificial neural networks (ANNs) are the imitation of the human brain. The natural brain is capable of learning novel things and adapting to a new and changing environment. The most wonderful ability of the brain is that it can analyze the information or data which is incomplete and unclear and the brain can make its judgment from that data. E.g. we can read the handwriting of other people although their way of writing may be fully different from the way we write. A few days old babies can identify their mother from smell, voice and touch. We can recognize a person which is known to us even from a blurred photo (Kukreja et al., 2016).

The brain is composed of cells which are called neurons. The combination or interconnection of these neurons builds up a neural network or brain. The human brain has approximately 8.6 x 1010 (86 billion) neurons and approximately 10000 connections with each other. ANN is the copy or imitation of natural or biological neural networks in which artificial neurons are interconnected in the same way as the brain neural network. A biological neuron has three parts: cell body, axon and dendrite. The function of the dendrite is the ability to receive electro-chemical signals into the cell body from other neurons. The cell body has a nucleus and other chemical molecules which are required for the support of cell. It is also called Soma. Axon works as a carrier which carries signal from one neuron to others. The link or connection between dendrites of two neurons or between neuron and muscle cells is called synapse (Kohli et al., 2014). Figure 1 displays the structure of a biological neuron.

4. CROW SEARCH ALGORITHM (CSA)

Crow search algorithm (CSA) is a bio-inspired population-based meta-heuristic optimizer which simulates the intellectual behavior of crows. Crow Search Algorithm was proposed in 2016 by Alireza Askarzadeh. It works on the idea of storing extra food by crows in some hiding places and the retrieval of this food when they need it. Crows are considered the most intelligent birds because of their large brain size.

Crows are living in groups or flocks. They hide their foods in some hiding places. They can remember these places to recall their hidden food even after several months. They follow each other to know about their food hiding places and to steal the hidden food. When a crow commits thievery, then for the sack of securing its food, it takes some precautionary steps like moving to some hiding places randomly for avoiding being pilfered by other crows. As a thief, using their expertise, they predict the actions of a thief and can decide the safest place for protecting their food from being theft. The above intelligent behaviors of crows are used as an optimization process in CSA.

Crow Search Algorithm has the following principles of crows like:

- They are living in groups or flocks.
- They remember the location of the places where they hide their food.
- They keep an eye on each other to commit thievery.
- They safeguard their stored food from being theft by a probability.

With a number of N crows in a d-dimensional search space, the location of each crow i at the iteration *iter* in the search environment is indicated by a vector (x):

Figure 1. Structure of a biological neuron

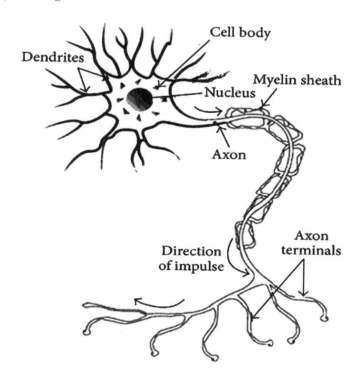

$$x^{i,iter} = [x_1^{i,iter}, x_2^{i,iter}, x_3^{i,iter}, ..., x_d^{i,iter}]$$

Vector (x) represents the values of the control variables which are random primary positions. Then at each iteration, they update their positions while searching for their best food source (solution to the optimization problem). For every iteration, this process is repeated till $iter_{max}$ is reached. Every crow has a memory $m^{i,iter}$ where they store their best food hiding places position.

Suppose, iteration *iter*, there may happen two conditions:

Condition 1: Crow *j* does not know that Crow *i* is following it. As a result, the food hiding place of crow *j* will be approached by crow *i*. In this scenario, the new location of crow *i* can be gotten as:

$$x^{i,iter+1} = x^{i,iter} + r_i * fl^{i,iter} (m^{j,iter} - x^{i,iter})$$

Where r_i is a random number between 0 and 1 with uniform distribution and $fl^{i,iter}$ denotes the flight length of crow *i* at iteration *iter*. Small values of *fl* result in local search (at the vicinity of $x^{i,iter}$) while global search (far from $x^{i,iter}$) is resulted by the large values of *fl*. Figure 3(a) indicates, when the value of *fl* chosen smaller than 1, the subsequent location of crow *i* is between $x^{i,iter}$ and $m^{j,iter}$ on the dashed line. As figure 3(b) shows, when the value of *fl* is chosen greater than 1, then the next location of crow *i* may exceed $m^{j,iter}$ on the dashed line.

Condition 2: Crow *i* is following Crow *j* but Crow *j* knows about it. Then as a result, for the sack of securing its stored food from being theft, crow *j* will make fool of crow *i* by going randomly to some other position in the search environment. Condition 1 and 2 can be shown as:

$$x^{i,iter+1} = \begin{cases} x^{i,iter} + r_i \, fl^{i,iter} * \left(m^{j,iter} - x^{i,iter}\right) & r_j \geq AP^{j,iter} \\ a \; random \; position & otherwise \end{cases}$$

In Crow Search Algorithm, the intensification and diversification are mainly controlled by the parameter of awareness probability (AP). A decrease in the value of AP leads CSA to search in the local region and a local optimal solution is carried out in this region. Using small values of AP increases intensification. Furthermore, increasing the AP values decreases the probability of conducting local search and CSA conducts a global search (randomization). As a result, diversification increases by using large values of AP.

Based on the fitness values of the new position, each crow's memory is also updated as:

$$m^{i,iter+1} = \begin{cases} x^{i,iter+1} & f\left(x^{i,iter+1}\right) \geq f\left(m^{j,iter}\right) \\ \left(m^{j,iter}\right) & otherwise \end{cases}$$

If the fitness value of a new position is better than the fitness value of a memorized one, then the crow updates its memory to the new position (Askarzadeh, 2016). Figure 2 displays the pseudo-code of CSA. Similarly, figure 3 shows the flowchart of CSA Condition 1.

5. PROPOSED METHODOLOGY

This study comprised of two core stages which are pre-processing phase and post-processing. Binary codification of DNA sequences and conversion of Binary DNA sequences into the windows of length 4, 8, and 12 is done in pre-processing phase, while in post-processing, the workflow can be broken down into two sub-steps which is learning of the model and its evaluation in terms of accuracy and MSE. Figure 4 shows the research flow graphically.

5.1 Collection of Benchmark Datasets

The cancer DNA sequences data is obtained from the NCBI database for training and testing the proposed hybrid model. NCBI is a platform where so many Databases are available containing any kind of molecular biology data like DNA sequences, Protein Sequences, Gene Expressions etc. Any kind of DNA sequence may be obtained from these databases e.g. the data about different diseases like Cancer, Diabetes etc. The data about Leukemia is collected here for this research, which is discussed below.

5.1.1 Acute Lymphoblastic Leukemia (ALL) DNA Sequence

The source of this DNA sequence is Homo sapiens which is the biological name for a human. The full definition of this sequence on NCBI is "Homo sapiens t(9;22) (q34,q11) reciprocal chromosomal translocation breakpoint, patient 6853 with acute lymphoblastic leukemia". FN869174 is the accession number of this sequence, through which, it can be accessed on NCBI. This DNA sequence has a total 464

Figure 2. Pseudocode of the CSA

```
Start
1.      Randomly initialize the position of a flock of N crows in the search space
2.      Evaluate the position of the crows
3.      Initialize the memory of each crow
4.      while iter < iter_max
            for i = 1: N (all N crows of the flock)
5.      Randomly choose one of the crows to follow (for example j)
6.      Define an awareness probability
            if r_j ≥ AP^{j,iter}
                    x^{i,iter+1} = x^{i,iter} + r_i × fl^{i,iter} × (m^{j,iter} − x^{i,iter})
            else
                    x^{i,iter+1} = a random position of search space
            end if
            end for
7.      Check the feasibility of new positions
8.      Evaluate the new position of the crows
9.      Update the memory of crows
        end while
    end
```

nucleotides. The individual nucleotides count of the DNA sequence is given below in table 1. Similarly, figure 5 shows the percent nucleotides count of ALL DNA sequence.

The individual nucleotides density and A-T and C-G combination density of the ALL DNA sequence is shown in figure 6.

5.1.2 Acute Myeloid Leukemia (AML) DNA Sequence

The source of this DNA sequence is Homo sapiens which is the biological name for a human. The full definition of this sequence on NCBI is "Homo sapiens t(8;16)(p11;p13) chimeric MOZ/CBP genomic DNA from acute myeloid leukemia patient (case 4)". AJ315158 is the accession number of this sequence, through which, it can be accessed on NCBI. This DNA sequence has a total 480 base pairs. The individual nucleotides count of the DNA sequence is given below in table 2. Similarly, figure 7 shows the percent nucleotides count of ALL DNA sequence.

The individual nucleotides density and A-T and C-G combination density of the AML DNA sequence is shown in figure 8.

Figure 3. CSA Condition 1 Flowchart

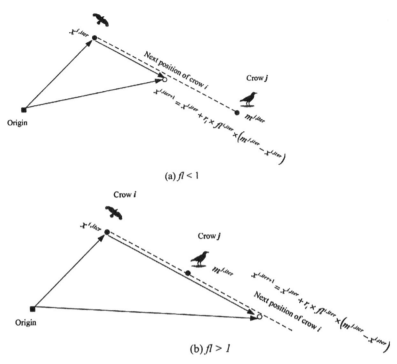

5.2 Data Preprocessing

Before the data is being mined, it is very important to be processed. This process is called the preprocessing of data. Data preprocessing is a vital step for enhancing the efficiency of data. It is one of the many data mining steps which deals with the transformation and preparation of the dataset into a format from which the needed features and parameters can easily be mined efficiently (Bhaya, 2017). Data preprocessing will be done in the following two steps.

5.2.1 Binary Codification of DNA Sequences

The binary codification of DNA sequences will be done for efficient machine readability. Binary codification of DNA sequences will be done according to some rules, which are given below:

Binary Coding Scheme ------- 2 1

Adenine (A) = 0 0 = 0

Thymine (T) = 0 1 = 1

Guanine (G) = 1 0 = 2

Figure 4. Step by step research process

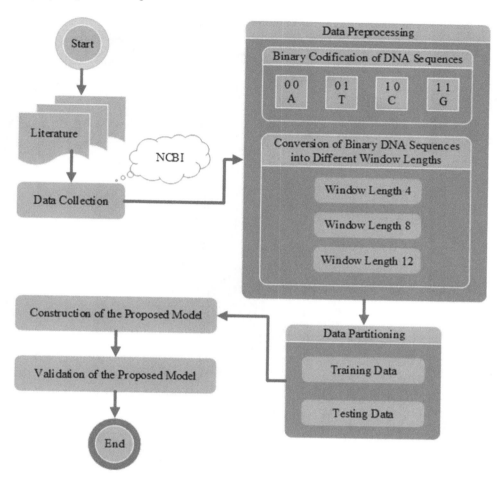

Cytosine (C) = 1 1 =3

In this way, the whole DNA sequences will be converted from Nucleotides form to Binary.
Suppose we have a DNA sequence "ATCCAGAC" which have 7 base pairs, then according to an above coding scheme, its binary version will look like "0 0 0 1 1 1 1 1 0 0 1 0 0 0 1 1".

Table 1. Individual nucleotide counts of all DNA sequences

Nucleotide	Count	Percentage
Adenine (A)	125	26.939655%
Cytosine (C)	109	23.491379%
Guanine (G)	99	21.336207%
Thymine (T)	131	28.232759%

Figure 5. Percent nucleotides counts of ALL DNA sequence

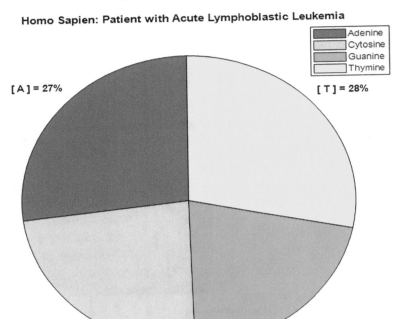

Figure 6. Nucleotides density of ALL DNA sequence

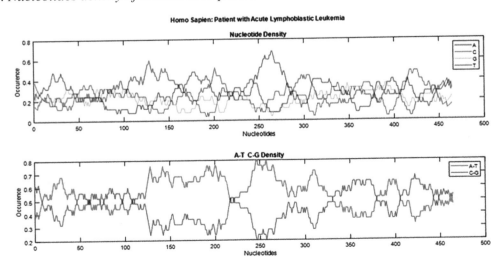

Table 2. Individual nucleotides count of AML DNA sequence

Nucleotide	Count	Percentage
Adenine (A)	134	27.916667%
Cytosine (C)	72	15.000000%
Guanine (G)	88	18.333333%
Thymine (T)	186	38.750000%

$$\frac{00}{A} \frac{01}{T} \frac{11}{C} \frac{11}{C} \frac{00}{A} \frac{10}{G} \frac{00}{A} \frac{11}{C}$$

5.2.2 Selection of Window Lengths

Observing a single nucleotide separately does not lead to good results using neural networks. The interaction between the nucleotides in a DNA sequence needs to be maintained in some way that a neural network can easily read and give promising results. For the aim of getting better results from neural

Figure 7. Percent nucleotides count of AML DNA sequence

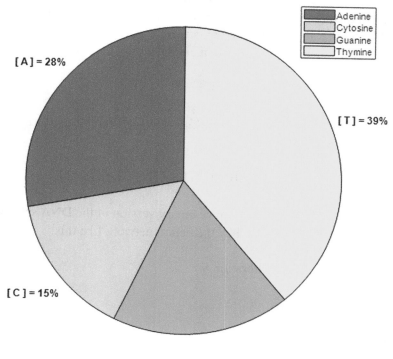

Homo Sapien: Patient with Acute Myeloid Leukemia

[A] = 28%

[T] = 39%

[C] = 15%

[G] = 18%

(Legend: Adenine, Cytosine, Guanine, Thymine)

Figure 8. Nucleotides density of AML DNA sequence

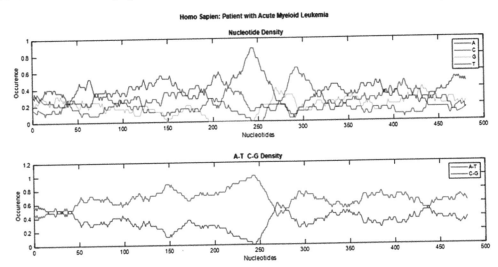

networks, windows of different lengths are considered (Hasic et al., 2017). This research considered windows of length 4, 8, and 12.

5.2.2.1 Window Length 4

While considering the window of length 4, the neural network will read a group of 8 binary digits at a time from the whole DNA sequence because one nucleotide is represented by two binary digits. Then it will go forward and will read the stream of the next 8 binary digits. In this way, the neural network will read the whole DNA sequence and will compute it stream by stream.

Suppose we have a DNA sequence having 30 nucleotides:

ATCCAGACTGTCCACAGCATTCCGCTGACC

Then using the above Binary Coding Scheme, it is converted into binary form which has 60 binary bits and looks like:

000111110010001101100111110011001011000101111110110110001111

According to the window of length 4, the above binary version of the DNA sequence is divided into streams of 8 binary bits. Then it will be read by the neural network like this:

Iteration 1 Iteration 2 Iteration 3 …….. Iteration 8

00011111 00011111 00011111 ……… 00011111

00100011 00100011 00100011 ……… 00100011

01100111 01100111 01100111 01100111

11001100 11001100 11001100 11001100

10110001 10110001 10110001 10110001

01111110 01111110 01111110 01111110

11011000 11011000 11011000 11011000

1111 1111 1111 1111

5.2.2.2 Window Length 8

While considering the window of length 8, the neural network will read a group of 16 binary digits at a time from the whole DNA sequence because one nucleotide is represented by two binary digits. Then it will go forward and will read the stream of the next 16 binary digits. In this way, the whole DNA sequence will be read by the neural network and will be computed stream by stream.

Using the window of length 8, the above binary sequence will be divided into streams of 16 binary bits. Then it will be read by the neural network like this:

Iteration 1 .... Iteration 2 .... Iteration 4

0001111100100011 0001111100100011 0001111100100011

0110011111001100 0110011111001100 0110011111001100

1011000101111110 1011000101111110 1011000101111110

110110001111 110110001111 110110001111

5.2.2.3 Window Length 12

While considering the window of length 12, the neural network will read a group of 24 binary digits at a time from the whole DNA sequence because one nucleotide is represented by two binary digits. Then it will go forward and will read the stream of the next 24 binary digits. In this way, the whole DNA sequence will be read by the neural network and will be computed stream by stream.

Using the window of length 12, the above binary sequence will be divided into streams of 24 binary bits. Then it will be read by the neural network like this:

Iteration 1 .... Iteration 3

000111110010001101100111 000111110010001101100111

11001100101100010111110 ……. 11001100101100010111110

110110001111 ……. 110110001111

5.3 Data Partitioning

In artificial neural networks, Data partitioning is a very important step. By the use of data partitioning, the best neural network models may be obtained (Rehman et al., 2011). First of all, the data for the classification problem is divided into two different subsets: Training data and testing data. The majority part of the data is used for training purposes of neural networks while a minimum portion of it is used to test the ANNs (Nawi et al., 2007). Table 3 displays the details of the DNA sequences used in this research.

5.4 The Proposed "Crow-ENN" Model

This research proposed a novel hybrid technique called Crow-ENN, which is the combination of Crow Search Algorithm (CSA) and Elman Neural Network (ENN) for Leukemia DNA sequences classification. In Crow-ENN, every position denotes a possible solution (i.e. the weight space and the corresponding biases for ENN optimization). The food source position and the weight optimization problem shows the quality of a solution. In the first iteration, the best biases and weights are initialized with CSA and after that those weights are given to the ENN.

The central theme of this hybrid model is that CSA is used at the beginning stage of searching for the optimum to choose the best initial weights. After this, ENN continues the training process using the best weights from CSA. Furthermore, in the next iteration, CSA will update the weights again with the best possible solution, it will continue passing the best weights to ENN until the final iteration of the network is encountered or either the MSE is reached.

The pseudocode for the Crow-ENN algorithm is given in figure 9. Similarly, figure 10 shows the flow diagram of the proposed hybrid Crow-ENN model. The performance of the proposed algorithm is shown in section "Results" and compared with other conventional models in terms of MSE and accuracy.

5.5 Verification of the Proposed Model

The performance evaluation of any model is been checked by some standard measures like sensitivity, specificity, accuracy, error rate, f-score, precision, recall, mean square error, etc. These measures have their values for every model. Different models are checked and compared with each other through these measures. The model with the best measures is then called the best model for a particular problem (Pow-

Table 3. Details of used DNA sequence

Dataset	No. of Nucleotides	Training Data	Testing Data
ALL DNA Sequence	464	70%	30%
AML DNA Sequence	480	70%	30%

Figure 9. Pseudo code of the Crow-ENN algorithm

```
    Begin
1: Initialize Crows Population size, Flight Length, Awareness Probability and ENN structure
2: Load the training and testing data
3: While MSE<stopping criteria
4: Pass the Best food source as weights to the network
5: Feed forward network runs using the weights initialized with CSA
6: Calculate the error using the Equation (3.10)
7: Minimize the error using by adjusting network parameter using CSA
8: Generate Crow food source (xⱼ) by going to another position of the search space.
                xᵢ = xⱼ
9: Evaluate the fitness of the food source, choose a random Crow i
        If
            a.    Xⱼ > Xᵢ        Then
            b.    xᵢ ← xⱼ
            c.    Xᵢ ← Xⱼ
        End if
10: CSA keeps on calculating the best possible weight at each iteration until the network is
    converged.
    End While
11: Post process Results and Visualization.
    End
```

ers, 2008). In the case of this research, the proposed model will be checked for its performance on the bases of its Accuracy and Mean Squared Error (MSE).

5.5.1 Accuracy

Accuracy is the most native measure of performance evaluation. The inverse of difference between the real answer and the simulation results gives the generalization accuracy which is denoted by the range of percentage boundaries. Accuracy is a great measure. The high accuracy of a model means that the model is best. (Nawi et al., 2007)

$$\text{Accuracy (\%)} = \frac{1 - \left| y_i - \hat{y}_i \right|}{UB - LB} * 100$$

y_i = Actual Value
$\hat{y}_i$ = Predicted Value
UB = Upper Bound of the activation function
LB = Lower Bound of the activation function

Figure 10. The proposed Crow-ENN Algorithm flowchart

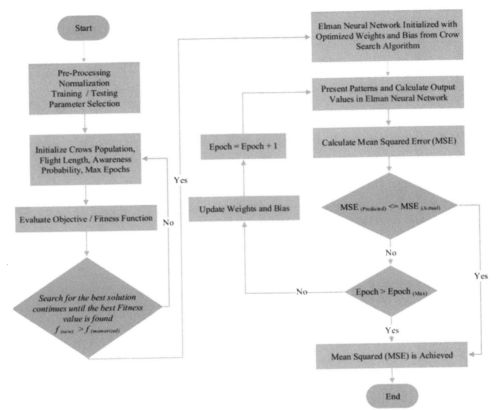

5.5.2 Mean Squared Error

Mean Squared Error (MSE) is the average of squared difference between the predicted value of an estimator and the actual values. (Kamble et al., 2017)

$$MSE = \frac{1}{n} \sum_{i=1}^{n} \left(y_i - \hat{y}_i \right)^2$$

n = Number of samples
y_i = Actual Value
$\hat{y}_i$ = Predicted Value

6. PRELIMINARY STUDY

The tool and system used in this research work to implement and analyze the proposed and other models contain these specifications. The operating system used in this research is Windows 8.1 Pro 64-bit (6.3, Build 9600). The used system is manufactured by Haier Information Technology (Shen Zhen) Co., Ltd. The model of system is Haier Y11C, BIOS is 1.23, processor is Intel(R) Core(TM) m3-7Y30 CPU @ 1.00GHz (4 CPUs), ~1.6GHz, memory is 8192MB RAM, available OS memory is 8110MB RAM, and the tool used for the implementation purpose is MATLAB R2018a (9.4.0.813654) 64-bit.

7. RESULTS

7.1 Results for [ALL] Window Length 4

The above table shows the results obtained from the six-different model which are used in this research work. The dataset of Acute Lymphoblastic Leukemia DNA sequence is being given as input to all the models in the form of the window of length 4. Crow-ENN is a proposed model amongst these and the rest are being evaluated for comparison purposes. Three of the models are hybrid and three are not. Table 4 demonstrates the accuracy and MSE for training and testing of the proposed and other models. All the models are being evaluated with 1000 iterations. The research used 70% of the data for training and 30% for testing all the models.

In this study, the most efficient and promising results for training are given by the proposed Crow-ENN model with the highest accuracy of 99.99034% and the lowest MSE of 0.000193%. In addition, Crow-ANN comes in the second position according to its accuracy rate of 97.95019% and MSE of 0.040996%. After this, ANN achieved the Accuracy of 97.82658% and MSE of 0.003539%. BPNN gives an accuracy rate of 97.50548% and MSE of 0.002684%. With the accuracy of 95.24661% and MSE of 0.095068%, Crow-BPNN got 5th position in the list. The lowest accuracy is achieved by ENN. ENN got 85.48019% of accuracy and 0.091912% of MSE.

During testing, the highest rate of 99.98836% accuracy with the lowest MSE of 0.000233% is been given by the proposed Crow-ENN model. Furthermore, ANN obtained the second-highest accuracy of 97.5173% with the MSE of 0.004436%. BPNN comes after ANN with the Accuracy rate of 97.354995% and MSE of 0.002941%. Crow-ANN and Crow-BPNN come at the fourth and fifth positions after BPNN

Table 4. Results of all models for [ALL] window length 4

Algorithms	Training		Testing	
	MSE	Accuracy	MSE	Accuracy
Crow-ENN	0.000193	99.99034	0.000233	99.98836
Crow-ANN	0.040996	97.95019	0.058214	97.08929
Crow-BPNN	0.095068	95.24661	0.087865	95.60675
ANN	0.003539	97.82658	0.004436	97.5173
BPNN	0.002684	97.50548	0.002941	97.35499
ENN	0.091912	85.48019	0.051795	89.5674

with the accuracies of 97.08929% and 95.60675% and with the MSEs of 0.058214% and 0.087865% respectively. ENN delivers the lowest accuracy of 89.5674% and the MSE of 0.051795%.

From the above results, it is concluded that Crow-ENN provides an optimal solution with the highest training accuracy of 99.99034% with the lowest MSE of 0.000193% on 70% of training data. While for 30% of testing data, it gives the highest accuracy of 99.98836% with the lowest MSE 0.000233%. Crow-ENN gives the most efficient results as compared to all other used models. Figure 11, figure 12 and figure 13 show graphically the testing Accuracy and MSE for each model used in this research.

7.2 Results for [ALL] Window Length 8

The above table displays the results of six various models that are used in this research. These results are obtained by giving as input the Acute Lymphoblastic Leukemia dataset in the form of the window of length 8 to all the six models. All the models are trained by 70% of the data and tested by 30% of the data. The performance of each model used in this study is been checked with 1000 iterations. As it can be seen that in the training performances of all models, Crow-ENN have performed very well and efficient in terms of both the accuracy and MSE. It has obtained the highest accuracy of 99.97562% with the lowest MSE of 0.000488%. The second highest accuracy is achieved by ANN which is 97.5319% with the MSE of 0.004557%. Crow-ANN attained 97.51947% of accuracy and 0.049611% of MSE. BPNN, Crow-BPNN, and ENN have reached the accuracies of 97.43696%, 94.88994% and 88.2631% respectively and their MSEs are 0.002892%, 0.102201%, and 0.057757% individually.

Using 30% of testing data, among all the used models, Crow-ENN has performed very efficiently by reaching the highest accuracy of 99.97585% with the lowest MSE of 0.000483%. The second highest accuracy is been achieved by Crow-ANN which is 98.84643% with the MSE of 0.023071%. BPNN obtained 97.6531% of accuracy and 0.002354% of MSE. At last, Crow-BPNN and ENN acquired the accuracies of 95.21757% and 88.63178 with the MSEs of 0.095649% and 0.056315% correspondingly. Figure 14, figure 15 and figure 16 displays graphically the testing accuracies and MSEs of each model.

7.3 Results for [ALL] Window Length 12

The table given above illustrates the training and testing performances of all the six models used in this research. 70% of the Acute Lymphoblastic Leukemia (ALL) DNA sequence dataset is used for training and 30% is used for testing all the models. The input to the models is given in the form of window length 12. The most efficient result in training is recorded from Crow-ENN with an accuracy of 99.97027% and MSE of 0.000595%. Cow-ANN obtained the second most efficient accuracy which is 98.1426% with the MSE of 0.037148%. ANN reached the accuracy of 97.5612% and the MSE of 0.00441%. BPNN comes at the fourth position according to its accuracy which is 97.34393% and its MSE is 0.00292%. Furthermore, Crow-BPNN achieved 95.21946% of accuracy with the MSE of 0.095611%. ENN got 88.15782% of accuracy and 0.0699% of MSE.

In the testing stage, Crow-ENN acquired an accuracy of 99.98085% with the MSE of 0.000383% which is the most promising result amongst all the six models. Crow-ANN comes after Crow-ENN with an accuracy rate of 98.5158% and MSE of 0.029684%. ANN achieved the third most efficient accuracy of 97.60209% with the MSE of 0.004324%. BPNN, Crow-BPNN, and ENN attained the accuracies of 97.35398%, 94.73091%, and 88.3004% with the MSE rates of 0.003045%, 0.105382%, and 0.059574% individually. Figure 17, figure 18 and figure 19 displays the Testing performance of each model graphically.

Crow-ENN

Figure 11. Graphical representations of Crow-ENN & Crow-ANN's performance for [ALL] WL 4

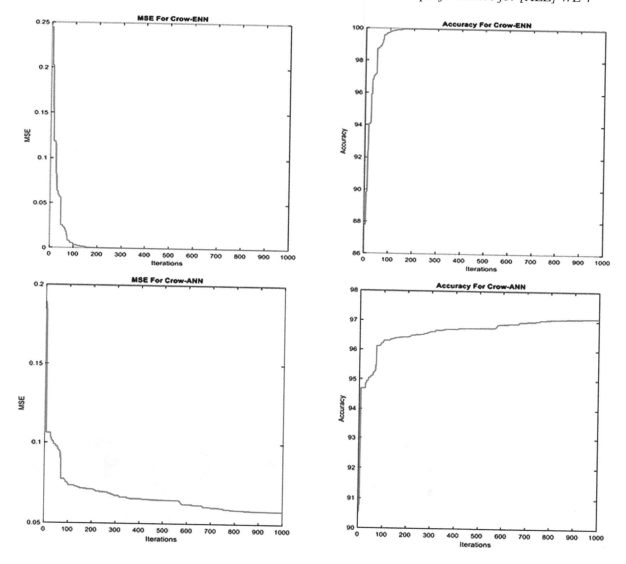

7.4 Results for [AML] Window Length 4

This table about the simulation results of all six models which are trained and tested with Acute Myeloid Leukemia (AML) DNA sequence with the window of length 4. All the given models are checked for their performance in terms of accuracy and Mean Squared Error (MSE). According to the training accuracy and MSE, Crow-ENN is the most efficient model amongst all used models. Crow-ENN obtained 99.98058% of accuracy with the MSE of 0.000388%. With the accuracy rate of 98.21847% and MSE of 0.035631%, Crow-ANN is in the second position. BPNN attained an accuracy of 97.44197% and the MSE of 0.002828% which puts it on the third position. ANN, Crow-BPNN, and ENN achieved the accuracies of 97.36177%, 94.93133%, and 86.3442% with the MSEs of 0.004734%, 0.101373%, and 0.082023% correspondingly.

191

Figure 12. Graphical representations of Crow-BPNN & ENN's performance for [ALL] WL 4

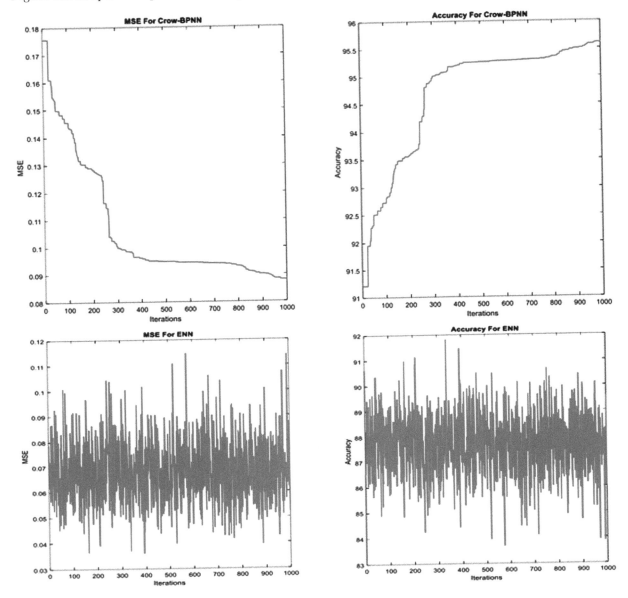

According to testing results, the most promising result is obtained by Crow-ENN with an accuracy of 99.98037% and MSE of 0.000393%. Crow-ANN comes after Crow-ENN according to its accuracy of 98.03103% and the MSE of 0.039379%. ANN acquired an accuracy rate of 97.56172% with the MSE of 0.004248%. BPNN is a little behind ANN having an accuracy of 97.22955% and MSE of 0.003245%. Furthermore, Crow-BPNN and ENN accomplished the accuracies of 95.25042% and 88.39997% with the MSEs of 0.094992% and 0.063512% respectively. Figure 20, figure 21 and figure 22 graphically show the simulation results of testing for all the six models.

Figure 13. Graphical representations of ANN & BPNN's performance for [ALL] WL 4

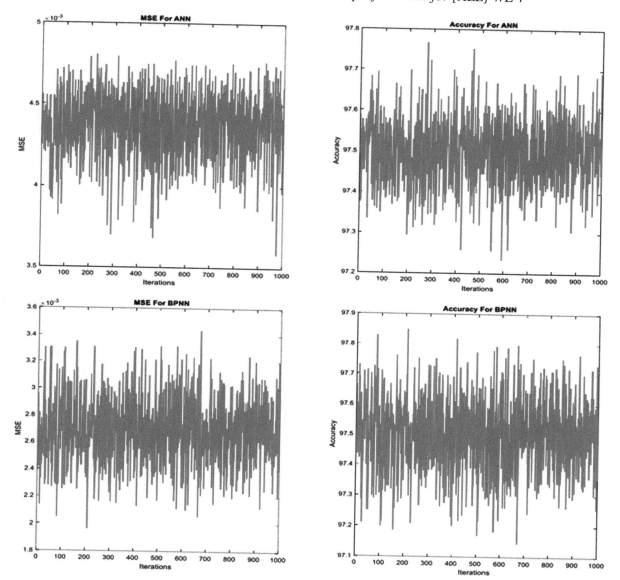

Table 5. Results of all models for [ALL] window length 8

Algorithms	Training		Testing	
	MSE	Accuracy	MSE	Accuracy
Crow-ENN	0.000488	99.97562	0.000483	99.97585
Crow-ANN	0.049611	97.51947	0.023071	98.84643
Crow-BPNN	0.102201	94.88994	0.095649	95.21757
ANN	0.004557	97.5319	0.004618	97.48637
BPNN	0.002892	97.43696	0.002354	97.6531
ENN	0.057757	88.2631	0.056315	88.63178

Figure 14. Graphical representations of Crow-ENN & Crow-ANN's performance for [ALL] WL 4

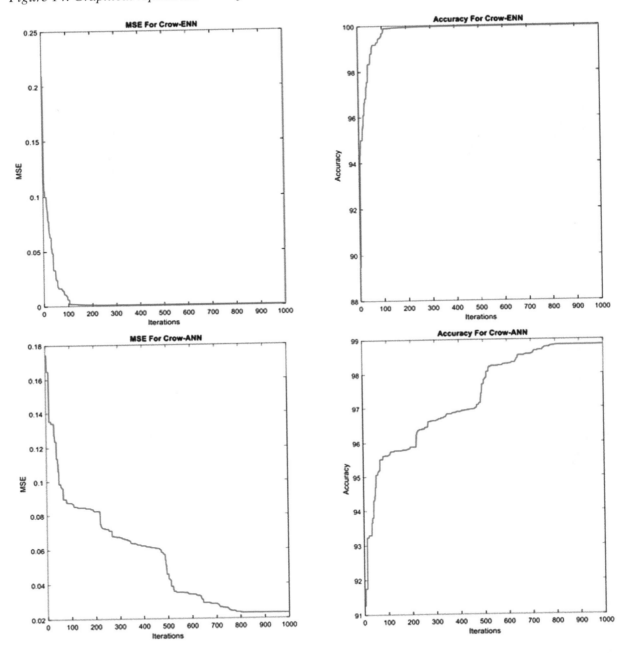

7.5 Results for [AML] Window Length 8

The above table displays the simulation results of all the six models using Acute Myeloid Leukemia DNA sequence window length 8 as input. In this research, 70% of the dataset is used for training and 30% is used for testing all the models. While training, amongst all the models, the most efficient performance is given by Crow-ENN by reaching an accuracy rate of 99.96704% and the MSE of 0.000659%. Crow-

Figure 15. Graphical representations of Crow-BPNN & ENN's performance for [ALL] WL 4

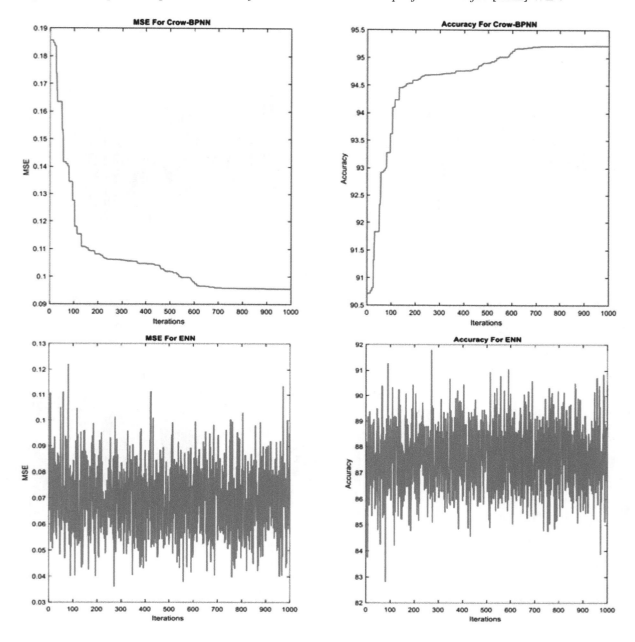

ANN obtained 97.66717% of accuracy and 0.046657% of MSE which takes it to the second position. 97.62648% of accuracy and 0.004186% of MSE is achieved by ANN. Furthermore, BPNN, Crow-BPNN, and ENN attained the accuracies of 97.54013%, 94.97907%, and 84.18195% with the MSEs of 0.002607%, 0.100419%, and 0.10759% respectively.

According to testing results, Crow-ENN has outperformed all the models by acquiring an accuracy rate of 99.98868% and the MSE of 0.000226%. Crow-ANN has the second-highest accuracy of 98.17621% and the MSE of 0.036476%. By reaching the accuracy of 97.68855% and the MSE of 0.002315%, BPNN

Figure 16. Graphical representations of ANN & BPNN's performance for [ALL] WL 4

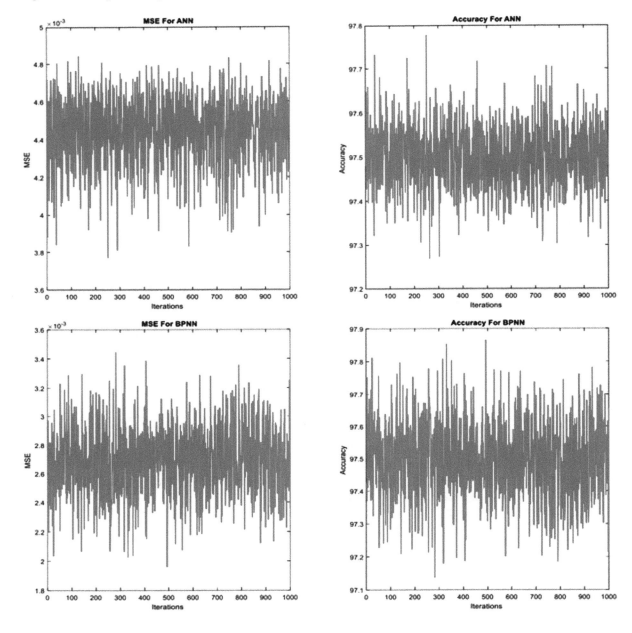

Table 6. Results of all models for [ALL] window length 12

Algorithms	Training		Testing	
	MSE	Accuracy	MSE	Accuracy
Crow-ENN	0.000595	99.97027	0.000383	99.98085
Crow-ANN	0.037148	98.1426	0.029684	98.5158
Crow-BPNN	0.095611	95.21946	0.105382	94.73091
ANN	0.00441	97.5612	0.004324	97.60209
BPNN	0.00292	97.34393	0.003045	97.35398
ENN	0.0699	88.15782	0.059574	88.3004

comes after Crow-ANN. Moreover, ANN, Crow-BPNN, and ENN procured the accuracies of 97.35031%, 94.87081%, and 87.08641% with the MSEs of 0.004602%, 0.102584%, and 0.07303% individually. Figure 23, figure 24 and figure 25 graphically demonstrate the testing result of all the six models.

7.6 Results for [AML] Window Length 12

Table 9 illustrates the outcomes of the simulation for all the six models using Acute Myeloid Leukemia DNA sequence window length 12 dataset as input. In this research, 70% of the dataset is used for training and 30% is used for testing the models. While training, the most efficient and promising result is recorded from Crow-ENN. It has reached the highest accuracy of 99.97892% with the MSE of 0.000422%. Crow-ANN comes after Crow-ENN by attaining the second-highest accuracy rate of 98.57264% and the MSE of 0.028547%. With the accuracy of 97.51589% and the MSE of 0.004298%, ANN comes behind Crow-ANN. BPNN acquired an accuracy rate of 97.36353% with the MSE of 0.002964%. Likewise, Crow-BPNN and ENN reached the accuracies of 94.35987% and 87.79394% with the MSEs of 0.112803% and 0.069281% correspondingly.

As for the testing results are concerned, with 99.96071% of accuracy and 0.000786% of MSE, Crow-ENN has outperformed all the used models. After this, Crow-ANN acquired the second highest accuracy rate of 98.64829% with the MSE of 0.027034%. BPNN and ANN are near to each other in terms of accuracies which are 97.54685% and 97.49836% and their MSEs are 0.002617% and 0.004555% individually. Moreover, Crow-BPNN and ENN attained the accuracies of 95.03498% and 87.46079% with the MSEs of 0.0993% and 0.071894% correspondingly. Figure 26, figure 27 and figure 28 exhibit graphically the simulation results for testing of all models.

8. CONCLUSION

Crow Search Algorithm (CSA) is a bio-inspired meta-heuristic optimizer which imitates the intelligent behavior of crows. It was proposed by Alireza Askarzadeh in 2016. It is a very useful algorithm and gives the global optimal solution for a problem in the very least amount of time with promising accuracy. These optimization techniques may be combined with artificial neural networks for improving their performance. This study combined Crow Search Algorithm with the Elman Neural network to enhance its performance and accomplish promising results for classification. This research used six different models

Figure 17. Graphical representations of Crow-ENN & Crow-ANN's performance for [ALL] WL 4

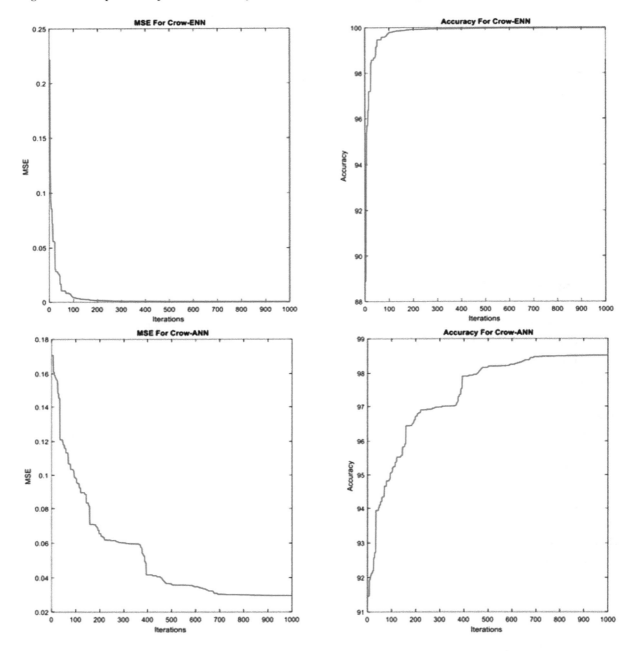

in which, one is a proposed hybrid model and the other five are comparable models. These models are used for the aim of DNA sequence classification. The Leukemia DNA sequences are preprocessed and each is converted into one dataset of windows of length four. Then the models are trained and tested by this dataset. After evaluating these models, their results indicate that Crow Search Algorithm with Elman Neural Network (Crow-ENN) achieved the highest accuracy rate of over 99% for 1000 iterations on every

Figure 18. Graphical representations of Crow-BPNN & ENN's performance for [ALL] WL 4

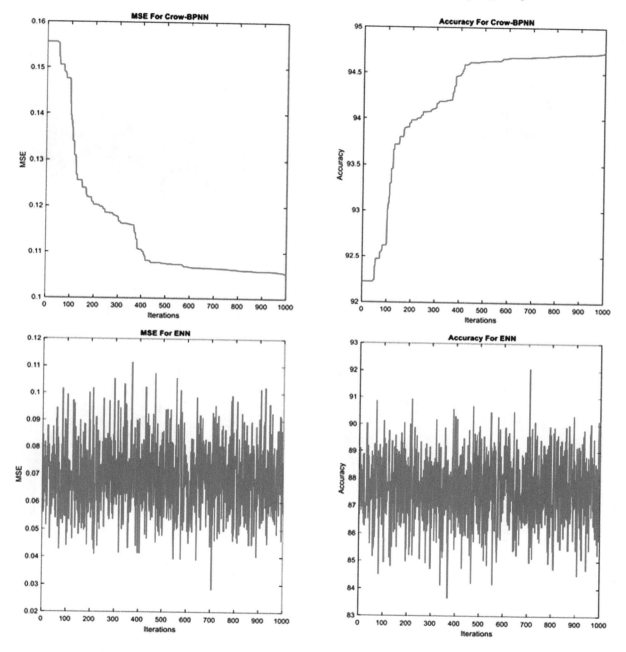

Figure 19. Graphical representations of ANN & BPNN's performance for [ALL] WL 4

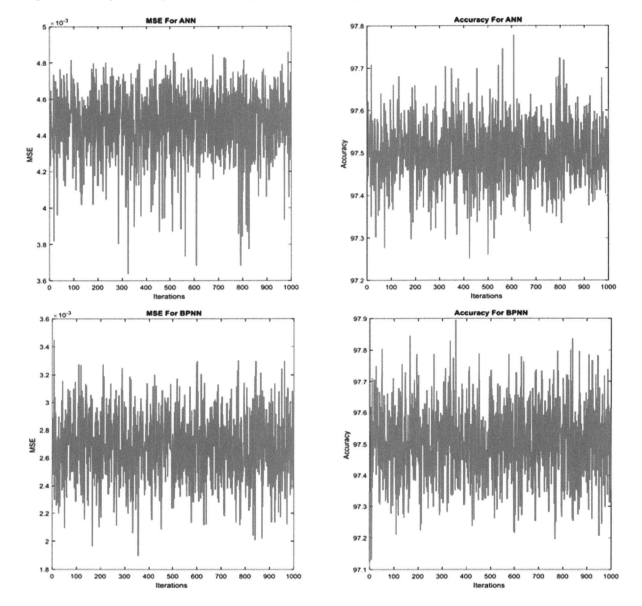

dataset amongst all other used models. Hence it is concluded that the proposed model "Crow-ENN" has outperformed all other five models and became the best classification model for DNA sequences.

9. FUTURE RESEARCH DIRECTION

After simulating and implementing the models successfully, it is seen that the proposed model "Crow-ENN" gives the most promising results with the accuracy over 99% in both training and testing for all

Table 7. Results of all models for [AML] window length 4

Algorithms	Training		Testing	
	MSE	Accuracy	MSE	Accuracy
Crow-ENN	0.000388	99.98058	0.000393	99.98037
Crow-ANN	0.035631	98.21847	0.039379	98.03103
Crow-BPNN	0.101373	94.93133	0.094992	95.25042
ANN	0.004734	97.36177	0.004248	97.56172
BPNN	0.002828	97.44197	0.003245	97.22955
ENN	0.082023	86.3442	0.063512	88.39997

Figure 20. Graphical representations of Crow-ENN & Crow-ANN's performance for [ALL] WL 4

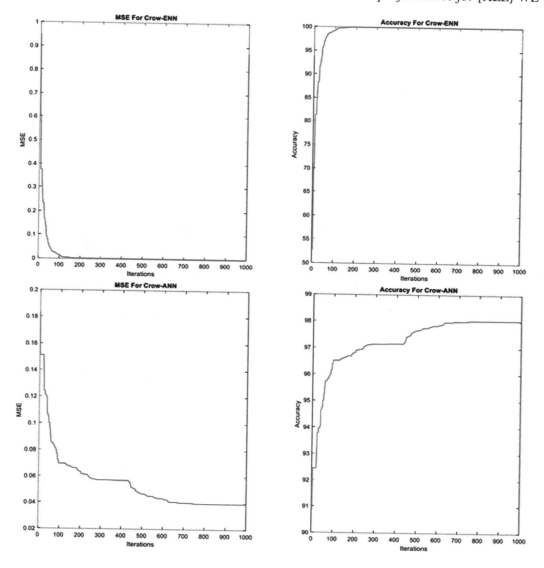

Figure 21. Graphical representations of Crow-BPNN & ENN's performance for [ALL] WL 4

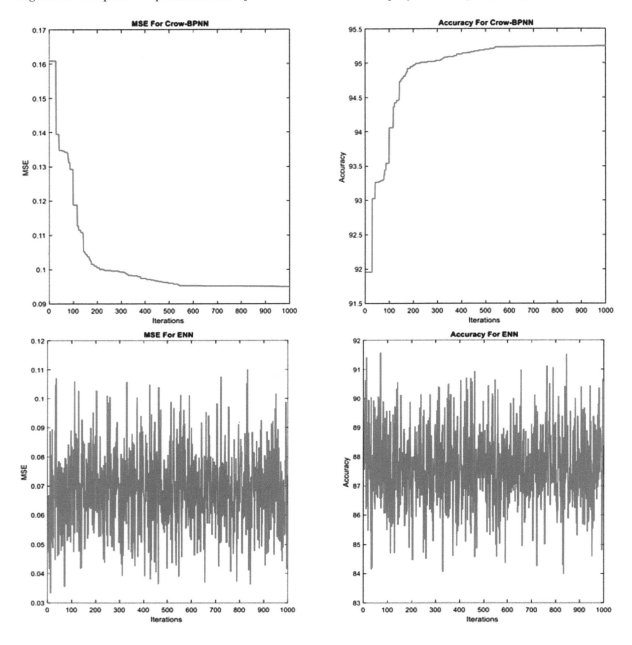

the datasets of leukemia DNA sequences. Its classification accuracy is very high amongst all other used models which indicates the importance and usefulness of meta-heuristic optimization algorithms in combination with artificial neural networks for improving their performance. Therefore, this study recommends the use of this kind of hybrid model for solving different sorts of classification problems with high accuracy and in a minimum amount of time and because of their high accuracy and low time consumption, they will also be very helpful in the future.

Figure 22. Graphical representations of ANN & BPNN's performance for [ALL] WL 4

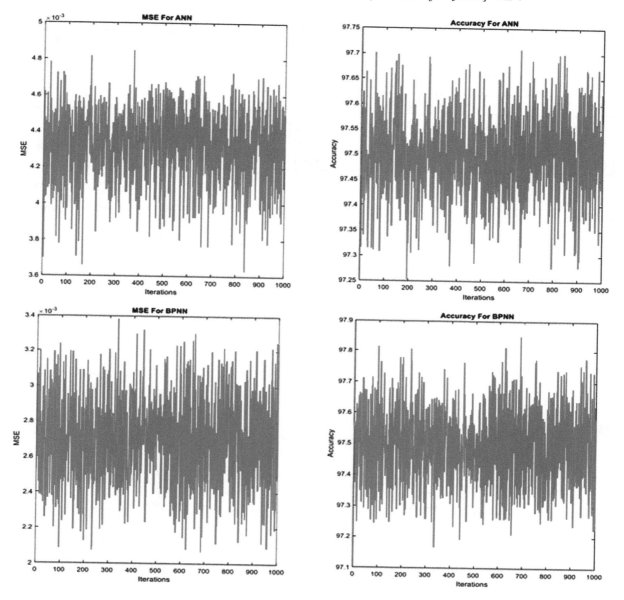

ACKNOWLEDGMENT

The author would like to thank the institute of computer sciences and information technology, faculty of management and computer sciences, the University of Agriculture Peshawar for supporting this research.

Table 8. Results of all models for [AML] window length 8

Algorithms	Training		Testing	
	MSE	Accuracy	MSE	Accuracy
Crow-ENN	0.000659	99.96704	0.000226	99.98868
Crow-ANN	0.046657	97.66717	0.036476	98.17621
Crow-BPNN	0.100419	94.97907	0.102584	94.87081
ANN	0.004186	97.62648	0.004602	97.35031
BPNN	0.002607	97.54013	0.002315	97.68855
ENN	0.10759	84.18195	0.07303	87.08641

Figure 23. Graphical representations of Crow-ENN & Crow-ANN's performance for [ALL] WL 4

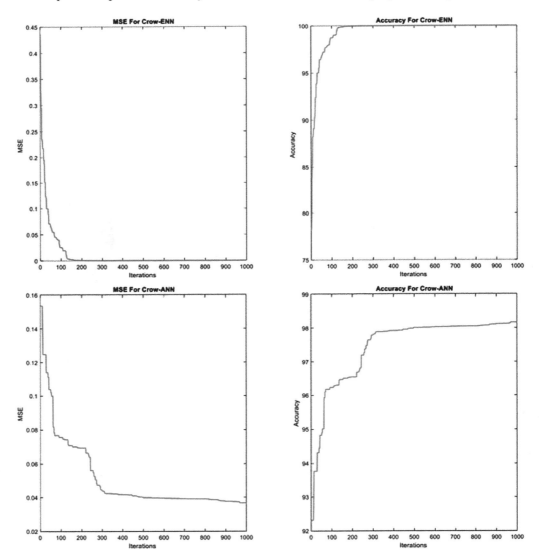

Figure 25. Graphical representations of ANN & BPNN's performance for [ALL] WL 4

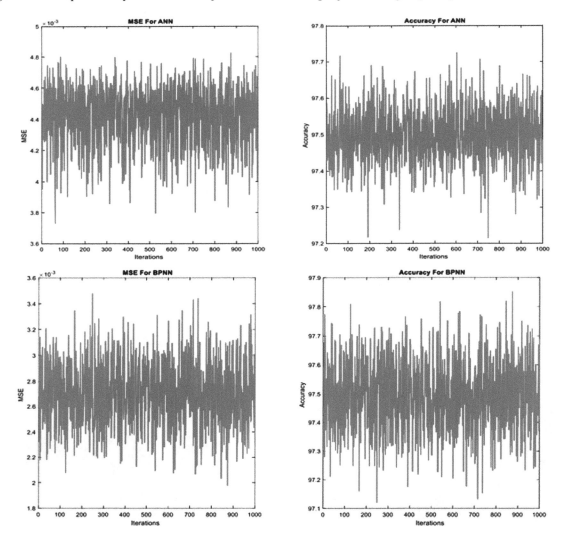

Table 9. Results of all models for [AML] window length 12

Algorithms	Training		Testing	
	MSE	Accuracy	MSE	Accuracy
Crow-ENN	0.000422	99.97892	0.000786	99.96071
Crow-ANN	0.028547	98.57264	0.027034	98.64829
Crow-BPNN	0.112803	94.35987	0.0993	95.03498
ANN	0.004298	97.51589	0.004555	97.49836
BPNN	0.002964	97.36353	0.002617	97.54685
ENN	0.069281	87.79394	0.071894	87.46079

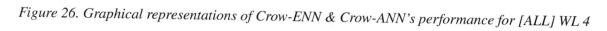

Figure 26. Graphical representations of Crow-ENN & Crow-ANN's performance for [ALL] WL 4

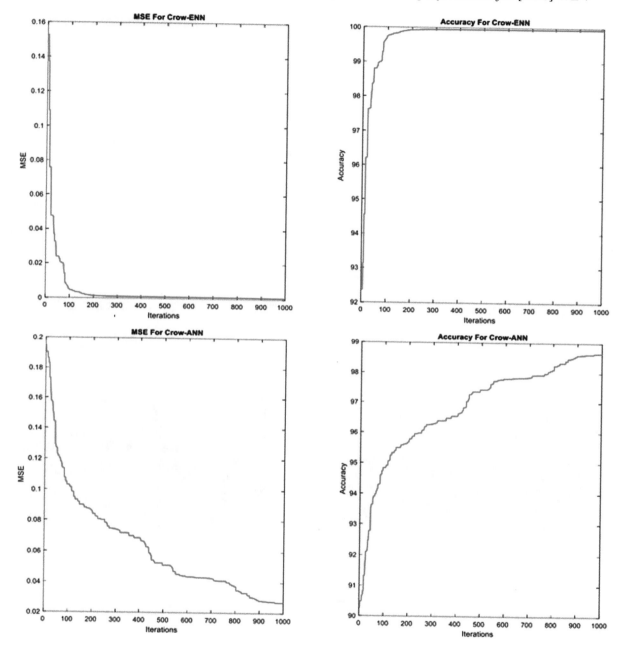

Figure 27. Graphical representations of Crow-BPNN & ENN's performance for [ALL] WL 4

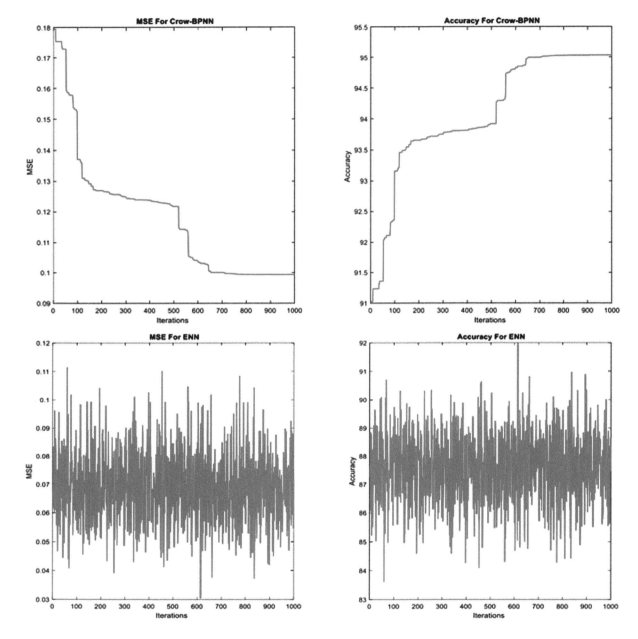

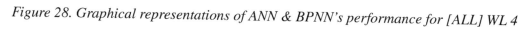

Figure 28. Graphical representations of ANN & BPNN's performance for [ALL] WL 4

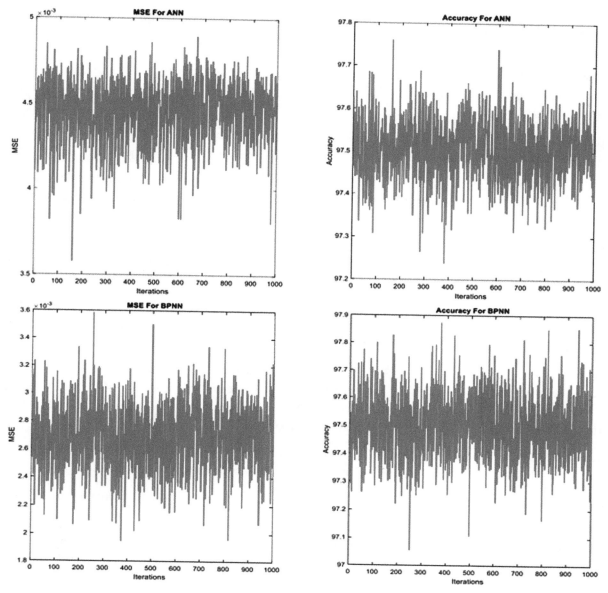

REFERENCES

Adetiba, E. (2015). Lung Cancer Prediction Using Neural Network Ensemble with Histogram of Oriented Gradient Genomic Features. *The Scientific World Journal*. doi:. doi:10.1155/2015/786013

Askarzadeh, A. (2016). A novel metaheuristic method for solving constrained engineering optimization problems: Crow search algorithm. *Computers & Structures, 169*, 1–12. doi:10.1016/j.compstruc.2016.03.001

Bhaya, W. (2017). Review of Data Preprocessing Techniques in Data Mining. *Journal of Engineering and Applied Sciences (Asian Research Publishing Network), 12*, 4102–4107. doi:10.3923/jeasci.2017.4102.4107

Bzhalava, Z., Tampuu, A., Bała, P., Vicente, R., & Dillner, J. (2018). Machine Learning for detection of viral sequences in human metagenomic datasets. *BMC Bioinformatics, 19*(1), 336. doi:10.118612859-018-2340-x PMID:30249176

Dakhli, A., Bellil, W., & Amar, C. B. (2016). Wavelet Neural Networks for DNA Sequence Classification Using the Genetic Algorithms and the Least Trimmed Square. *Procedia Computer Science, 96*, 418–427. doi:10.1016/j.procs.2016.08.088

Giang, N., Tran, V. A., Ngo, D. L., Phan, D., Lumbanraja, F., Faisal, M. R., ... Satou, K. (2016). DNA Sequence Classification by Convolutional Neural Network. *Journal of Biomedical Science and Engineering, 09*(05), 280–286. doi:10.4236/jbise.2016.95021

Hasic, H., Buza, E., & Akagic, A. (2017, May). A hybrid method for prediction of protein secondary structure based on multiple artificial neural networks. In *Proceedings of the 2017 40th International Convention on Information and Communication Technology, Electronics and Microelectronics (MIPRO)* (pp. 1195-1200). IEEE. doi:10.23919/MIPRO.2017.7973605

Kamble, V.B., & Deshmukh, S.N. (2017). Comparison Between Accuracy and MSE, RMSE by Using Proposed Method with Imputation Technique. *Orient. J. Comp. Sci. and Technol., 10*(4).

Kassim, N. A., & Abdullah, A. (2017). *Classification of DNA Sequences Using Convolutional Neural Network Approach*. Academic Press.

Kesavaraj, G., & Sukumaran, S. (2013). A study on classification techniques in data mining. In *Proceedings of the 2013 Fourth International Conference on Computing, Communications and Networking Technologies (ICCCNT)* (pp. 1-7). IEEE. 10.1109/ICCCNT.2013.6726842

Kohli, S., Miglani, S., & Rapariya, R. (2014). Basics of Artificial Neural Network. *International Journal of computing science and Mobile computing, 3*(9), 745-751.

Kukreja, H., Bharath, N., Siddesh, C. S., & Kuldeep, S. (2016). An introduction to artificial neural network. *International Journal Of Advance Research And Innovative Ideas In Education, 1*(5), 27–30.

Kumar, A. (2016). Artificial neural network model for effective cancer classification using microarray gene expression data. *Neural Computing & Applications*. doi:10.100700521-016-2701-1

Libbrecht, M. W., & Noble, W. S. (2015). Machine learning applications in genetics and genomics. *Nature Reviews. Genetics, 16*(6), 321–332. doi:10.1038/nrg3920 PMID:25948244

Mehmood, M. (2014). Use of Bioinformatics Tools in Different Spheres of Life Sciences. *Journal of Data Mining in Genomics & Proteomics*, *5*. doi:10.4172/2153-0602.1000158

Nawi, N. M., Ransing, R. S., & Ransing, M. R. (2007). An improved conjugate gradient based learning algorithm for back propagation neural networks. *International Journal of Computational Intelligence*, *4*(1), 46–55.

Patel, M., Mehta, D., Patterson, P., & Rawal, R. (2016). Applying Back Propagation Algorithm for classification of fragile genome sequence. *IOSR Journal of Computer Engineering*, *18*(5), 1–10. doi:10.9790/0661-1805010110

Powers, D. M. W. (2008). Evaluation: From precision, recall and f-factor to roc, informedness, markedness and correlation. *J Mach Learn Technol*, *2*, 2229–3981.

Rehman, M. Z., Nawi, N. M., & Ghazali, M. I. (2011). Noise-Induced Hearing Loss (NIHL) Prediction in Humans Using a Modified Back Propagation Neural Network. International Journal on Advanced Science. *Engineering and Information Technology.*, *1*, 185–189. doi:10.18517/ijaseit.1.2.39

Sarhan, A. M. (2009). Cancer classification based on microarray gene expression data using DCT and ANN. *Journal of Theoretical & Applied Information Technology*, *6*(2).

Tan, K. K., Le, N. Q. K., Yeh, H. Y., & Chua, M. C. H. (2019). Ensemble of Deep Recurrent Neural Networks for Identifying Enhancers via Dinucleotide Physicochemical Properties. *Cells*, *8*(7), 767. doi:10.3390/cells8070767 PMID:31340596

Wen, J., Liu, Y., Shi, Y., Huang, H., Deng, B., & Xiao, X. (2019). A classification model for lncRNA and mRNA based on k-mers and a convolutional neural network. *BMC Bioinformatics*, *20*(1), 469. doi:10.118612859-019-3039-3 PMID:31519146

Zaman, S., & Toufiq, R. (2017). Codon based back propagation neural network approach to classify hypertension gene sequences. In *Proceedings of the 2017 International Conference on Electrical, Computer and Communication Engineering (ECCE)* (pp. 443-446). Academic Press. 10.1109/ECACE.2017.7912945

Zheng, X., Xu, S., Zhang, Y., & Huang, X. (2019). Nucleotide-level Convolutional Neural Networks for Pre-miRNA Classification. *Scientific Reports*, *9*(1), 628. doi:10.103841598-018-36946-4 PMID:30679648

ADDITIONAL READING

Bertoni, G., & Verbeeck, J. (2008). Accuracy and precision in model based EELS quantification. *Ultramicroscopy*, *108*(8), 782–790. doi:10.1016/j.ultramic.2008.01.004 PMID:18329173

Hussain, K., Salleh, M. N. M., Cheng, S., & Shi, Y. (2019). Metaheuristic research: A comprehensive survey. *Artificial Intelligence Review*, *52*(4), 2191–2233. doi:10.100710462-017-9605-z

Jang, H. J., & Cho, K. O. (2019). Applications of deep learning for the analysis of medical data. *Archives of Pharmacal Research*, 1–13. PMID:31140082

Krawetz, S. A., & Womble, D. D. (Eds.). (2003). *Introduction to bioinformatics: a theoretical and practical approach*. Springer Science & Business Media. doi:10.1385/1592593356

Lesk, A. (2019). *Introduction to bioinformatics*. Oxford University Press.

Lewis, R. J. (2000, May). An introduction to classification and regression tree (CART) analysis. In *Proceedings of the Annual meeting of the society for academic emergency medicine* (Vol. 14). Academic Press.

Li, J., Cheng, J. H., Shi, J. Y., & Huang, F. (2012). Brief introduction of back propagation (BP) neural network algorithm and its improvement. In *Advances in computer science and information engineering* (pp. 553–558). Berlin, Heidelberg: Springer. doi:10.1007/978-3-642-30223-7_87

Lin, W. M., & Hong, C. M. (2010). A new Elman neural network-based control algorithm for adjustable-pitch variable-speed wind-energy conversion systems. *IEEE Transactions on Power Electronics*, *26*(2), 473–481. doi:10.1109/TPEL.2010.2085454

Rajkomar, A., Dean, J., & Kohane, I. (2019). Machine learning in medicine. *The New England Journal of Medicine*, *380*(14), 1347–1358. doi:10.1056/NEJMra1814259 PMID:30943338

Zurada, J. M. (1992). *Introduction to artificial neural systems* (Vol. 8). St. Paul: West publishing company.

KEY TERMS AND DEFINITIONS

Accuracy: Accuracy is the most native measure of performance evaluation. It is concerned with the closeness of an outcome to the true or actual value. It is a great measure. The high accuracy of a model means that the model is best.

ANN: ANN is a machine learning model that works on the mechanism of the human brain. ANN is composed of processing units which are called neurons. Artificial neuron tries to imitate the behavior and structure of a natural or biological neuron.

Bioinformatics: Bioinformatics is a field of science, which uses statistics, mathematics and computer science in molecular biology for storing, analyzing and retrieving biological data.

BPNN: The BPNN is a multilayer feed-forward neural network that is trained according to an error backpropagation algorithm. The learning process of the backpropagation algorithm is done in two steps, Operating signal forward propagation, and Error signal backpropagation.

Classification: Classification is kind of supervised machine learning which is used to classify every element in a dataset into one of the predefined set of groups or classes based on some similarities or homology. There are many machine learning techniques used for classification like Decision Trees, Support Vector Machine, Artificial Neural Networks, and Bayesian Classification etc.

Crow-ANN: It is a hybrid model that is developed by combining the Crow Search Algorithm and Artificial Neural Network (ANN).

Crow-BPNN: It is a hybrid model that is developed by combining the Crow Search Algorithm and Back Propagation Neural Network (BPNN).

Crow-ENN: This is the proposed hybrid meta-heuristic model which is the combination of an Optimization technique called Crow Search Algorithm and a type of Neural Network called Elman Neural Network.

Crow Search Algorithm: Crow Search Algorithm (CSA) is a bio-inspired meta-heuristic optimizer which simulates the intelligent behavior of crows. CSA was proposed by Alireza *Askarzadeh* in 2016. It is a population-based algorithm that works on the following four principles: Crows live in the form of groups or flocks, Crows memorize the position of their food hiding places, Crows follow each other to do thievery, Crows protect their caches from being pilfered by a probability. CSA has been developed based on intelligent behaviors and used them as an optimization process.

DNA: DNA stands for "Deoxyribonucleic Acid" is a carrier molecule of genetic information. It can be found in the nucleus of any cell. DNA contains all the information which are necessary for the duplication of life. The DNA structure is like a double helix comprising of two long strands. Each strand is made up of four types of nucleotides: Adenine (A), Cytosine (C), Guanine (G), and Thymine (T).

Elman Neural Network: Elman Neural Network (ENN) is a feedback neural network that is enhanced by Elman in 1990. ENN is based on the study of the backpropagation neural network (BPNN). The physical layout of the Elman neural network is divided broadly into 4 layers: the input layer, the hidden layer, the Undertake layer, and the output layer. The purpose of undertake layer is to memorize the hidden layer output. As it is based on a backpropagation neural network, the output of the hidden layer connects with its input via the delay and memory of undertake layer.

Leukemia: Leukemia is cancer of the body's blood-forming tissues, including the bone marrow and the lymphatic system. Many types of leukemia exist. Some forms of leukemia are more common in children. Other forms of leukemia occur mostly in adults. Leukemia usually involves white blood cells.

Machine Learning: Machine learning is a subfield of AI, which is concerned with designing and development of computer algorithms which get improved with experience.

Meta-heuristic: A meta-heuristic is a generic or higher-level heuristic that is more general in problem-solving. Meta-heuristic computing is adaptive computing that applies general heuristic rules in solving a category of computational problems.

MSE: Mean Squared Error (MSE) is the average of the squared difference between the predicted value of an estimator and the actual values.

Chapter 10
Psychology With Mahnoor App:
Android–Based Application for Self Assessment, Psychology Dictionary, and Notes

Abu Baker
Khyber Coded, Pakistan

Furqan Iqbal
Stuttgart Technology University of Applied Sciences, Germany

Mahnoor Laila
University of Peshawar, Pakistan

Annas Waheed
University of Peshawar, Pakistan

ABSTRACT

One in four people in the world will be affected by mental or neurological disorders at some point in their lives. Around 450 million people currently suffer from such conditions, placing mental disorders among the leading causes of ill-health and disability worldwide, according to the World Health Organization. Keeping in mind the above facts, Self Assessment Psychology Dictionary and Notes app has been designed and developed to educate psychology students and psychological patients. With the help of this application the user can do different physiological tests like Hads Mood, Internet Addiction Test, The Robertson Emotional Distress Scale, Beck Anxiety Inventory and Zung Self-Rating Anxiety Scale. The application has a smart algorithm that calculates the result on the basis of the user inputs. The application also generates the certificate for the user to share and use it for further treatment. The application provides detail information about psychology and psychologist. Apart from that, the application has a psychology dictionary of psychology-related topics.

DOI: 10.4018/978-1-7998-2521-0.ch010

1. INTRODUCTION

Psychology is the study of mind and without mind the invention of science and technology was impossible. Psychology plays a pivotal role in the medical sciences when combining with technology. The use of technology has been drastically developed over the past few decades. Peoples use technology for various purposes such as Scientific Research, Engineering, Medical Appliances, Agriculture, Showbiz, Entertainment and so on. Advancement in mobile technology students and society give preference to technology for the sake of easiness and reliability and use their smartphones for learning aim also.

The use of cellular technology in health care has been identified as M. Health (Donor et al., 2013; Lu Luxton, MacKinnon, Bush, Michigan & Rieger, 2011), which involves the use of large-scale mobile devices Such as smartphones, tablets, personal digital assistants and so on. Recent portable devices Many scholars have stated this Potential Benefits of Mobile Healthcare Overcoming Potential Barriers Cost, transportation, lack of medical care, lack of insurance or The long waitlist (Zeph et al., 2014; Dolan, Gonzalez, & Campbell, 2014; He Heffner, Wellardga, Mercer, Kentz, & Breaker, 2015; Lu Luxton, Hansen, & Steinfeld, 2014; Ro Rupak et al., 2015; Lui, Marcus, & Barry, 2017).

Through psychology, people can better understand how the body and mind work. In the twenty-first-century peoples are involved in depression, anxiety, distress and sometimes they want to test it but due to busy life and time-consuming system of doctors, they are unable to do so. For that reason, it is comfortable to just install the application from play store and test different psychological level. This knowledge can be helpful in making decisions and avoiding stressful situations. It can help with time management, setting goals and achieving goals and leading an efficient life. In addition, the insights you gain as a psychologist or psychology student can be crucial to better understanding your relationships and those around you. Whether you are dealing with friends, family, colleagues, or your significant other, understanding the human mind and behavior can help you build stronger and more successful relationships (Philippe, 2017).

Using this application "Self Assessment Psychology Dictionary and Notes" users can get complete guidance of psychology dictionary, notes and psychological test name it self-assessment for every person. The previous work is done related to self-assessment and psychology in different ways some or online and other websites also exits which are paid and unpaid. The specialty of this application is that it combines the multiple features at one platform which is the best package for the students of psychology, those are new to psychology and want to study it at a specific level.

According to the importance of psychology and psychological test, the application "Self Assessment Psychology Dictionary and Notes App" is developed in the manner to give benefits to the students and learners of psychology and also to the general people who want to check their different psychological level such as anxiety, distress, internet addiction, and moods. The student can use it either for dictionary aim or for notes. All the relevant study material is grouped together in one application in a portable form. Users can download it from Google Play and use it everywhere offline. The dictionary is made according to the need for psychology students and applicable everywhere. Users can just type the initial word the application will recommend the suggested word to complete the search. However, the different chapters related to the psychology field are added to the application. The application also provides history and a period of psychologists to help the students to know about the history of psychology.

2. BACKGROUND

Psychology is now facing new challenges arising from the evolution of digital technology, the internet, and mobile phones. These new horizons change our way of communicating, they also understand the world and the living. Compared to traditional personal diagnostics in the context of psychology (such as paper and pencil tests), online assessment offers some of the strengths and advanced features that make it attractive. (Buchanan, 2004) With the rapid development in the field of technology, everything transforms from manual to automatic and becomes easy for the user. In the past knowledge was only gained from the teachers and books without these resources it was never possible to learn something new. With the passage of time, the internet is introduced and learner takes advantage of it by searching and accessing required materials. All books are accessible in pdf format and other lectures also. Besides these development developers and researchers are working to enhance the method of learning new tips and tricks are introduced to maximize the ratio of readability. Regarding these developments, smartphones are a very important factor which plays a crucial role. In the early invent of smartphones, it was only used for calling and searching purposes. Nowadays different applications are developed to help peoples and easy their work. Some are using for gaming and advertising purpose while others for educational purposes.

Traditionally, the staff at a clinic or hospital examine a patient's health (eg blood pressure, height, weight, temperature, etc.). However, when using mobile applications as a connection between patients and health care providers, self-monitoring of health may be influenced by public bias. Therefore, the reliability of self-reporting becomes an essential factor in mobile health care. Based on the literature on "technical identity" and "technical self-efficacy", we propose the following ideas: Understanding mobile technology directly affects the reliability of self-report, and self-perceived utility.

Tests and assessments are two separate but related components of a psychological evaluation. Psychologists use both types of tools to help them arrive at a diagnosis and a treatment plan. Testing involves the use of formal tests such as questionnaires or checklists. These are often described as "norm-referenced" tests. That simply means the tests have been standardized so that test-takers are evaluated in a similar way, no matter where they live or who administers the test.

Most of the time for psychological test the traditional ways are used to book an appointment of a beloved doctor and go physically. With the help of this application, it becomes a piece of cake to note down the psychological illness and remove it. No technical expertise is required just for using an application and select the self-assessment and then chose the desired one in the listed when the test starts there will be a question and related answer selects those which suit you.

Online tests, such as traditional psychological tests, are characterized by several methods. Indeed, multiple-choice tests, such as objective testing techniques (see Anastasi, 1997), are most commonly published on the Internet, as they can be mechanically and automatically evaluated without direct human intervention. Despite this clear preference, other test methods, including test techniques and open formats, are available and available on the Internet. The first multiple-choice tests that were published on the Internet were tests that measure intellectual ability and application to be very popular because of the accuracy or falsity of test items. However, several factors should be considered in these tests. First, these tests must be professionally developed, following clear scientific and ethical guidelines, and generally, based on empirical psychological issues ("Psychological testing,").

The application of "Self Assessment Psychology Dictionary and Notes" has numerous benefits in one place. Those users who are a scholar of psychology can use it as a note and for dictionary purposes. While the other feature testing is applicable to everyone. In a busy life, people often don't have enough time to visit the doctor clinics and checkup their mental problems. For this matter, the application is developed to assist people who have psychology related problems. The application can be download from the play store and installed without paying the single penny. The usage of this application is easy for everyone for technical users and non-technical users.

3. OBJECTIVE

It is an undeniable fact that technological gadgets play an important role in the development of medical science. With the help of applications and other devices, it's become easy the way of diagnosing the problems. This application "Self Assessment Psychology Dictionary and Notes" has a significant role in medical science. People can use it for different purposes such as psychology notes, Dictionary and testing different psychological tests. The detail of the application is discussed in this chapter. Users can get the complete steps and ideas about how to use it.

4. MOTIVATION

Many exciting things are happening today in the world of technology. Psychologists are influenced by technological advancements in many ways, however, the impacts of technology on psychology can be beneficial (psychology.) (guide) Psychology is one of the top studying subjects and scholars access it by using different sources of study. Sometimes it becomes difficult to find the abstract material about the specific subject. Secondly, the most trending topic nowadays is psychological self-assessment and people give priority to it rather than going for physical evaluation to the doctor. The idea is come to the mind to prepare an application that combines both the feature psychology study and test in one single application to assist the student and newly learner and general people who want to check their different psychological levels. Furthermore, the application is developed user-friendly for access to society and upload it on play store for free of cost.

5. APPLICATION SCOPE

The aim of this application is to give numerous facilities at one place to the user. It provides helps to the students of psychology and also for those people who want to test psychological self-assessment. The motivation behind this application is to build a convenient application which is useful for students and local peoples can also take benefits. Therefore one of the most important factors of this application is a self-assessment test which is equally beneficial for the scholar and non-scholar for every gender and aged peoples. In this application, all the essential things about psychology are gathered at one plate form either it is in the form of dictionary, notes or self-assessment.

6. PROBLEM STATEMENT

Most of the time people have depression, anxiety and other types of disease and they want to check about these diseases but due to busy life and long procedure of testing system, they are unable to do. As a result, this disease may lead to significant illness. One of the big issue in physical appearance for the doctor is that sometimes at doctor clinic patient view other patients those have serious problems it has a bad impact on other patient and they fell guilty and become more illness. Another problem is searching for psychology relevant topics and a dictionary. Sometimes the user wants to find the abstract level of psychology notes and material and dictionary and it is difficult to find it in books and on the internet.

7. PROPOSED SOLUTION

Psychology is a vast field with many advances and branches. Previous work is done in a different manner with different functionality. Psychology is the study that is necessary for every field student because it is the basic need. Regarding the problem statement application "Self Assessment Psychology Dictionary and Notes" is developed to solve the issue of students, learners, and people to check different psychological tests. The richest point of this application that it is built in a convenient way that is accessible and usable for all category people.

8. Self Assessment Psychology Dictionary and Notes App Significant

a) Performance

This system should provide quick response devices and ensure its performance in terms of accuracy and precision.

b) Usability

"Self Assessment Psychology Dictionary and Notes" is an easy-to-use. Its functionality and design are absolutely user-friendly and simple.

c) Reliability

This application boast of accuracy and precision in terms of performance and work on a different device without error.

d) Error Tolerance and Security

Errors will be handled in a smart way and the application will not stop unexpectedly. This application is more secure because of offline data storage. Without the internet, the user can use this application securely.

9. APPLICATION LIMITATION

Following are the "Self Assessment Psychology Dictionary and Notes" limitation.

a) Platform Dependent

"Self Assessment Psychology Dictionary and Notes" is platform dependent and only runs on ANDROID devices. Other mobile operating systems like IO'S, Windows Phones did not support this application.

b) Limited Self-assessment

One of the limitations is that it gives only a few self-assessment tests. In some time users want to test other than the given tests.

c) Knowledge Restriction

The application focus only on psychology-related knowledge and psychological self-assessments.

10. ENTITIES IDENTIFICATION

The following entities are identified in ANDROID application "Self Assessment Psychology Dictionary and Notes":

- Dictionary
- Notes
- Self-assessment

a) Use-Case Diagram

The following Figure 1 specifies that the application user can do all this task. The user can access the Psychology Dictionary, psychology notes. Users can also assist themselves through an application.

b) Application Flow

The application flow is very simple the user just clicks on the application and the main window will appear on which different modules such as Dictionary, Notes, and Self-Assessment have. The user can access every module easily. The application flow diagram is shown in Figure 2 given below.

Figure 1. Use-case diagram

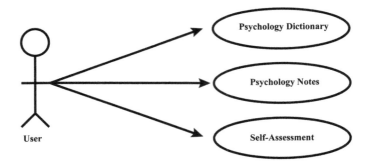

11. MODULES OF SELF ASSESSMENT PSYCHOLOGY DICTIONARY AND NOTES APP

In this section, we will discuss in detail each and every module of the "Self Assessment Psychology Dictionary and Notes." It is an ANDROID based mobile application that comprises the following modules.

a) Splash Screen

When a user clicks on the application the splash screen appears for a few seconds without performing any task. It just shows the logo and name of the application. The splash screen is shown in Figure 3 below.

b) Home Screen

Every application has a home screen and performs the main role in the application. From the main screen, you can go where you want. For the sake of easiness for a user, the overall dictionary is placed on the main screen alphabetic wise. In this application from the main screen, you can go to the module such as Dictionary, Notes, and Self-assessment. The graphical representation of the home screen of "Self Assessment Psychology Dictionary and Notes" is shown in Figure 4 given below.

Figure 2. Application flow

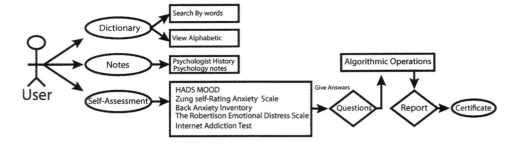

Figure 3. Splash screen

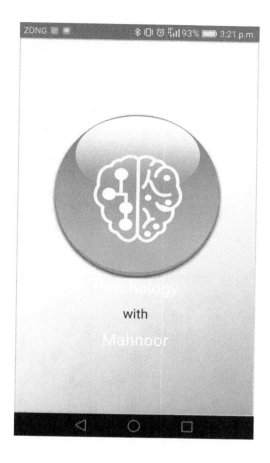

c) Psychology Dictionary Screen

In the dictionary screen, the user can search the psychology-related words. For the dictionary purpose, you can see all the words alphabetic wise on the main screen and also by clicking on the dictionary and search you're desired of a word. The graphical representation of the psychology dictionary screen is shown in Figure 5 given below.

d) Psychology Notes Screen

The notes are included for the students of psychology. The best thing about the notes is that it is

Made for the students of the initial stage to study at a specific level. It is also offline and it can be read by everywhere. Other important things are that also the history of psychology scientist is aided in familiar with history. The graphical representation of the psychology notes screen is shown in Figure 6 given below.

Figure 4. Home screen

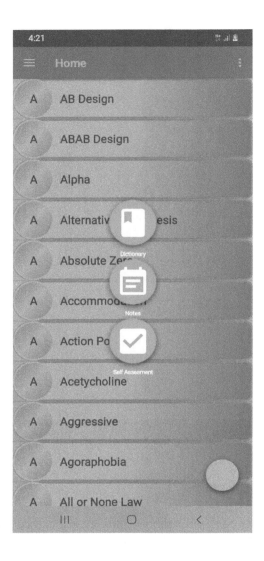

e) Psychologist History Screen

Knowing the background of the subject is necessary for that purpose the section psychologist history is aided. In this screen, the user can see the scientist's background and their work. The graphical representation of the psychologist history screen is shown in Figure 7 given below.

f) Psychology Notes Screen

The notes are included according to the important topics of psychology. These topics give a brief overview of psychology. The graphical representation of the psychology notes screen is shown in Figure 8 given below.

Figure 5. Dictionary screen

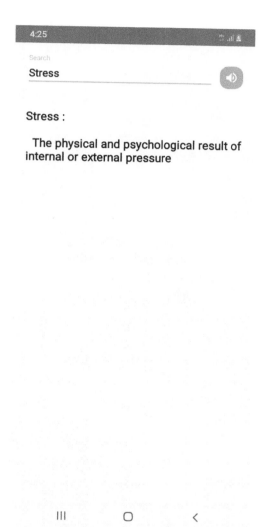

g) Self-Assessment Screen

The self-assessment is the unique feature of this application. From the self-assessment user can go to different psychological tests such as Hads Mood, Zung Self-Rating Anxiety Scale, Beck Anxiety Inventory, The Robertson Emotional Distress Scale and Internet Addiction Test. Users can select the test and start it without any technical expertise and just click on a suitable answer. After the completeness of the test, a report will be issued to the user and also the certificate which can be easily shareable everywhere. The graphical representation of the self-assessment screen is shown in Figure 9 given below.

Figure 6. Notes screen

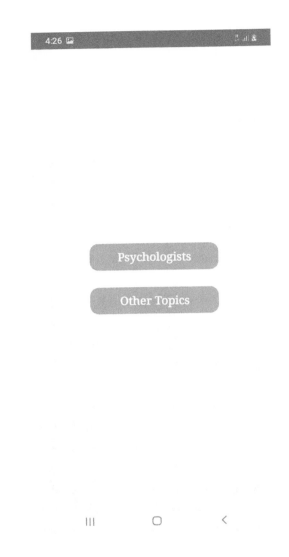

h) Report

When the user gives a test and completes the questions at the end the report is generated by an algorithm that is used in this application. The report gives an overview of the test that indicates the level of that disease and user notify for taking further action against it. The graphical representation of the report screen is shown in Figure 10 given below.

i) Certificate Generated Screen

After giving the test the user sees the report and the pdf form result card is also prepared which shows the guarantee of your test. The test is automatically generated by an algorithm and it is made by Hypnotherapist Miss. ***Mahnoor Laila***. The generated certificate is dynamic for every user. The name of

Figure 7. Psychologist history screen

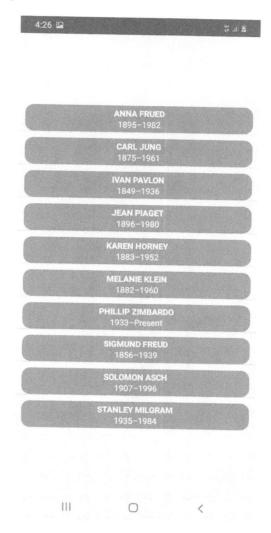

the user, test and their result will be displayed on the certificate. The graphical representation of the certificate screen is shown in Figure 11 given below.

12. TOOLS AND TECHNIQUES

Here is the list of tools and equipment which are used to develop the proposed ANDROID application for Psychology:

1. **Android Studio:** Android Studio is the official integrated development environment for Google's ANDROID operating system. Android Studio is a tool for ANDROID application development.

Figure 8. Psychology notes screen

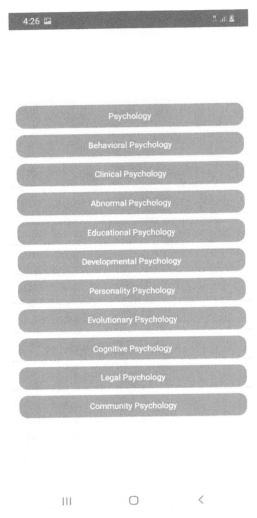

2. **MS Project:** Microsoft Project is the world's most popular project management software developed and sold by Microsoft. The application is designed to assist project managers in developing plans, assigning resources to tasks, tracking progress, managing budgets and analyzing workloads.
3. **Adobe Photoshop:** Adobe Photoshop software is the industry standard in digital imaging and is used worldwide for design, photography, video editing and more. Almost all professional graphic designers use Adobe PhotoShop for designing.

13. SYSTEM REQUIREMENTS

The hardware and software requirements are.

Figure 9. Self-Assessment screen

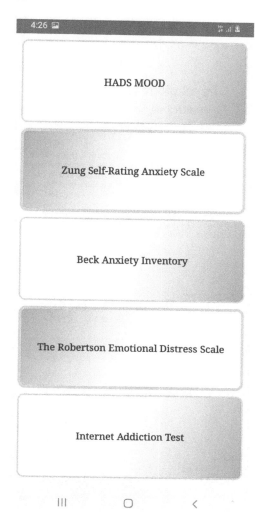

1. **Operating System:** ANDROID.
2. **CPU:** No such CPU specification.
3. **Memory:** Minimum 2 GB RAM.
4. **ANDROID Version Support:** 4.0 to 9.0.

14. FUTURE RESEARCH DIRECTIONS

The application is initially built for psychology topics, notes, and self-assessment. However, the self-assessment is also limited with few tests according to the needs of the users. In the future, the dictionary will be expanded to other medical science topics also. The application will also provide the solution and treatment for self-assessment. Later on the research, the application should be available for IOS and Windows Phone respectively.

Figure 10. Report generated screen

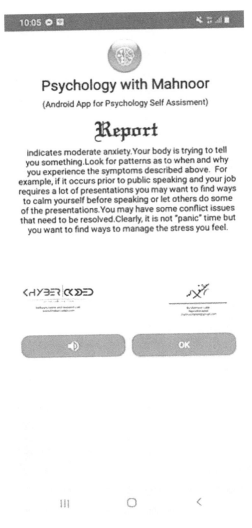

15. CONCLUSION

"Self Assessment Psychology Dictionary and Notes" is a useful application for psychology students as well as for those who want to assist different psychological levels. The application is made of abstract level according to the need of the user to access the subject materials easily. To test the psychological level which is a big problem for those who do it by manually going to the doctor's clinic. These issues are resolved and now it became comfortable to give the self-assessment test at home. Since the entire system is computerized, the user can use it for free. This system is user-friendly, and anyone can use it anytime through mobile. This application can be modified in the future so that to make it more efficient and effective.

Figure 11. Certificate generated screen

Psychology With Mahnoor
(Android App for Psychology Self
Assistant)

Certificate

To Whom It May Concern

This is certify that Mr/Miss ABU BAKAR
HADS_MOOD report is that Your Anxiety
is Abnormal And Depression is Abnormal
This certification is automatic system
generated based on user data provided.
 This certification is being issued for what
ever purpose it may serve.

Issued on:2019-09-23

KHYBER CODED

Software,Game and research Lab
www.KhyberCoded.com

By Mahnoor Laila
Hypnotherapist
mahnoorlaila4@gmail.com

REFERENCES

Anastasi, A., & Urbina, S. (1997). *Psychological testing*. Prentice Hall/Pearson Education.

Barak, A. (2011). Internet-based psychological testing and assessment. In *Online Counseling* (pp. 225–255). Academic Press.

Lui, J. H. L., Marcus, D. K., & Barry, C. T. (2017, February 20). Evidence-Based Apps? A Review of Mental Health Mobile Applications in a Psychotherapy Context. *Professional Psychology, Research and Practice*, *48*(3), 199–210; Advance online publication. doi:10.1037/pro0000122

Online Psychology Degree Guide. (n.d.). What Technology Advances Are Affecting Psychology Studies? Retrieved From https://www.onlinepsychologydegree.info/faq/what-technology-advances-are-affecting-psychology-studies/

Philippe, R. (2017). The importance of psychology. Owlcation. Retrieved From https://owlcation.com/social-sciences/Psychology-and-its-Importance

Philippe, R. (n.d.). The Importance of Psychology. Owlcation. Retrieved from https://owlcation.com/social-sciences/Psychology-and-its-Importance?

Psychological testing. (n.d.). Retrieved from https://psycnet.apa.org/record/1998-07223-000

ADDITIONAL READING

Asmundson, G. J., Koster, E., Purdon, C. L., van Straten, A., & Zvolensky, M. J. (2019). Four decades of excellence: An overview of the past, present, and future of clinical psychology review. *Pergamon-Elsevier.*

Capterra. (2017). Requirements Management Software. Retrieved from http://www.capterra.com/requirements-management-software/

Dowling, N., Merkouris, S., Dias, S., Rodda, S., Manning, V., Youssef, G., & Volberg, R. (2019). The diagnostic accuracy of brief screening instruments for problem gambling: A systematic review and meta-analysis. *Clinical Psychology Review*, *74*, 101784. doi:10.1016/j.cpr.2019.101784 PMID:31759246

McLeod, S. A. (2019). What is psychology? Simply Psychology. Retrieved from https://www.simply-psychology.org/whatispsychology.html

Roeckelein, J. E. (2006). *Elsevier's dictionary of psychological theories*. Elsevier.

Roundupreviews. (2017). Measuring Project Risk. Retrieved from http://roundupreviews.com/us/measuring%20project%20risk

Saltzman, M. (2016). Why you might want to own a 'burner phone.' USA Today. Retrieved from https://www.usatoday.com/story/tech/columnist/saltzman/2016/09/17/whats-a-burner-phone/90382874/

Shi, R., Sharpe, L., & Abbott, M. (2019). A meta-analysis of the relationship between anxiety and attentional control. *Clinical Psychology Review*, *72*, 101754. doi:10.1016/j.cpr.2019.101754 PMID:31306935

KEY TERMS AND DEFINITIONS

Abstract Material: The data which is in a specified form and has only topic-relevant material.

Beck Anxiety Inventory: The Becker Dread Scale is an emergency measure commonly used by physicians in outpatient and patient settings. It is commonly used as a treatment for physicians, psychologists, and psychiatrists.

Depression: Depression is an emotional disorder that causes constant sadness and loss of interest. Also known as major depression or clinical depression, it affects how you feel, think, and behave and can cause a variety of emotional and physical problems.

Disability: Disability is a condition that makes it difficult for individuals to perform certain activities or interact with the world around them.

HADS Mood: Hads stand for (Hospital Anxiety Depression Scale) it detect anxious and depressive states.

ILL Health: Health is an abnormal condition and the person feels unhealthy called ill health.

Internet Addiction: Internet addiction is the test in which users know how much time they spent while they are online.

Medical Science: In medicine, examines how the human body functions. Based on basic biology, it is generally divided into thematic areas.

MHealth: It is the abbreviation of mobile health used for mobile health technology.

Psychology: Psychology is the science of behavior and thought. Psychology involves the study of emotions and thoughts, as well as conscious and conscious phenomena.

Psychological App: The application which is used for psychology purpose is called psychological application.

Psychology Dictionary: The dictionary which is made for the psychology field and has specific psychology words.

Psychologist History: Psychologist is the scientist of psychology and history is background and wok for psychology.

Self-Assessment: The assessment which is performed by own without the help of others is called the self-assessment.

The Robertson Emotional Distress Scale: The Robertson distress scale is the technique for finding the distress level.

Zung Self-Rating Anxiety Scale: This is a method of checking levels of anxiety in patients who have anxiety-related symptoms.

Chapter 11
Insulin DNA Sequence Classification Using Levy Flight Bat With Back Propagation Algorithm

Siyab Khan
 https://orcid.org/0000-0003-4455-9466
The University of Agriculture, Peshawar, Pakistan

Abdullah Khan
The University of Agriculture, Peshawar, Pakistan

Rehan Ullah
 https://orcid.org/0000-0003-0738-9269
The University of Agriculture, Peshawar, Pakistan

Maria Ali
The University of Agriculture, Peshawar, Pakistan

Rahat Ullah
University of Malakand, Pakistan

ABSTRACT

Various nature-inspired algorithms are used for optimization problems. Recently, one of the nature-inspired algorithms became famous because of its optimality. In order to solve the problem of low accuracy, famous computational methods like machine learning used levy flight Bat algorithm for the problematic classification of an insulin DNA sequence of a healthy human, one variant of the insulin DNA sequence is used. The DNA sequence is collected from NCBI. Preprocessing alignment is performed in order to obtain the finest optimal DNA sequence with a greater number of matches between base pairs of DNA

DOI: 10.4018/978-1-7998-2521-0.ch011

sequences. Further, binaries of the DNA sequence are made for the aim of machine readability. Six hybrid algorithms are used for the classification to check the performance of these proposed hybrid models. The performance of the proposed models is compared with the other algorithms like BatANN, BatBP, BatGDANN, and BatGDBP in term of MSE and accuracy. From the simulations results it is shown that the proposed LFBatANN and LFBatBP algorithms perform better compared to other hybrid models.

1. INTRODUCTION

In the field biological sciences the analysis of humans DNA is a key factor and it is essential to know and understand about the DNA, and its functionality because DNA having all the genetic information related to the functioning and reproduction of an organism (Nguyen et al., 2016). It is the genetic material of the cell (Chao, 2006). DNA is fundamentally made up of four types of similar chemicals called Adenine, Guanine. Thiamine, and Cytosine which are repeated millions and billions of times in the genome, called nucleotides or base pairs of the DNA sequence. Adenine makes a bond with Thiamine and Guanine made bond with cytosine (Chao, 2006). In order to understand and decode the biological information a new field came into being called Bioinformatics (Hapudeniya, 2010). Bioinformatics is a newly evolving research area in the 21st century, which combines numerous fields like biology, Mathematics, computer science and statistics etc. Problem in the field of Bioinformatics is hard because the ratio of data in Bioinformatics is growing exponentially (Hapudeniya, 2010). For extracting of knowledge of the huge amount of biological data to various advanced computer technologies, algorithms are needed to be used (Hapudeniya, 2010). In this regard various statistical and computational methods are attempted, Data mining methods like rule learning (RL), Naïve Bayes (NB), nonlinear integral classifier (NIC) are used for DNA sequence classification (Nurul Amerah Kassim1, 2017). The decision tree is used for the classification of DNA sequence (Tansim, 2018a). The traditional statistical and data mining techniques for the classification of DNA sequence classification having limitations with respect to accuracy. In order to solve the problem of low accuracy, advanced computational methods like machine learning, and hybrid methods with neural network are used for DNA sequence classification (Nurul Amerah Kassim1, 2017). An artificial neural network is a computational model (Wu-Catherine, McLarty, & biochemistry, 2000). The concept of neural networks is primarily taken from the biological neural system. Artificial neural network mimics the human brain, which is made up of small units called neurons. Each neuron has its cell body few short dendrites and single elongated axon (Hapudeniya, 2010). Numerous researchers work in deep neural network for DNA and proteins problems (Eickholt & Cheng, 2013). Various nature inspired metaheuristic optimization techniques are also used in the field of Bioinformatics to solve problems like cuckoo search methods are used for multiple DNA sequence alignment, which is one of the core issues in the field of Bioinformatics (Kartous, Layeb, & Chikhi, 2014). Therefore, this research proposed a new hybrid metaheuristic method levy flight Bat algorithm for the classification of insulin DNA sequences of a healthy homosephian (Human). In the proposed model Bat algorithm are hybrid with Levy flight and artificial neural network and Back propagation neural network in order to improve the accuracy and explains the role of optimization techniques with neural networks.

The remaining section of the paper is organized as follows. Section 2 will discuss the background. While section 3 will explain the methods and material, section 4 will explain proposed algorithm. And similarly, the next section 5 will elaborate the result and discussion. Finlay section 6 will conclude the results respectively.

2. BACKGROUND

There are numerous categories which are used for the problem of classifications in which of them the first one model based, similar to the Markov model (HMM), sequence-sequence classification and further statistical models like linear regression, logistic regression etc. Used for the classification of the biological sequences like DNA, protein and RNA, etc. in the past. In the mentioned models the biological sequences are classified on the origin of the highest alignment score. The only alignment score is not there, also some additional parameters to check for the improved classification (Xing, Pei, and Keogh, 2010).

The other category is known as featured based selection. In this approach, the biological sequences are transformed into a sequence of features and attributed vectors and then the conventional classification methods are applied to classify the sequences into the chosen classes. But converting the sequences into the features and attributes the sequence, lots its original shape and nature (Xing et al., 2010).

Furthermore, the third category is the sequence distance-based classification. The distance function which measures the similarity between sequences, which shows the value of the classification meaningfully. Diverse techniques are exercised like KNN, SVM with local alignment, but all these are slow in learning approaches and does not pre-compute a classification model (Xing et al., 2010). Data mining, Artificial neural network (ANN) and machine learning methods like KNN (Chaurasiya, Chandulah, Misra, & Chaurasiya, 2010), Rule Learning, Naïve Bayes, Decision Tree, Neural Network, SVM (Leung et al., 2009), Genetic algorithm, (Xing et al., 2010). etc. are used to classify the DNA sequences. All the above revised methods having the restrictions and limitations with respect to accuracy and mean square error. With the passage of time and improvements in technology all these approaches are dominated by the machine learning and deep learning methods in order to attain improved consequences with in the less expanse of time and resources.

Wu, Berry, Shivakumar, and McLarty (1995), explains the developed neural network technique for the classification of protein sequences in his article neural network for protein sequences classification, sequence encoding with singular value decomposition. This study has the ability to classify the unknown protein sequences in to a full-scale system. This system classifies the protein sequences into their respective families. Three-layered neural network has been used feed forward, back propagation. By a hashing method a protein sequences are fixed into a neural input vector which used to count n-gram words. New SVD (singular value decomposition) technique that has the ability to compress the n-gram input vector and capture semantics of n-gram words that advance the generalization ability of the network. This system is used to reduce the search time and help to organize the protein sequences. This research work classifies the protein sequences with the accuracy of 90%.

(Tansim, 2018b) analyzes the implementation of the famous machine learning algorithm called decision tree ID3 for the aim of DNA sequence Classification. The implementation of the decision algorithm is done with the available data and use different criteria for the evaluation purpose. After the successful implementations of the decision tree the accuracy result obtained for testing is 88%.

Hasic, Buza, and Akagic (2017) proposed A hybrid Method for Prediction of Protein secondary structure in his research article and also present a hybrid method grounded on multiple artificial neural network with the use of consensus function and relate the approach with other effective methods. The finding of a universal algorithm for protein secondary structure prediction is not an easy problem to solve. In this research work a hybrid multiple neural network ensemble approach is used which shows promising results of improving the accuracy. The proposed method is based on multiple neural network, which is trained and achieves the accuracy of 65% for Protein secondary structure prediction. However, in this paper the hybrid method shows some encouraging results which enhances the accuracy of the existing algorithms. The accuracy of the existing methods lies up to 60% where the proposed method shows the accuracy up to 65%.

Zaman and Toufiq (2017) proposed a neural network method to classify the hypertension gene order using back propagation neural network. Hypertension is a disease which is mostly caused for death every year, according to an American heart association published a report on 17th December 2014. In the field of bioinformatics various data mining and machine learning methods like SVM and ANN are uses for the classification of this sort of problems. Codon frequency has been used in this research work which can classify the hypertension gene sequences. Predicting the hypertension disease form the genome order to cure this disease initially. According to this prediction the researchers can then prevent and do cure correctly. Different number of samples are tested such as 30, 50 and 80 on back propagation neural network system and gained the accuracy of 57.1, 75% and 90%.

3. MATERIALS AND METHODS

The study of this research project comprises of two phases, one is the pre-processing phase and the other one is post-processing phase. In the pre-processing phase the work focuses on the removing of all the unwanted materials form the data and the conversion of data into standard form according to the model. The data sets used in this research project is collected from one of the world largest biological data database known as NCBI. The data sets are insulin DNA sequences of a healthy Human, which are in FASTA format. It is a text-based format of the DNA sequences as shown in Figure 1. In the preprocessing steps initially, alignment of the DNA sequences is performed with the online tool called omega clustal in order to reduce the number of mismatches and increase the number of matches in the DNA sequence. Sequence having a greater number of matches are considered as the best sequence. Following is the Binarization representation of the DNA sequence base pairs. Adenine (A)= 0 0 1, Thymine (T)= 0 1 0, Cytosine (C)= 0 1 1, Guanine (G)= 1 0 0 and Gap (N)= 1 0 1.

While in the second step Binarization of the DNA sequences are done on the basis of the above mentioned binarization schema for the purpose of machine readability. Because DNA sequences are in character form as earlier mentioned and also shown in Figure 1. While, in the post processing step the clean data are fed into the proposed model. The proposed hybrid model is a merger of an optimization method called bat algorithm with levy flight random walk and artificial neural network and Back propagation neural network The proposed model starts with a random search of bat algorithm and picks the best value from the specified location by the levy flight and then fed, those best values to the training algorithm and finally generates the output results.

Figure 1. View of DNA sequence

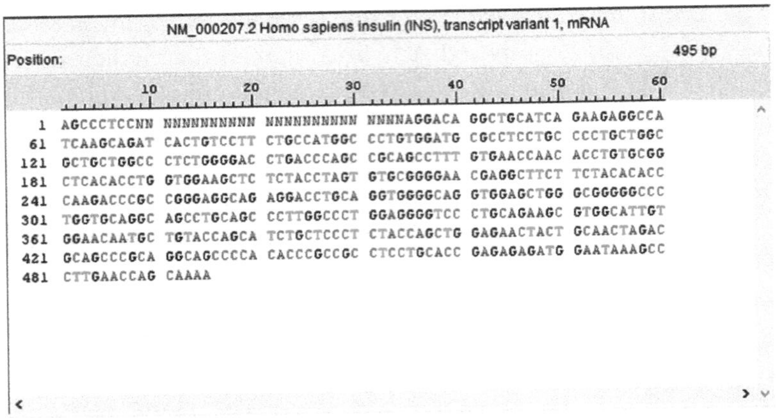

3.1 Artificial Neural Network (ANN)

Commonly used model of machine learning is Artificial Neural Network (ANN). Artificial Neural Network is actually modeled is a computational model and copy the way human brains works. The human brains are made up of a small unit called neurons. Each neuron contains a cell body, few short dendrites and a long single axon. Each neuron connected to several neurons by the dendrites and axons. Dendrites receives signals from neurons and work as in input to the neuron. Because of this input electric pulse of the cell body increase or decrease and if reaches to a threshold an electric pulse sent down to axon and this output become output for many other neurons (Hapudeniya, 2010). Similarly, the Artificial Neural Networks are made up of the above-mentioned mechanism. There are units in the ANN called neurons these units are connected to other by link and every link is associated with a weight. Like the biological neurons accepts input from the neurons through the input links each unit of the network compute the values and generate an output (Hapudeniya, 2010).

3.2 Multi-Layer Perceptron (MLP)

The most commonly used ANN structure is the multilayer feed forward neural network (MLFFNN) also known as multilayer perceptron (MLP). The multi-layer perceptron's having more than two layers of neurons are said to be multiple layer perceptron (MLP). The MLP comprises of the input layer and one or more hidden layers and an output layer. Generally, the transfer function of the hidden layer is sigmoid, logistic in function. One-layer neurons are normally connected to the neurons of the other layer and are said fully connected network. MLP has the ability to classify the data sets by the use of plans that split the data into discreate parts.(Popescu, Balas, Perescu-Popescu, & Mastorakis, 2009)

3.3 Bat Algorithm

Bat algorithm, as described form the name it shows that it is one of the natures encouraged algorithms. Bat algorithm was designed by Xin-She Yang in 2010 and it is found one of the well-organized and effective optimization techniques (Lin, Chou, Yang, Tsai, & Technology, 2012). Alike to other all metaheuristic algorithms, Bat employ new random walk feature called echolocation. The searching manner of the micro bats are determined by echolocation. With the help of echolocation random walk Bats interconnects efficiently and perceive very quickly the optimal solution with continuously changes occurring in the emission and loudness. The basic theme of BAT algorithm is pattern on the given below three rules:

- The natural behavior Bats, it uses echolocation to sense and calculate the distance, and also aware of the difference between prey and all the background obstacles in some magical way.
- Bat sails with a random velocity of (v_i) on a position (x_i) having static frequency (f_{min}) the varying wavelength λ and loudness A_0 to search for the prey. The wavelength is adjusted routinely of their released pulses and the adjust rate of the release of pulses, $r \in [0,1]$ depends on the nearness of the target.
- Regardless of the fact that the loudness can change in many ways, (yang. 2010a). It is considered that the loudness varies from a large positive, A_0 to a minimum constant value of A_{min}.

The early position x_i, Velocity vi, and frequency fi are prepared for Bat bi the mathematical demonstration for the original Bat algorithm is given as. (Lin et al., 2012)

$$fi = f_{min} + \left(f_{max} - f_{min}\right)\beta \tag{1}$$

$$vi^t = vi^t + \left(xi^{t-1} - x^*\right)fi \tag{2}$$

$$xi^t = xi^{t-1} + vi^t \tag{3}$$

where β denotes to a randomly produced number within the break of [0,1]. xi^t reveals the value of a conclusion variable j for Bat i at a time t. The result of fi in equation (1) is used to operate the speed and range of the movement of the Bats. x^* variable displays the present global best location which is situated after equating all the solutions among the all n Bats (Fister, Yang, Fong, & Zhuang, 2014).

3.4 Selection of Window Length

When the neural network reading the nucleotides of the DNA sequence while reading the single nucleotides it does not give promising results. For the purpose of achieving good results the window length selection size is considered. Following are different windows length selection size (Hasic et al., 2017).

3.4.1 Window Length Size 5

In this window length size, it will be reading a stream of five nucleotides from the whole DNA sequence computing these nucleotides and then slides to read the next five nucleotides of the DNA sequence and in this way the whole DNA sequence will be read. The following DNA sequence will be reading with the window size of 5.

ACCCCGCGAGATATTTTATATATGTGCGCA

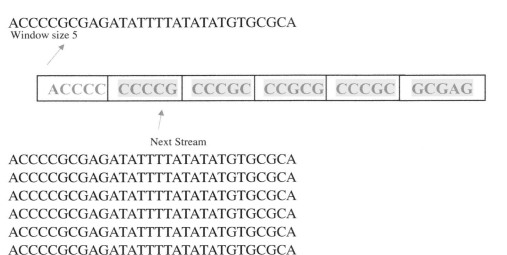

ACCCCGCGAGATATTTTATATATGTGCGCA
ACCCCGCGAGATATTTTATATATGTGCGCA
ACCCCGCGAGATATTTTATATATGTGCGCA
ACCCCGCGAGATATTTTATATATGTGCGCA
ACCCCGCGAGATATTTTATATATGTGCGCA
ACCCCGCGAGATATTTTATATATGTGCGCA

Thus, in this way the whole DNA sequence will be read.

3.4.2 Window Length Size 10

Here in this research project the window length size mean, it will be reading a stream of ten nucleotides from the whole DNA sequence computing these nucleotides and then slides to read the next ten nucleotides of the DNA sequence and in this way the whole DNA sequence will be read and executed. as shown given below.

ACCCCGCGAGATATTTTATATATGTGCGCA

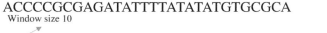

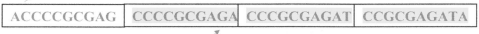

ACCCCGCGAGATATTTTATATATGTGCGCA
ACCCCGCGAGATATTTTATATATGTGCGCA
ACCCCGCGAGATATTTTATATATGTGCGCA

3.4.3 Window Length Size 15

In this window length size, it will be reading a stream of fifteen nucleotides from the whole DNA sequence computing these nucleotides and then slides to read the next fifteen nucleotides of the DNA sequence and in this way the whole DNA sequence will be read.as shown given below.

ACCCCGCGAGATATTTTATATATGTGCGCA

Window length 15

| ACCCCGCGAGATATT | CCCCGCGAGATATTT | CCCGCGAGATATTTT |

Next Stream

ACCCCGCGAGATATTTTATATATGTGCGCAACCCCGCGATTTTATATATGTGCGC
AACCCCGCGAGATATTTTATATAGGCAACCCCGCGAGAACCCCGCGAGATATTT
ATATATGTGC

4. DATA SET

The Data for the aim of classification of DNA sequences are taken from National Center for Biology information's NCBI which is the DNA sequence of insulin of a healthy human being. The Number of base pairs or nucleotides and the partitioning details for classification is given below in Table 1. Figure 2 shows the density of nucleotides and as well as show the bond of A with T and C with G Density in the DNA sequence. Table 1 shows the description of the dataset.

4.1 Partitioning of Data

The partitioning of data is extremely essential part in neural networks in order to obtain best neural network model result. The finest neural networks models can be gained using the partitioning of the data (Rehman, Nawi, & Ghazali, 2011). Initially in first step the data is split into testing and training two different subsets for the purpose of classification. The 70% portion of datasets are used for the training purpose while 30%, of the datasets are used for the purpose of training. It is to be noticed that the complexity of data is decreased with the help of analytical techniques by sampling the dataset into similar subsets. These parallel subsets have a smaller amount effect on the data complexity in the neural network design and useful in neural network evaluation process. Data partitioning is mentioned in Table 2

4.2 Preprocessing of Data

Data preprocessing is another important step in any research work, which is a data mining technique which has the quality to remove all the unwanted noise, unnecessary materials and inconsistency from data and convert the data into a standard form according to the machine for further processing. In data preprocessing section the raw data are converted into meaningful and understandable form for the promising results. In this research the preprocessing of the data is explain as in the below steps which consist of Alignment of DNA sequences, Binarization of DNA Sequences and Selection of different Window length size.

4.3 Alignment of DNA Sequence

DNA sequences alignment is the arrangement of two or more than two sequences according to another sequence. The sequence can be DNA, Protein, Genome, Gene, Nucleic Acid or Nucleotides etc. the following two parameters are looking in sequence alignment:

Table 1. Description of datasets

Data Set	Total Instances	Training Sample	Testing Sample	Window Length	Inputs	Classes
DNA sequence of Insulin Variant2 (V2)	495	70%	30%	5	25	5
DNA sequence of Insulin Variant2 (V2)	495	70%	30%	10	50	5
DNA sequence of Insulin Variant2 (V2)	495	70%	30%	15	75	5

Figure 2. Nucleotides density of the DNA sequence

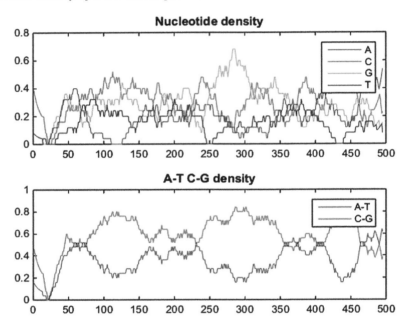

- Match
- Mismatch

The best and suitable align sequence is the one which gives maximum number of matches. The sequence having maximum number matches are more similar and the other having a smaller number of matches are less similar. The researcher need alignment for the sequence similarity or homology of the sequence. In this research pair wise global alignment will be used to achieve the most suitable DNA sequence.

4.4 Binarization of DNA Sequence

While working on the DNA sequences initially the researcher has to convert the DNA sequence into a binary form. Because DNA sequence is like text data is shown in Figure 1, DNA sequences are sequences of consecutive letters with no space. In a DNA sequence there is no term of word. Thus, use a way to convert a DNA sequences into a sequence of words into the binary number 0 and 1 form in order to apply the same representation technique for text data without losing position information of each nucleotide in sequences.

4.5 Insulin Variant 2 DNA Sequence

The given DNA sequences contained 495 nucleotides or base pairs which are the various combinations of A, T, C, G and N where N represent the Gap. The Gap occurs after the alignment if the number of the both the DNA sequences are not same in number, the gap makes the nucleotides base pairs equal in number of the DNA sequences. In Figure 3 Variant V2 shows the physical view of the DNA sequence. Figure 4 shows the base count of the DNA sequence base count shows the number of occurrences of each nucleotide base pair in DNA sequence.

5. PROPOSED LFBatBP ALGORITHM

This study proposed levy flight Bat with a neural network (NN), and back propagation (BP) algorithm which is used for the classification of an insulin DNA sequence of human. In the proposed LFBatBP model first the Bat population is initialized. Then the BP network structure is constructed. Similarly, the BP network is trained with input value. The initial weights, and bias values are initialized i.e. the weights and the bias values are initialized with levy flight Bat algorithm and then those weights are passed into the BP. All the weights are computed and compared in the backward pass. In the coming pass Bat will update the weights until to reach the best possible solution and Bat will continue to search the best weights until the last pass or epoch of the network is reached or the MSE is achieved. The MSE can be considered as the performance index for the proposed hybrid LFBatBP. And the proposed model is given in Figure 5.

Figure 3. View of DNA sequence

```
NM_001185097.1 Homo sapiens insulin (INS), transcript variant 2, mRNA
Position:                                                           495 bp
            10         20         30         40         50         60
  1 AGCCCTCCAG GACAGGCTGC ATCAGAAGAG GCCATCAAGC AGGTCTGTTC CAAGGGCCTT
 61 TGCGTCAGAT CACTGTCCTT CTGCCATGGC CCTGTGGATG CGCCTCCTGC CCCTGCTGGC
121 GCTGCTGGCC CTCTGGGGAC CTGACCCAGC CGCAGCCTTT GTGAACCAAC ACCTGTGCGG
181 CTCACACCTG GTGGAAGCTC TCTACCTAGT GTGCGGGGAA CGAGGCTTCT TCTACACACC
241 CAAGACCCGC CGGGAGGCAG AGGACCTGCA GGTGGGGCAG GTGGAGCTGG GCGGGGGCCC
301 TGGTGCAGGC AGCCTGCAGC CCTTGGCCCT GGAGGGGTCC CTGCAGAAGC GTGGCATTGT
361 GGAACAATGC TGTACCAGCA TCTGCTCCCT CTACCAGCTG GAGAACTACT GCAACTAGAC
421 GCAGCCCGCA GGCAGCCCCA CACCCGCCGC CTCCTGCACC GAGAGAGATG GAATAAAGCC
481 CTTGAACCAG CAAAA
```

Figure 4. Base count of DNA sequence in percentage

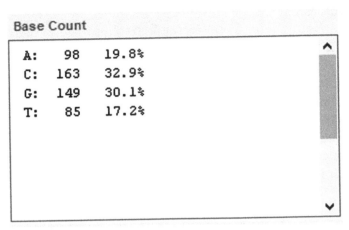

6. RESULTS

This portion of the results and discussion comprises of all the outcome which are obtained from all the six models using numerous window lengths such window length five, window length ten and window fifteen, in which two are proposed and four of them are comparable models.

6.1 Preliminaries Studies

In this portion of the research work, the machines used for the aim of simulations are equipped with an Intel core i7 turbo processor having the strength of 2.9 GHz, seventh generation and having 8GB RAM. The tool used for the intent of implementations of a proposed algorithm MATLAB R2014b on operating system windows10pro. The proposed Bat Algorithm with Levy flight back propagation neural network is tested on the benchmark data, the data are the DNA sequences which are taken from the world famous and large biological database called NCBI which acronym for National Center for Biotechnology Information. The proposed algorithms used in this section are given below:

1. Bat with Levy Flight Artificial Neural Network algorithm (BatLFANN).
2. Bat with levy Flight Back Propagation algorithm (BatLFBP).

The performance of the proposed algorithms which are used in this research work are equate with following given four neural network algorithms merged with optimization algorithms on two data sets with two different variants and three separate window sizes:

1. Bat with Artificial Neural Network algorithm (BatANN).
2. Bat with Back Propagation Neural Network algorithm (BatBP).
3. BAT with Gaussian Distribution Artificial Neural Network algorithm (BatGDNN).
4. BAT with Gaussian Distribution Back Propagation algorithm (BatGDBP).

Figure 5. Flow chart of the proposed model

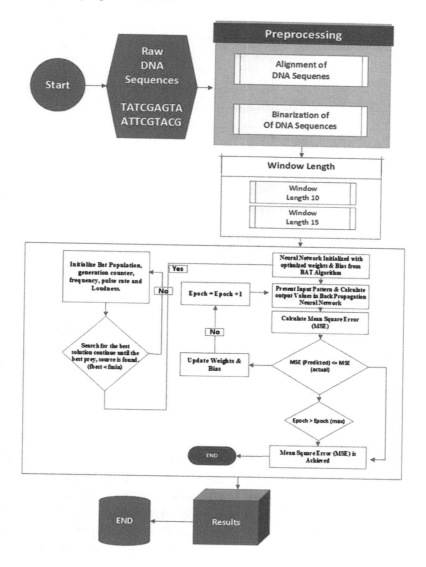

While performing the experimental performance parameters are used such as Accuracy and mean square error (MSE). The evaluation of the proposed algorithms is done on one data set of the DNA sequence which are two variants of insulin DNA, having different window length size like window length five, window length ten and window length fifteen. The maximum number of epochs are performed for this experimental work are 1000. Table 2 show the description of preliminary study.

6.2 Results Performance for Insulin DNA Sequences on Window

This portion of the article comprises of the outcome or results which are obtained from the proposed hybrid BatLFANN and BatLFBPNN model and the rest of comparable models using numerous window

Table 2. Description of preliminaries study

Parameters	Description	Network Structure			
		Algorithms	Widow Length 5	Window Length 10	Window Length 15
Operating System	Windows10	BatANN	5 - 5 – 5	10 – 5 – 5	15 – 5 – 5
Processor	2.9 GHz	BatBP	5 - 5 – 5	10 – 5 – 5	15 – 5 – 5
RAM	8 GB	BatGDNN	5 - 5 – 5	10 – 5 – 5	15 – 5 – 5
Target error	0.0001	BatGDBP	5 - 5 – 5	10 – 5 – 5	15 – 5 – 5
Max Epochs	1000	BatLFNN	5 - 5 – 5	10 – 5 – 5	15 – 5 – 5
IDE	MATLAB R2014b	BatLFBP	5 - 5 – 5	10 – 5 – 5	15 – 5 – 5

lengths such window length ten and window length fifteen, in order to evaluate the performance of the machines with respect to mean square error and accuracy.

6.3 Results Performance for WL 5

This DNA sequence of insulin data set is taken from NCBI of a multicellular organism, the source of this DNA sequence is a healthy homosephian (Human being). The number of base pairs in the DNA sequence is 469 originally which then become 495 after the alignment, 26 gaps are added to the DNA sequence to equate with other variant V2. The accession number of "Homo sapiens insulin (INS), transcript variant 1, mRNA" is Nm_000207. With the help of this number, the sequence can be traced easily in the large database like NCBI.

The input to the algorithm is given in the window length of five of a variant 1 dataset, which gives the output in a single number. The above given Table 3 illustrates the performance of various algorithms consists of numerous results which are finally obtained from numerous hybrid algorithms which are applied to the DNA sequence of Insulin Variant 1 (V1) data set with a window length five. The values in the tables illustrates the accuracy and MSE for the proposed hybrid models and other traditional hybrid models. Here in this research work the most efficient result is given by the proposed BatLFANN and BatLFBP with the accuracy rate of 99.93408%, 99.54337 and low MSE of 0.000659 and 0.004566 on

Table 3. Performance of proposed models for DNA sequence Variant2 (V2) on WL 5

Algorithm	Training Data		Testing Data	
	Accuracy	MSE	Accuracy	MSE
BatANN	99.09948	0.009005	98.32182	0.016782
BatBP	98.66667	0.013333	99.02543	0.006746
BatGDANN	99.02225	0.001777	99.00318	0.002968
BatGDBP	98.83873	0.011613	98.95178	0.010482
BatLFANN	99.93408	0.000659	99.82853	0.001715
BatLFBP	99.54337	0.004566	99.32621	0.006738

70% training datasets. Furthermore, BatGDBP comes behind BatLFANN with respect to accuracy and MSE. BatLFBP delivers the accuracy of 99.54337% with 0.004566 of MSE for the 70% of training datasets. Similarly, BatGDANN attains the accuracy of 99.02225% with MSE of 0.001777 for the 70% of training data performance wise it comes after BatGDANN. BatANN ensure the accuracy of 99.09948% and MSE of 0.009005. Finally, BatBP gives the accuracy of 98.6667% and MSE of 0.013333.

While for the testing data sets the proposed hybrid algorithms BatLFANN and BatLFBP attains the accuracy rate of 99.82853%, 99.32621%, with MSE of 0.001715, 0.006738 respectively. The rest algorithms like BatANN, BatBP, BatGDANN and BATGNBP attains the accuracy of 98.32182%, 99.02543%, 99.00318%, 98.95178% and MSE of 0.016782, 0.006746, 0.002968, 0.010482 respectively. From the above results concluded that BatLFANN and BatLFBP gives best optimal solution 99.93408% and 99.54337 on 70% of training datasets which almost near to actual result whereas, also BatLFANN and BatLFBP gives promising outcome of 99.82853% and 99.32621 on the 30% testing datasets with an MSE of 0.001715and 0.006738. Furthermore, Figure 6 shows graphical representation of MSE convergence performance for testing dataset of each hybrid algorithms.

6.4 Result Performance for WL 10

The above-mentioned Table 4 having numerous results which are obtained from the proposed hybrid algorithms and from the comparable hybrid models. The input presented to the hybrid algorithms in window length ten of DNA sequence Variant V2. These numerical values in the mentioned table explains the performance of the proposed and comparable models with respect to accuracy and mean square error. The proposed hybrid algorithms BatLFANN and BatLFBP provide the accuracy of 99.78454% and 99.86547% on the amount of 70% of training data with the MSE of 0.002155 and 0.001345 respectively. Moreover, the comparable hybrid algorithms like simple BatANN and BatBP obtained the accuracy of 99.52942%, 99.20104% with the MSE of 0.004706, 0.00799, BatGDNN and BatGDBP gives the performance in the form of accuracy is 99.13334% and 99.33164% and MSE of, 0.00166 and 0.006684 respectively for the measure of 70% of training datasets.

Moreover, for the aim of testing 30% of the data are taken and the result given in the form of accuracy and MSE by the proposed hybrid algorithms BatLFANN and BatLFBP is 99.84617%, 99.41922% and MSE of 0.001538 and 0.005808. whereas, rest of the hybrid algorithms like simple BatANN, BatBP, BatGDNN, and BatGDBP attains the performance for 30% of the testing datasets is 99.42687%, 99.45103%, 99.20948%, and 97.9337% and MSE of 0.005731, 0.00549, 0.007905, and 0.020663. it is to be concluded from the above explanations of the results that BatLFANN and BatLFBP gives better performance on the training and as well as on the testing side among all the models used in this simulation work. Graphical representation of each hybrid algorithm performance is given below in Figure 7 which shows the performance through the graph line.

6.5 Result Performance for WL 15

The input to the algorithm is given in the window length of fifteen which gives the output in a single term. The above given Table 5 consists of numerous results which are finally obtained from various hybrid algorithms which are applied to the DNA sequence of Insulin Variant 2 (V2) data set. The values in the tables illustrates the accuracy and MSE for the proposed hybrid models and other comparable hybrid models which is run 1000 times for each data set and the result at 1000nd epoch is taken. Here in

Figure 6. MSE graphs for WL five for dataset Variant2 (V2) of the used algorithms

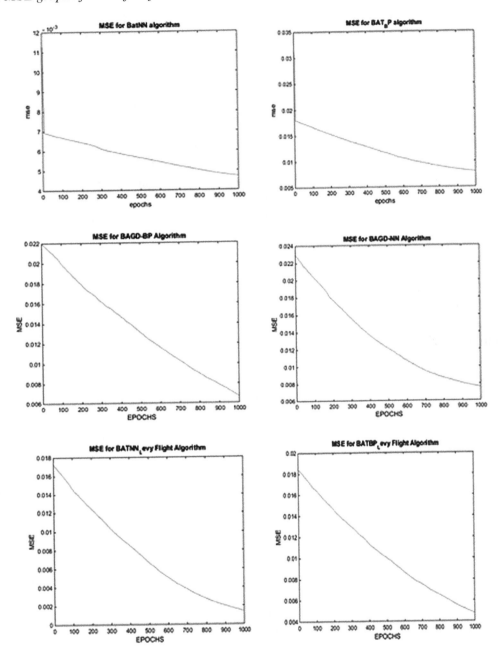

this research work the most efficient result is given by the proposed hybrid algorithms BatLFANN and BatLFBP in term of accuracy and MSE for 70% of the training datasets is 99.81884% and 99.99388% and MSE of 0.001821 and 0.009061. Furthermore, simple BatNN, BatBP BatGDANN, BatGDBP gives the accuracy of 99.79166, 99.33333%, 99.18282% and 99.69282% and MSE of 0.002083, 0.006667, 0.001172 and 0.003072 respectively.

Table 4. Performance of Proposed Model for DNA sequence Variant2 on WL 10

Algorithm	Training Data		Testing Data	
	Accuracy	MSE	Accuracy	MSE
BatANN	99.52942	0.004706	99.42687	0.005731
BatBP	99.20104	0.00799	99.45103	0.00549
BatGDNN	99.13334	0.001667	99.20948	0.007905
BatGDBP	99.33164	0.006684	97.9337	0.020663
BatLFANN	99.78454	0.002155	99.84617	0.001538
BatLFBP	99.86547	0.001345	99.91922	0.005808

While for the testing data sets the proposed hybrid algorithms BatLFANN and BatLFBP attains the accuracy rate of 99.90332 and 99.90011, with MSE of 0.000967 and 0.007999 respectively. The rest of the algorithms like simple BatANN, BatBP, BatGDANN and BatGDBP attains the accuracy of 98.9333%, 98.74074%, 99.66967%, 9.43485% and MSE of 0.010667, 0.012593, 0.003303, .005651 respectively. From the above results concluded that BatLFANN and BatLFBP gives best optimal solution on training and as well as on the testing datasets as compared to other hybrid models, which almost near to actual result. Graphically Figure 8 illustrates these results.

7. CONCLUSION

Recently, in the past decade one of the natures inspired metaheuristic optimization algorithms came under the radar and became famous because of his best performance, optimal solution and best results, among all these algorithms BAT algorithm is the most used model for the optimization. It is popular because of its disposition towards the convergence of its most desirable points in the search circle while using echolocation behavior when the Bats are on its random walk. Furthermore, these metaheuristic optimization algorithms are also hybrid with the neural network models to achieve better optimal solutions. This research work targeted the hybridization of the metaheuristic optimization techniques with Artificial Neural Network (ANN) and Back Propagation Neural Network (BPNN) to achieve a high level of results and accuracy for the task of classification. In this research work levy flight BAT algorithm is hybrid with ANN and BPNN. Total six numbers of hybrid algorithms are used for the aim of DNA sequence classification, two of them are proposed hybrid algorithms and the rest four are comparable hybrid algorithms. The performance of the proposed models is compared with the other algorithms like BatANN, BatBP, BatGDANN and BatGDBP in term of (MSE) and accuracy. From the simulations results it is shown that the proposed LFBatANN and LFBatBP algorithms perform better as compared to other hybrid models.

ACKNOWLEDGMENT

The researchers would like to thank Institute of Computer Sciences & Information Technology (ICSIT) The University of Agriculture Peshawar (AUP) Pakistan for supporting this project.

Figure 7. MSE graphs for WL ten for dataset Variant2 (V2) of the used algorithms

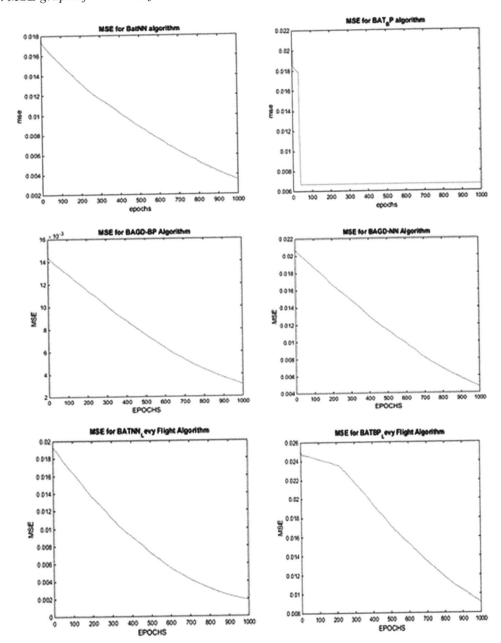

Table 5. Performance of proposed model for DNA sequence Variant2 on WL 15

Algorithm	Training Data		Testing Data	
	Accuracy	MSE	Accuracy	MSE
BatANN	99.79166	0.002083	98.93333	0.010667
BatBP	99.33333	0.006667	98.74074	0.012593
BatGDNN	99.18282	0.001172	99.66967	0.003303
BatGDBP	99.69282	0.003072	99.43485	0.005651
BatLFANN	99.81884	0.001812	99.90332	0.000967
BatLFBP	99.99388	0.009061	99.90011	0.007999

Figure 8. MSE graphs for WL fifteen for dataset Variant2 of the used algorithms

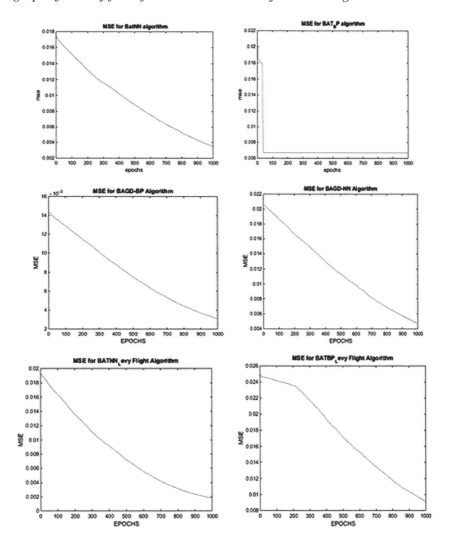

REFERENCES

Siddiquee, M.A. & Tasnim, H. (2018). A Comprehensive Study of Decision Tre es to Classify DNA Sequences. *University of New Mexico.*

Amerah, Nurul Kassim1, a. D. A. A. (2017). Classification of DNA Sequences Using Convolutional Neural Network Approach. *Innovations in Computing Technology and Applications, 2,* 6.

Chao, K.-M. (2006). *Basic Concepts of DNA, Proteins, Genes and Genomes. Graduate Institute of Biomedical Electronics and Bioinformatics (Department of Computer Science and Information Engineering).* Taiwan: Graduate Institute of Networking and Multimedia National Taiwan University.

Chao, K.-M. (2006). *Basic Concepts of DNA, Proteins, Genes and Genomes.* Taiwan: National Taiwan University.

Chaurasiya, M., Chandulah, G. B., Misra, K., & Chaurasiya, V. K. (2010). Nearest-neighbor classifier as a tool for classification of protein families. *Bioinformation, 4*(9), 396–398. doi:10.6026/97320630004396 PMID:20975888

Kassim, N. A., & Abdullah, D. A. (2017). Classification of DNA Sequences Using Convolutional Neural Network Approach. *Innovations in Computing Technology and Applications, 2,* 6.

Eickholt, J., & Cheng, J. (2013). DNdisorder: Predicting protein disorder using boosting and deep networks. *BMC Bioinformatics, 14*(1), 88.

Fister, I., Yang, X.-S., Fong, S., & Zhuang, Y. (2014). Bat algorithm: Recent advances. *Paper presented at the 2014 IEEE 15th International Symposium on Computational Intelligence and Informatics (CINTI).* IEEE Press. 10.1109/CINTI.2014.7028669

Hasic, H., Buza, E., & Akagic, A. (2017). A hybrid method for prediction of protein secondary structure based on multiple artificial neural networks. *Paper presented at the 2017 40th International Convention on Information and Communication Technology, Electronics and Microelectronics (MIPRO).* Academic Press. 10.23919/MIPRO.2017.7973605

Kartous, W., Layeb, A., & Chikhi, S. (2014). A new quantum cuckoo search algorithm for multiple sequence alignment. *Journal of Intelligent Systems, 23*(3), 261–275.

Leung, K., Lee, K., Wang, J., Ng, E. Y., Chan, H. L., Tsui, S. K., ... Sung, J. J. (2009). Data mining on dna sequences of hepatitis b virus. *IEEE/ACM Transactions on Computational Biology and Bioinformatics, 8*(2), 428–440.

Lin, J. H., Chou, C. W., Yang, C. H., & Tsai, H. L. (2012). A chaotic Levy flight bat algorithm for parameter estimation in nonlinear dynamic biological systems. *Computer and Information Technology, 2*(2), 56–63.

Nguyen, N. G., Tran, V. A., Ngo, D. L., Phan, D., Lumbanraja, F. R., Faisal, M. R., ... Satou, K. (2016). DNA sequence classification by convolutional neural network. *Journal of Biomedical Science and Engineering, 9*(05), 280–286. doi:10.4236/jbise.2016.95021

Nguyen, N. G., Tran, V. A., Ngo, D. L., Phan, D., Lumbanraja, F. R., Faisal, M. R., ... Satou, K. (2016). DNA sequence classification by convolutional neural network. *Journal of Biomedical Science and Engineering*, *9*(05), 280–286. doi:10.4236/jbise.2016.95021

Popescu, M.-C., Balas, V. E., Perescu-Popescu, L., & Mastorakis, N. (2009). Multilayer perceptron and neural networks. *WSEAS Transactions on Circuits and Systems*, *8*(7), 579–588.

Rehman, M. Z., Nawi, N. M., & Ghazali, M. I. (2011). Noise-Induced Hearing Loss (NIHL) prediction in humans using a modified back propagation neural network. *International Journal on Advanced Science. Engineering and Information Technology*, *1*(2), 185–189.

Wu, C., Berry, M., Shivakumar, S., & McLarty, J. (1995). Neural networks for full-scale protein sequence classification: Sequence encoding with singular value decomposition. *Machine Learning*, *21*(1-2), 177–193. doi:10.1007/BF00993384

Wu, C. H., & McLarty, J. W. (Eds.). (2012). *Neural networks and genome informatics*. Elsevier.

Xing, Z., Pei, J., & Keogh, E. (2010). A brief survey on sequence classification. *ACM Sigkdd Explorations Newsletter*, *12*(1), 40–48. doi:10.1145/1882471.1882478

Zaman, S., & Toufiq, R. (2017). Codon based back propagation neural network approach to classify hypertension gene sequences. *Paper presented at the 2017 International Conference on Electrical, Computer and Communication Engineering (ECCE)*. Academic Press. 10.1109/ECACE.2017.7912945

ADDITIONAL READING

Du, K. L., & Swamy, M. N. S. (2016). Search and optimization by metaheuristics. In Techniques and Algorithms Inspired by Nature. Birkhauser: Basel, Switzerland. doi:10.1007/978-3-319-41192-7

Hapudeniya, M. (2010). Artificial neural networks in bioinformatics. *Sri Lanka Journal of Bio-Medical Informatics*, *1*(2), 104. doi:10.4038ljbmi.v1i2.1719

KEY TERMS AND DEFINITIONS

Accuracy: the parameter for evaluating the performance of the machine or models which finds that how much the measured results are near to the actual value. Accuracy calculate all the correct prediction observation divided by the total observation number or actual number.

Artificial Neural Network: a computational model and copy the way human brains works. There are units in the ANN called neurons these units are connected to other by link and every link is associated with a weight.

Back Propagation Neural Network: the most famous supervised learning artificial neural network algorithm presented by Rumelhart Hinton and Williams in 1986 mostly used to train multi-layer perceptrons. It is an algorithm which is used for optimization and applied to the Artificial Neural Network

(ANN) to accelerate the network convergence to global optima during training process. Like ANN BPNN composed of an input layer, one or more hidden layers and an output layer of neurons.

Bat Algorithm: It is a nature or bioinspired algorithm working on the behavior of bats. Bat algorithm is working on the basis of echolocation behavior of the bats.

Bioinformatics: The field of bioinformatics is an interdisciplinary field in which different fields like computer science, biology, math's are combined and used for the analysis and processing of the biological sequences like DNA, RNA, protein, etc.

Binarization: A way to convert a DNA sequence into a sequence of binary numbers, 0 and 1, in order to apply a representation technique for data without losing position information of each nucleotide sequence.

Classification: Classification is a technique in which the data are grouped into a given number of classes on the basis of some similarity and constraints. The main aim of the classification technique is to shrink the measure of the error.

Levy Flight: It is a random walk which having the probability distribution with heavy tailed. Levy flight is or levy motion is a category of non-Gaussian random process whose random walks are attracted from the levy stable distribution.

Machine Learning: Machine learning is the sub field of Artificial intelligence which is a huge and multipurpose field in the modern technological world. Machine learning is related with the development and design of the computational system that can adopt themselves and learn. In machine learning the computational system learns on the basis of the training data.

Mean Square Error: In statistics the mean square error initials are (MSE) of an estimator (it is a procedure for estimating an unobserved quantity) which has the ability to measure the average of all the square of errors. It is used to verify the accuracy in the classification results.

Metaheuristics: It is a type of approximate algorithm and is composed of two Latin words meta and heuristic, meta means upper limit and heuristic signifies the art of determining new approaches. It is designed on the map of heuristic and leads to an optimal solution

Multi-Layer Perceptron: more than two layers of neurons are said to be multiple layer perceptron (MLP). The MLP comprises of the input layer and one or more hidden layers and an output layer.

Sequence Classification: is the technique in which various biological sequences are classifying into their respective classes on the basis of some similarities and constraints.

Optimization: the process in which there are various alternatives and the selection of best alternatives among them all is an optimization.

Chapter 12
UBERGP:
Doctor Home Consultancy App

Abu Baker
Khyber Coded, Pakistan

Furqan Iqbal
Stuttgart Technology University of Applied Sciences, Germany

Lala Rukh
The University of Agriculture, Peshawar, Pakistan

ABSTRACT

For successful life human being needs good health but illness is a part of life. The crowd in the hospitals, long waiting of doctor appointments makes the patients more disturb. Sometimes the patient sees the other serious patients in hospitals which makes him mental sick. Also due to busy life schedules, the peoples have not enough time to visit the doctor's clinics for small health problems which may lead to a serious disease. In this regard, the application UberGP is developed to assist the patients to connect with the doctor on phone to phone consultancy or book appointment to come doctor at home. This application has numerous benefits in case of time saving and quick appointment system at home or office. This study provides the detail documentation and usage of the UberGP Application.

1. INTRODUCTION

In the engaged life and increasing rate of diseases, there is an overwhelming response of patients. For avoiding unnecessary wait and giving priority to patients the online appointment for a phone to phone and home-based consultancy is introduced. The medical science is a vast field and now with advanced technological gadgets and mobile applications, it becomes easier for the user. The technologist every day comes with new ideas to assist the affected people. In a modern healthcare management system, an online appointment scheduling system has become more popular. It facilitates and minimizes waiting time for patients (Yin, Zhang, Ye, & Xie, 2019). The online appointment scheduling system is a system

DOI: 10.4018/978-1-7998-2521-0.ch012

through which a user can access the doctor's website through the internet, and the patient can easily make their appointments. Furthermore, the patient can also provide more detail of their illness to the doctor. The doctor aware of the patient's situation and prepares himself for patient consultancy. In this way, an online appointment management system can help the doctor, the office staff, and the patients. There are several online appointment scheduling software in the market, some of which are rich functionalities, easy to set up and cheap. For doctors, online appointment scheduling brings a lot of value to add services and benefits, like engaging the patient, making the patient feel appreciated, and being able to store patients data securely for future reference. But the big and useful advantage is that online appointment scheduling has a low cost (Nazia & Ekta, 2014).

The research on appointment scheduling has a long history, starting with the work of (Bailey, 1952). Their most famous result is the so-called Bailey-Welch appointment schedule, which states that some patients should be scheduled for an appointment in the morning time and some in the evening time in a day. The patient should have evenly spaced throughout the day, to offset the bad effects of no-shows and patient lateness. They also stated that an appointment system is a trade-off between doctors' and patients' waiting times. Although outpatient clinic's average internal waiting times are long, doctors frequently have idle time. Patients who do not show up or who are late for their appointments cause idle time for doctors, leading to temporary underutilization of the outpatient clinic's capacity. Gaps in the appointment schedules also cause the underutilization of the doctor's time.

What makes the appointment booking problems. The booking preferences are different for each patient, and they change over time for the same patient. For example, some patients are willing to see any available doctor if they can have an appointment sooner whereas others prefer to wait until a slot becomes available. Some patients are able to visit the clinic only within a short time because of job-related constraints or personal schedules. Finally, changes in work schedules, marital status, and family size can alter a patient's booking pattern.

In our proposed system the initial step toward the consultancy and for booking the appointment patient will pay the initial service fee which is mandatory. By booking the appointment patient will select the category either phone to phone or face to face home-based consultancy. The doctor will receive the notification of appointment and patient detail of disease and can check also the previous history in the database. After that, at the specified time the doctor ready to go or ready to call the patient and the doctor can see the location to track one another. When the doctor reached the patient receives the notification is ready for a checkup. The invoice will be made upon the time consumption and paid online from the account. The doctor can also generate a certificate and refer the pharmacy for the medicine.

What does the popularity of online consultancy mean for the future of healthcare? This change has positive and negative effects. Many of these changes are positive for patients, allowing them to engage with physicians better, interact with health care providers, meet individual needs and reduce costs. Make it better. However, not every health problem can be solved by a virtual doctor. They cannot perform surgeries, cannot sew, test or accept specialized equipment that requires video chat or messaging services. In any case, online medical care can never completely replace personal treatment. In addition, every online doctor and medical service has its own strengths and weaknesses.

In the hospitals, the patient's comfortability is not like at a home. Furthermore, some time for small problems like general checkups, tests or taking some suggestions from the doctor on the phone the user has no time to do it physically to the doctor clinic. *At the alarming rate of disease patients due to certain reasons unable to visit the doctor clinics.* For this reason, the proposed "UberGP General Physician Home Consultancy System" is developed to make it easy to talk with the doctor on phone or do a test by delivery service or book appointment to come doctor to the patient door. It has many benefits for patients as well as for the doctor. The first and big benefit is to eliminate the waiting problem and the second is the wastage of appointments and third is to treat the patient in their office or home. Regarding these facts and problems for the proposed solution, this system is developed.

UBERGP providing all the services that you could need from a General Physician (GP) clinic ("We Will Bring The Health Care Where It's Convenient For You," 2019). The "UberGP General Physician Home Consultancy System" is the combination of mobile applications and web-based applications which is developed for patient-doctor phone consultancy and face to face consultancy at home. First of all the patient need to install the UberGP patient and doctor application from Google Play or App Store and log in as a patient or doctor. When patients need consultancy they contact the doctor either face to face consultancy or on phone consultancy by pressing the Book Appointment button in the UberGP mobile application. When the patient book appointment all doctors in their area will receive a notification message of appointment. The patient will enter the consultancy type, their disease, comments about the disease and pay the service charges with PayPal payment. Then the doctors within their zone will receive a notification. One doctor will assign who accepts the patient request.

The doctor press the Ready to Go button from his appointments screen and will start driving to reach on the exact time, and on the Global Position System (GPS) Location which could be traced by the patient that where the doctor is coming. Furthermore, the businessman and busy people want to test the blood etcetera they can do it remotely sitting in their office by using the UberGP mobile application.

2. BACKGROUND

The appointment refers to the time period specified in the timetable for a specific patient visit. "Service time" refers to the time the doctor actually spends on the patient. In the manual system, the patient goes physically first to book the appointment. The appointment number is allocated manually and recorded by pen and paper. At the exact time of appointment, the patient is called by appointment number which is another problem that may lead to mismanagement by calling the wrong appointment number. The average waiting time for walk-in patients yearly has increased to 45 minutes per patient. In an online doctor appointment system, no prioritization made and paperwork needs to be done in order to register a visit (Hylton Iii & Sankaranarayanan, 2012). Furthermore, in the manual system from appointment to the nurse checking essential requirements such as blood pressure, the Sugar level is noted on the peace of paper. The doctors also see the previous record and create a new one on paper. To conclude the record is on risk in case of lost or destroying. Which is also one of the big issues. (Teke, Londh, Oswal, & Malwade, 2019) proposed the Clinic management system which is a computerized patient record system. Their main purpose is to reduce the burden of doctors and nurses and improve patient records management. Their proposed system integrates clinical, scheduling, electronic medical records, charting and data reporting components for clinics.

The Internet's role in health care is growing rapidly. Increasingly, the Internet is used by patients to find medical facilities or doctors, to research specific medical conditions, and to support networks specific to health. The Pew Internet & American Life Project 2008's Tracking Survey found an increase in the number of Americans that look online for health information from 25% in 2000 to 61% in 2008. Among those who use the Internet for health care information, the majority (60%) access "user-generated" information, including reading others' health experiences, and consulting rankings or reviews of health care facilities or health care providers. To date, Internet ratings of physicians have received much interest from media and doctors, but little academic scrutiny. The one prior academic study of physician ratings, restricted to selected physicians in a small geographic area, revealed that Internet data on physicians is highly variable, with an absence of user-generated information on most (López, Detz, Ratanawongsa, & Sarkar, 2012).

In some cases, the appointment is received on the same day while in some cases it is necessary to wait for the assigned date. While in the online system user just need the Internet for booking the doctor's appointment. Due to various reasons and a busy schedule of work, the patient can often miss their appointment. With this respect, the patient needs a home-based doctor consultancy.

3. OBJECTIVE

In this study, the detailed overview discussed "UberGP General Physician Home Consultancy System" which connects doctors and patients in a smart way for consultancy. The main aim of this study is to assist the patient and connect them to the doctor through mobile technology. The "UberGP General Physician Home Consultancy System" is developed with the advanced features of the online booking system and doctor consultancy. It also defined the scope of the "UberGP General Physician Home Consultancy System" and how the user gets benefits from it.

4. MOTIVATION

The Internet makes life easy. From home, users can just place the order online and within minutes it will be at their doorstep. The Internet not only beneficial in business and education but also have an important role in medical science. In the digital era, most of the work done by the internet in the medical field as well as in other fields too. There is a lot of online doctor-patient application that exists but those are only related to the appointment. There was a need for a complete setup which is in the best favor of patient and doctor. The motivation behind this study is to provide detail information about the online home base doctor consultancy system so you can take benefits from them. The "UberGP General Physician Home Consultancy System" is one of the best systems in the medical field which is the complete platform for the patient and doctor from start to the end of the consultancy. That's why the "UberGP General Physician Home Consultancy System" is discussed in detail.

5. PROBLEM STATEMENT

In every place, the patient is prioritized and a plethora of research is done that how to assist the patient in a better way. Many systems are made to make the patient treatment in an easy way such as an online appointment system, an online consultancy with the doctor on a voice call or video call or finding the disease in the software by checking the symptoms and getting the result about the problem. Furthermore, in this system, the doctors also referring to the medicine list and store etcetera. In the old system, the doctor and patient have no valid record in the database However, the complete requirement of the patient does not meet in these projects. For this purpose, the "UberGP General Physician Home Consultancy System" is the best fit to meet the need of the patient and doctor.

6. PROPOSED SOLUTION

According to the above facts for the proposed solution the "UberGP General Physician Home Consultancy System" is developed. In this system, the doctor and patient are connected through mobile applications. The patient book the appointment for a test, phone to phone consultancy or home-based consultancy and doctor receive notification of appointment and accept it in the available time. If the patient did the previous checkup with this application or doctors then they can see their history of treatment which can help to know the background of treatment. This system can access data from a database and also generate the certificates for the patient.

7. APPLICATION SCOPE

The "UberGP General Physician Home Consultancy System" has various facilities. It facilitates patients, doctors and pharmacies. The patient getup the service of the doctor, the doctor commits a successful appointment and the pharmacy sales their pharmaceuticals. The patient can also get these services remotely by phone to phone consultation or giving test while sitting in the office. Further, in the case of home-based consultancy the patient and doctor trace the location of one another in mobile applications. It can give relaxation to the patient that he is viewing the location that the doctor is on the way. One of the big scopes of this application is that it saves the record of a patient for further service and treatment. The application also generates the certificate for legal circumstances authorized and signed by the doctor.

8. SIGNIFICANCE

a) Performance

The application ensures its performance in terms of accuracy and precision.

b) Usability

The usage of this application is simple and user-friendly everyone can use it without knowing the technical knowledge.

c) Reliability

The *UberGP* is reliable and works accurately on different devices without the error.

d) Error Tolerance and Security

Errors will be handled in a smart way and the application will not stop unexpectedly. The patient data is kept secretly and applicable for further treatment.

e) Platform Dependencies

"UberGP General Physician Home Consultancy System" is not platform dependent. Almost all platforms like ANDROID, IOS devices and all web browsers can run the UberGP applications.

9. LIMITATIONS

The following are the "UberGP General Physician Home Consultancy System" limitations.

a) Internet Connection Failure:

UberGP is an online mobile application and needs an internet connection for its smooth functioning. The application stops working when the internet connection fails.

b) Normal Consultancy

It provides consultancy to the only normal patient and doesn't offer the emergency service for serious patients.

c) Centralized Database

All data are stored in a centralized server in a single database. If that server gets down then the "UberGP General Physician Home Consultancy System" will not work.

10. ENTITIES IDENTIFICATION

The following entities are identified in the UberGP Application:

1. Appointment
2. Consultation
3. Invoice
4. Certificate
5. Tracing Doctor

Figure 1. Use Case diagram of UberGp app

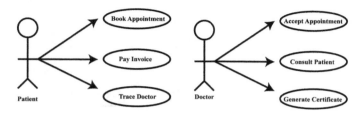

11. USE-CASE DIAGRAM

Figure 1 specifies that the application user-patient can perform all these tasks. The mobile applications have two user patients and a doctor. First of all the patient book appointment and doctor accept it. Secondly, the patient pays the initial service fee. The doctor starts travel for consultancy and the patient can track him/her by using the application map. At the end of the consultancy, the doctor generates a certificate for the patient.

12. APPLICATION FLOW

The application flow is made easy to use it without any technical expertise. The patient needs to login on their portal and select the category of consultancy and add some notes about their disease. As the patient book appointment, the doctor will receive the notification of appointment and he will accept it and it will be automatically added to the doctor's schedule. The initial service charges will also be provided by the patient at the time of booking. The doctor can see the previous history of the patient and the treatment. In case of the phone to phone consultancy at the exact appointment time doctor will call the patient or go physically to the patient. When the doctor starts rides the patient can track it that where the doctor is actually coming. At the end of consultancy, the patient pays the consultancy fee if the total time of doctor on consultancy is ten minutes then no consultancy fee either wise the consultancy fee will be charged with respect to time. In the end, a signed certificate will be generated by the application. The application flow is shown in Figure 2.

14. MODULES OF UBERGP APPLICATION

In this section, we will discuss in detail each and every module of UberGp application It is an ANDROID based mobile application that has the following modules.

1. Login Screen

When a user clicks on the application the login screen appears user (Patient or Doctor) can register himself and can log in through this screen. User can also recover their password if he/she forgets their password. When a user clicks on the Register button the registration screen appears, the user can provide their basic information like name, father name, date of birth, contact, address, zone, city and country.

Figure 2. Flow diagram of UberGp app

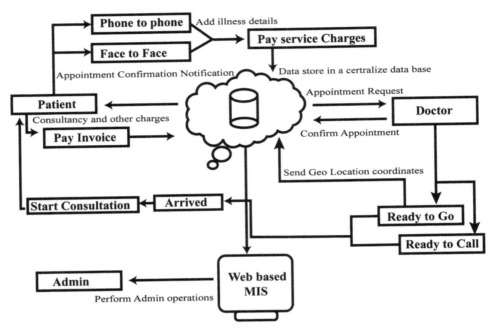

Users can also upload their profile image. All information can be stored in a database on an online server. The Login Screen is shown in Figure 3.

2. Patient Dashboard Screen of UberGP Patient Application

Every application has a home screen and performs the main role in the application. From the main screen, you can go where you want. For the sake of easiness for the patient can book their appointment by selecting consultancy types like Face to Face or Phone Consultancy and service type. The patient can also view their notifications. The graphical representation of the Patient Dashboard screen of UberGP is shown in Figure 4 given below.

3. Book Appointment Screen

In this screen, the patient can submit their medical form for consultancy. From this screen, the patient can book an appointment for himself, family and friends. The patient can also change the consultancy location by changing the user registered address and contact information. If the patient clicks on the *Next* button the application first check for doctors availability in the provided patient zone and time slot if the doctors available then the next payment screen appear otherwise doctor not availability message show to the user. The medical form screen is shown in Figure 5.

Figure 3. Login screen

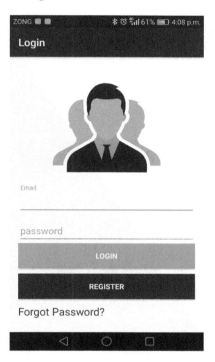

Figure 4. Patient dashboard screen

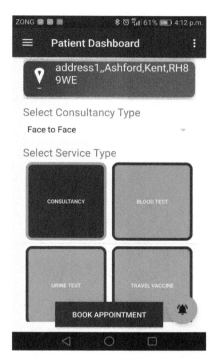

Figure 5. Medical form screen

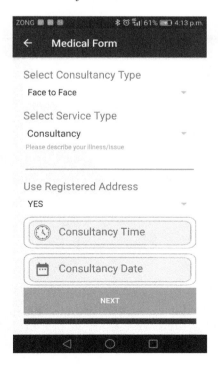

Figure 6. Payment screen

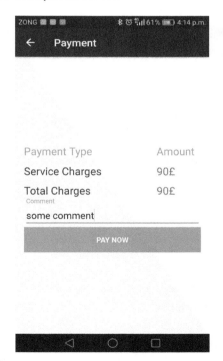

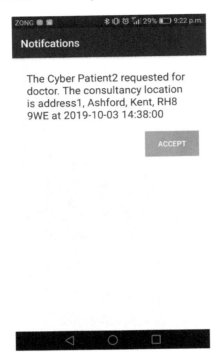

Figure 7. Doctor notification screen

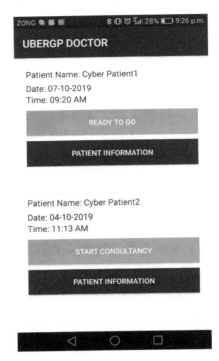

Figure 8. Doctor bookings screen

4. Patient Payment Screen

After the submission of medical form this screen appears having patient, consultancy service charges amount displayed. The user first pays this amount using PayPal payment. After payment, the push notification automatically sends to all doctors of the user-provided zone. The patient payment screen is shown in Figure 6.

5. Doctor Notifications Screen

In this screen the doctor all notification displays like a patient request for consultancy, the patient pay their invoice and patient download their medical certificates. If the doctor accepts a request for patient consultancy than a push notification also sends to a patient like a doctor assign for your consultancy. The doctor notification screen is shown in Figure 7.

6. Doctor Bookings Screen

This screen is a very important screen of doctor application which have all bookings having multiple functionalities on the first button. If the doctor is ready for consultancy on specified booking time and date then he/she must click on Ready to Go or Ready to Call button. The Ready to Call in that case when patient consultancy type is Phone Consultancy, a push notification having a message the doctor is ready to call you for phone consultancy send to a patient than the doctor can call the patient and start a consultancy. Ready to Go in that case when patient consultancy type is Face to Face, a push notification

Figure 9. Patient information screen   *Figure 10. Patient consultancy screen*

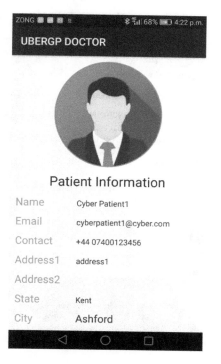 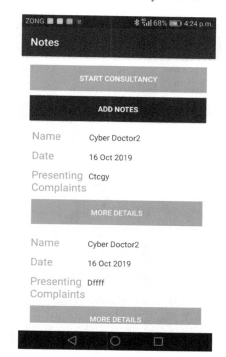

having a message like a doctor is coming towards you and Track button appears, the patient can track doctor through Google Map. When the doctor reaches the patient address than an Arrived button can click and the patient than receiving notification of the doctor's arrival. After these steps, a Start Consultancy button appears on the screen, by clicking on that button the Notes screen opens. Every booking also has a Patient info button which displays patient information on the next screen. The doctor booking screen is shown in Figure 8.

7. Patient Information Screen

On this screen the patient all information displayed like their personal info, photo, contact information and booking information. The patient information screen is shown in Figure 9.

8. Patient Notes

With this screen, a doctor can view the patient's past medical history can also add notes about the patient. When this screen opens the start consultancy time starts, the consultancy screen opens when the doctor clicks on the Start Consultancy button and Patient Notes Detail Screen open when More Detail button clicked. The patient notes screen is shown in Figure 10.

Figure 11. Patient notes detail screen

Figure 12. Prescription screen

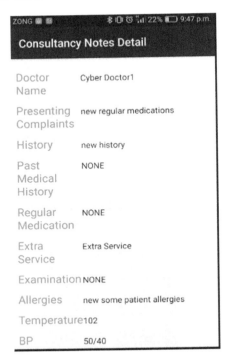

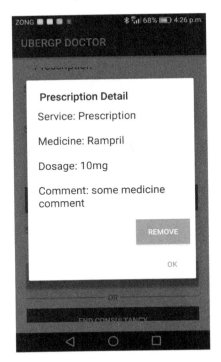

9. Patient Notes Detail Screen

From this, screen the doctor can view the patient's past medical history which can help them in consultancy. The patient notes detail screen is shown in Figure 11.

10. Prescription Screen

In this screen, the doctor can add medicine and their dosage to the prescription list and also recommend pharmacy on patient suggestions. The prescription screen is shown in Figure 12.

11. Consultancy Screen

This is the most important screen of the UberGP application. The doctor can select multiple services like prescription, medical test, and medical certificates and can add to the list by clicking on the Next button. When the doctor clicks on the End Consultancy button the consultancy time end and calculates an amount for the invoice. If the calculated time is less than 10 minutes than there is no consultancy amount because the patient already paid the service charges amount. The consultancy screen is shown in Figure 13.

Figure 13. Consultancy screen

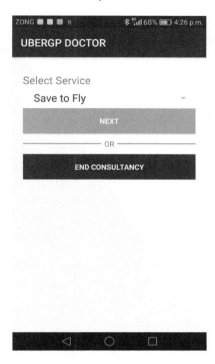

Figure 14. Invoice screen

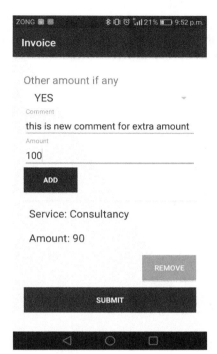

Figure 15. Doctor Home screen

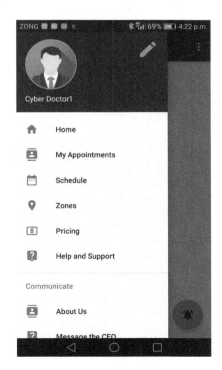

12. Invoice Screen

From this screen, the doctor can generate an invoice for the patient. The doctor can add another amount also to invoice if he/she consult more than one patient on a single booking. If consultancy and other amounts are greater than zero than Submit the Invoice button appear otherwise home screen appears. When the doctor clicks on the Submit button the patient receives notification having the Pay Invoice button. The patient pays their invoice and their booking marked as completed and the doctor receives notification message of the patient payment invoice. The invoice screen is shown in Figure 14.

13. Doctor Home Screen

This is the main screen of the doctor's UberGP application. The doctor can update their own information, view their appointment list, add their schedule and add their zones for consultancy. The doctor can view also other important information like about us, pricing, CEO message and help and support. The doctor's home screen is shown in Figure 15.

10. TOOLS AND TECHNIQUES

Here is the list of tools and equipment which are used to develop the proposed system:

- **Android Studio:** It is the platform for developing the android mobile application.
- **MS Project:** Microsoft Project is a tool used for project management. The MS Project is designed to help managers schedule timetables, allocate resources for tasks, track progress, manage budgets, and analyze workloads.
- **Adobe Photoshop:** It is the tool for designing the pages and pictures etcetera.

11. SYSTEM REQUIREMENTS

The hardware and software requirements are:

- Operating System: ANDROID, IOS.
- CPU: No such CPU specification.
- Memory: Minimum 2 GB RAM.
- Versions: ANDROID 4.0 to 10 and Swift 6.0.

12. FUTURE RESEARCH DIRECTION

The UberGp application is initially developed for normal diseases home consultancy no emergency case is entertained. In the future, it should be included the emergency response center like ambulances and special medical teams. Furthermore, in future research, the app should be capable to find the medical specialist for the patient-specific disease. Few tests are included and in the future, it will be expanded to more medical tests.

18. CONCLUSION

Treatment is the basic need of every gender and person and it is necessary to make it easy as possible. In this regard, the UberGp application is developed to consult the patient at their door. The patient often at the hospital sees serious patient discouraged. Another problem is waiting which is also removed now the patient track the doctor. The business class people who have no much time also get benefit from this service by phone consultancy, test by delivery or office-based consultancy. This system is easy to use, and anyone can use it anytime through mobile or personal computer. This application will be enhanced further in the future so that to make it more reliable and effective for the user.

REFERENCES

Bailey, N. T. J. (1952). A study of queues and appointment systems in hospital out-patient departments, with special reference to waiting-times. *Journal of the Royal Statistical Society. Series B. Methodological*, *14*(2), 185–199. doi:10.1111/j.2517-6161.1952.tb00112.x

Hylton Iii, A., & Sankaranarayanan, S. (2012). Application of intelligent agents in hospital appointment scheduling system. *International Journal of Computer Theory and Engineering*, *4*(4), 625.

López, A., Detz, A., Ratanawongsa, N., & Sarkar, U. (2012). What patients say about their doctors online: A qualitative content analysis. *Journal of General Internal Medicine*, *27*(6), 685–692. doi:10.100711606-011-1958-4 PMID:22215270

Nazia, S., & Ekta, S. (2014). Online appointment scheduling system for hospitals–an analytical study. *Int J Innov Res Sci Eng Technol*, *4*(1), 21–27.

Teke, A., Londh, S., Oswal, P., & Malwade, S. S. (2019). Online Clinic Management System. *International Journal (Toronto, Ont.)*, *4*(2).

We Will Bring The Health Care Where It's Convenient For You. (2019). UberGP. Retrieved from http://www.ubergp.co.uk/

Yin, L., Zhang, A., Ye, X., & Xie, X. (2019). Security-Aware Department Matching and Doctor Searching for Online Appointment Registration System. *IEEE Access: Practical Innovations, Open Solutions*, *7*, 41296–41308. doi:10.1109/ACCESS.2019.2904724

ADDITIONAL READING

Azzez, S. S., Abdulah, D. M., Piro, R. S., & Alhakem, S. S. M. (2019). Sleep severity and fatigue manifestations in relation to the doctor–patient relationship. *Sleep Medicine, 58*, 13–17. doi:10.1016/j.sleep.2019.02.015 PMID:31042620

Diamond-Brown, L. (2016). The doctor-patient relationship as a toolkit for uncertain clinical decisions. *Social Science & Medicine, 159*, 108–115. doi:10.1016/j.socscimed.2016.05.002

Forrest, N., Wilson, V., Doran, A., & Macormack, S. (2017). 99: Nurse led helpline and online support service. *Lung Cancer (Amsterdam, Netherlands), 103*, S45. doi:10.1016/S0169-5002(17)30149-6

Grossman, L. (2009). The net doctor will see you now. *New Scientist, 203*(2718), 20–21. doi:10.1016/S0262-4079(09)61951-5

Hoff, T. J. (2017). *Saving the Doctor-Patient Relationship and Raising Expectations.* Oxford Scholarship Online. doi:10.1093/oso/9780190626341.003.0007

Roberts, C. (2006). Doctors and Patients in Multilingual Settings. In Encyclopedia of Language & Linguistics (pp. 741–748). Academic Press. doi:10.1016/b0-08-044854-2/02349-x

Yang, Wu, H., & Lu, N. (2017). Online written consultation, telephone consultation and offline appointment: An examination of the channel effect in online health communities. *International Journal of Medical Informatics, 107*, 107–119. doi:10.1016/j.ijmedinf.2017.08.009

Yang, Y., Zhang, X., & Lee, P. K. (2019). Improving the effectiveness of online healthcare platforms: An empirical study with multi-period patient-doctor consultation data. *International Journal of Production Economics, 207*, 70–80. doi:10.1016/j.ijpe.2018.11.009

KEY TERMS AND DEFINITIONS

Doctor: someone who is qualified in medicine and treats people who are ill.

Doctor Appointment: It is an arrangement to meet the doctor and patient at a particular time in the clinic.

Doctor Home Consultancy: The doctor's service which is provided at home is called doctor home consultancy.

Disease: an abnormal condition that badly affects the structure or function of an organism.

Emergency: An abnormal and dangerous situation that comes unexpectedly and must be dealt with immediately.

General Physician (GP): a physician who provides routine health care and treats many different diseases and injuries.

Global Position System (GPS): a satellite-based radio navigation system that provides the geographical location.

HealthCare: the various services for the prevention or treatment of diseases and injuries.

Internet: the global network of computers and devices which are connected with each other in the world through dedicated routers and servers.

Patient: a person who is under medical care or treatment.

Prescription: a piece of paper on which a doctor writes medicine for the patient.

Pharmacy: The science and art concerned with the preparation and standardization of drugs. Its scope includes the cultivation of plants that are used as drugs, the synthesis of chemical compounds of medicinal value, and the analysis of medicinal agents.

Relaxation: when the body and mind are free from tension and anxiety.

Tracking: The process of determining or searching for someone or place.

Treatment: The process which cures a disease.

Chapter 13

Optimizing Learning Weights of Back Propagation Using Flower Pollination Algorithm for Diabetes and Thyroid Data Classification

Muhammad Roman

The University of Agriculture, Peshawar, Pakistan

Siyab Khan

ⓘD https://orcid.org/0000-0003-4455-9466

The University of Agriculture, Peshawar, Pakistan

Abdullah Khan

The University of Agriculture, Peshawar, Pakistan

Maria Ali

The University of Agriculture, Peshawar, Pakistan

ABSTRACT

A number of ANN methods are used, but BP is the most commonly used algorithms to train ANNs by using the gradient descent method. Two main problems which exist in BP are slow convergence and local minima. To overcome these existing problems, global search techniques are used. This research work proposed new hybrid flower pollination based back propagation HFPBP with a modified activation function and FPBP algorithm with log-sigmoid activation function. The proposed HFPBP and FPBP algorithm search within the search space first and finds the best sub-search space. The exploration method followed in the proposed HFPBP and FPBP allows it to converge to a global optimum solution with more

DOI: 10.4018/978-1-7998-2521-0.ch013

efficiency than the standard BPNN. The results obtained from proposed algorithms are evaluated and compared on three benchmark classification datasets, Thyroid, diabetes, and glass with standard BPNN, ABCNN, and ABC-BP algorithms. The simulation results obtained from the algorithms show that the proposed algorithm performance is better in terms of lowest MSE (0.0005) and high accuracy (99.97%).

1. INTRODUCTION

A back-propagation (BP) neural network can resolve complex arbitrary nonlinear planning problems; therefore, it can be applied to a varied problem. However, as the model magnitude rises, the time becomes increased to train BP neural. Additionally, the classification exactness shrinkages as well. A parallel design proposed to enhance the classification exactness and runtime efficiency of the BP neural network algorithm. The HFPBP and FPBP algorithms used to optimize the BP neural network's original weights and thresholds and improve the exactness of the classification procedure. This research proposed a novel hybrid flower pollination based back propagation (HFPBP) algorithm with altered activation function and flower pollination back propagation (FPBP) algorithm with log-sigmoid activation function. The proposed HFPBP and FPBP algorithm firstly find the best search space. The investigated technique allows the convergence of global optimum resolution with more efficacy than the conventional BPNN algorithm. The proposed algorithm assessed and equated on three benchmark classification datasets, thyroid, diabetes, and glass, with conventional and proposed which is clearly shows that the proposed model performance is better than conventional with respect to low MSE (0.0005) and high accuracy (99.97%).There are a lot of successes which are achieved by artificial neural network in various field that are such as health sciences engineering and the one field cognitive science which is unable to unnoticed due to admirable capability in intellectual complex nonlinear plotting bond and generate trainer mock-ups (Alsmadi, Omar, & Noah, 2009).Gradient descent based back propagation algorithm are used to training of ANNs. Unfortunately, training of ANNs leading some drawbacks such as local minimum value, lower accuracy and time-consuming convergence speed Aydin (2014). To reduce these problems, the naturally enthused algorithms which are representing met heuristic algorithms are consumed to training ANNs. In illustration of research, different researchers used 2nd order stochastic learning method for the aim of training Artificial neural network mock-ups (Basheer et al., 2000). Another algorithm called Krill Herd which is also practiced for the training of ANNs (Bi et al., 2005). Bat-inspired algorithm is also used by some other researchers to adapt optimizing ANNs mock-up (Castellani & Rowlands, 2009). They used to adapt editions of bat algorithm for increasing the performance of Artificial Neural Networks. And all the given adapted structures of bat-algorithm guides to enhance performance of convergence. Metaheuristic algorithms are grouped into two techniques one is single and the other is population-based. The training of an artificial neural network which is based on a single based metaheuristic technique, it is started on one resolution, integrates with its locality to discover most excellent answer (Celik, Koylu, & Karaboga, 2016). The algorithm which is based on the Population open number of resolutions as well as produce a sequence of answers; it is not ending till it meet the condition. The algorithm based on Population similarly categorizes the evolutionary-algorithm and SI algorithm. EA include heritable algorithm that is applied in recently for a consuming Artificial Neural Network efficiency. Other researchers suggested other approaches that are giving a physics idea to instigate gravitational search technique as well biological enthused flower-pollination technique. For a suggested algorithm illustrates from the investigation outcomes, enhanced classification accuracy (Chiroma et al., 2016).

From the social conduct of animals which have a very common task consist of many trainings, the swarm intelligence algorithm inspired from that. For instance, numerous researchers used ACA for the training aim of Artificial Neural Network.

For the training purpose of the ANNs many researchers used ant colony optimization (ACA) as well as modified ACA (Chiroma et al., 2015). Also, many researcher's cast-off animal nature inspired Multiverse model for global optimization (Coppin, 2004). One of the successful algorithms PSO, which are proposed by Kennedy and Eberhard are vital used for training of AANs. (Cunningham & Delany, 2007). Modified form of PSO shows rich efficiency for resolving meek issues, but it is not better for another method (Dreiseitl & Ohno-Machado, 2002). Furthermore, many researchers assumed algorithm hinge on a Gaussian technique as well as ambiguous thought to improve e ideal weightiness for the Feed Forward Neural Network (FFNN) and advance FFNN structure and all the layers of the networks. Let's assume that Gaussian's technique which enhanced PSO convergence. For a significance, the adjusted variables initially didn't influence on the speediness of PSO algorithm. The code after fuzzy reasoning operated to remove redundancies from weights in Artificial Neural Network architecture. The researcher practices a dataset of iris problem to investigate the accomplishment of assumed algorithm (Dunham, 2006). In addition, the original and the other modifies version also has been used for solving different problems from the real-life. (Chatterjee, 2016) Suggest (NNPSO) a classification technique in direction for the assumption to break down the potential in RC structure. The researchers suggest a PSO based method for the aim to fix a package of connected weights in the neural network model with fewer RMSE rate (Engelbrecht, 2007). PSO improved the speeding up operator which advanced the adapted inertia weight and to enhance the weights and the threshold of BP for the model of ANN. All the alterations directed, and it increases the proportion of the convergence speediness. For training ANN Shuffled Leaping Frog Algorithm (SFLA) is exercised on total ten datasets. All the data were taken from a famous dataset repository called UCI browser. Both performances of SFLA and BP algorithm are compared in a tool called WEKA which is a data mining tool contains of an input set which is signified input component of the model of ANN. The 2nd layer consists of hidden neurons, which considered to be hidden layer. Hidden layer linked entirely with the layer of output. The 3rd layer said to be an output layer and assumed reply layer of the model. Neurons are represented activation functions which are assumed output layer which analyzing the desired last and final output of the ANN. All the nodes are connected in an organized way in the ANN model by synaptic weights. Firstly, all the assigned weights, random and update time to time throughout the learning phase to the training algorithm completion. For problems like classification, the model like ANN needs to leans until to accomplished demand of outcomes That's why, dataset is provided to ANN model until they reach and in order to learn ANN or train ANN model. (Eom, Jung, & Sirisena, 2003).

2. THE PROPOSED METHOD

The proposed hybrid flower pollination back propagation algorithm (HFPBP), a possible solution is represented by best pollen (i.e., "The initialized weight space and conforming values of biases for neural network optimization"). The Quality of the solution expressed population size and the weight optimization problem with FPA biases initialized, then these weights approved for the neural network. The calculated weight of the neural network equated with respect to the best results. The coming round FPA will able to upgrade weights with the finest conceivable result, FPA shall remain penetrating better weights up to the last round of the network is touched or the MSE is accomplished. Figure 1 illustrates HFPBP flowchart.

The calculated matrix value of the weight is as under:

$$Wx = \sum_{x=1}^{n} a.\left(rand - \frac{1}{2}\right) \tag{1}$$

$$Bx = \sum_{x=1}^{n} a.\left(rand - \frac{1}{2}\right) \tag{2}$$

In the above Eq. (1) $W_x = i^{th}$ is the weight value, rand is between the range of [-1, 1], a is constant parameter, similarly in Eq. (2) Bx is the bias value of the matrix. Now the combine list of the matrix is as under:

$$W^s = \left[W_x^1, W_x^2, W_x^3, \ldots\ldots W_x^{n-1}\right] \tag{3}$$

Now from the Back-Propagation procedure, MSE simply computed for each and every weight matrix in W^s. Multilayer feed forward network considered for the proposed method is:

For each hidden layer's unit j:

$$h_j = f\left(\sum_{i=1}^{N} W_{x(ji)} neti + B_{xj}\right) \tag{4}$$

The total output of t unit for the output layer is given as under:

$$Y_t = f\left(\sum_{t=1}^{M} W_{x(jt)} h_j + B_{xt}\right) \tag{5}$$

where, Y_t is network output, f is transfer function, $W_{x(jt)}$ represents the weights matrix and Y_t is the net output. The work of the network is to acquire connotation between a definite set of output and input pairs,

$$\left\{ \left(net_1, T_1 \right), \left(net_2, T_2 \right), \left(net_3, T_3 \right), \ldots, \left(net_t, T_t \right) \right\}$$

According to the back-propagation method the weight and bias values are computed. One-layer sensitivity can be calculated from its prior one and the calculation of the sensitivity continues from the last layer of the network and in regressive direction. The sensitivity calculated for each unit t in the output layer as:

$$err_t = Y_t \left(1 - Y_t \right) \left(T_t - Y_t \right) \tag{6}$$

For each unit j in the hidden layer:

$$Err_j = h_j \left(1 - h_j \right) \sum_k err_t W_{x(jt)} \tag{7}$$

Biases and Weights changed to output as given below:

$$\Delta W_{k(jt)} = W_{x(jt)} + \eta Err_j h_j \tag{8}$$

$$\Delta B_{k(jt)} = B_{x(jt)} + \eta Err_j h_j \tag{9}$$

The input weights for the HFPBP calculated as:

$$\Delta W_{k(jt)} = W_{x(jt)} + \eta Err_j net_i \tag{10}$$

$$\Delta B_{k(jt)} = B_{x(jt)} + \eta Err_j net_i \tag{11}$$

Error calculation of the proposed method is as follows:

$$E = \left(T_t - Y_t \right) \tag{12}$$

The network performance index calculated using the following Eq:

$$V\left(x \right) = \frac{1}{2} \sum_{t=1}^{R} \left(T_t - X_t \right) \left(T_t - Y_t \right) \tag{13}$$

$$V_F\left(x\right) = \frac{1}{2}\sum_{t=1}^{R} E^T \cdot E \tag{14}$$

Calculation of the Mean Square Error as the performance index is as under:

$$V_\mu\left(x\right) = \frac{\sum_{j=1}^{N} V_F\left(x\right)}{P_i} \tag{15}$$

where the network output is Y_t, and $E=(T_t-Y_t)$ the calculation of errors for the tth input $V_\mu(x)$ is the average efficiency, $V_F(x)$ is the error for the tth input, performance index is $V_\mu(x)$, and the number of pollens is P_i. The average MSE calculated as under:

$$MSE_i = \left\{ V_\mu^1\left(x\right), V_\mu^2\left(x\right), V_\mu^3\left(x\right)\ldots\ldots V_\mu^n\left(x\right) \right\} \tag{16}$$

Pollen search method is replacing Mean Square Error, it is found when all the input processed for each population of the pollen. So, the pollen search pollen calculated as:

$$X_j = Min\left\{ V_\mu^1\left(x\right), V_\mu^2\left(x\right), V_\mu^3\left(x\right)\ldots\ldots V_\mu^n\left(x\right) \right\} \tag{17}$$

The remaining MSE assumed other pollen gametes. The newest solution x_i^{t+1} for global pollination i is created by means of levy flight, according to the following Equation (18):

$$x_i^{t+1} = x_i^t + x_r L\left(g_* - x_i^t\right) \tag{18}$$

where x_i^t is pollen i, x_r is a scaled parameter, L is levy distribution and g_* is the fittest solution. A new solution x_i^{t+1} for local pollination I generated as given below:

$$x_i^{t+1} = x_i^t + x_r\left(x_j^t - x_k^t\right) \tag{19}$$

Other flower pollen gametes movement x_i towards sx_j drawn from Eq. (20).

$$X = \begin{cases} x_i^t + x_r\left(x_j^t - x_k^t\right) & if\ x_r\left[0,1\right] > p\alpha \\ x_i^t & otherwise \end{cases} \tag{20}$$

The flower pollen gamete can move from x_i towards x_j through Levy flight as:

$$\nabla X_i = \begin{cases} x_i^t + levy\left(\lambda\right) \sim x_r \left(\dfrac{U_j}{\left|V_j\right|^{\frac{1}{\mu}}}\right) \\ x_i^t \qquad\qquad otherwise \\ \left(X - X_{best}\right) \quad if\ x_r\left[0,1\right] > p\alpha \end{cases} \tag{21}$$

where, ∇X_i is the best pollen gametes, selected through levy flight from position x_i towards x_j. For each layer the weight and bias value:

$$W_x^{n+1} = W_x^n - \nabla X_i \tag{22}$$

$$B_x^{n+1} = B_x^n - \nabla X_i \tag{23}$$

2.1 Proposed Algorithm Pseudo Code

The Given table illustrates the pseudo code for the proposed algorithm. Table 1 shows the pseudo code for the proposed hybrid model.

3. DATASETS

The following three datasets used in this research work, which discussed in details as under.

A) Thyroid Dataset

Thyroid dataset obtained from UCI machine-learning repository, this dataset based on thyroid disease (Quinlan, 1986). Thyroid dataset consists of 7200 patterns, 21 inputs, 5 hidden nodes, and 3 outputs. Each case consists of 21 attributes, which is assigned to one of the 3 classes, such as hyper, Hypro and the normal role of the thyroid gland. The target error is set to the value of 0.00001.

B) Diabetes Dataset

The dataset of diabetes taken from UCI; it is based on the Pima Indian diabetes. The dataset comprises of all information's due to a chemical variation in the body of a female whose difference causes diabetes (Smith et al., 1988). Diabetes dataset comprises a total of 768 patterns, 8 inputs, 5 hidden nodes and 2 outputs. The target error for this dataset is set to 0.00001.

Figure 1. The proposed HFPBP flowchart

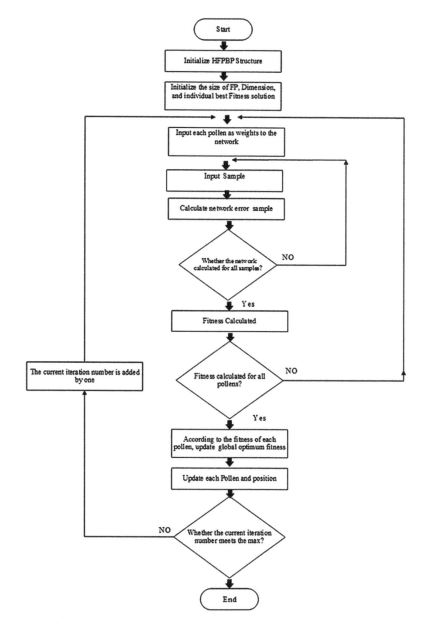

C) Glass Dataset

For criminal investigation the glass dataset used for the separation of glass splinters, this dataset consists of six classes. It is consisting of vehicle windows, containers, building windows, tableware and headlamps (Evett & Spiehler, 1988). This dataset comprises of 214 parameters, 9 inputs and 6 outputs. The target error for this dataset is set to 0.00001.

Table 1. Proposed algorithm pseudo code

1. Population size Initialization of FP, & structure of BPNN.
2. Loading of training data.
3. While MSE<ending criteria.
4. Pollen is pass as weights to the network.
5. Weights runs the Feed Forward Network.
6. The layers sensitivity computed from its prior layer, also the calculation of the sensitivity begins form the last layer of the network and move in back direction.
7. Bias and Weights values are updated Via Eq. (8) to (11).
8. Calculate the error using the Eq. (12).
9. The FP used to reduce error by correcting network parameters.
10. create flower pollen gametes from random pollen.
11. for *i*=1:*n* (all n flowers in the population).
12. If *rand<p*.
13. Draw a (d-dimensional) step-vector *L*, which obeys a levy distribution.
14. Global pollination via $x_i^{t+1} = x_i^t + L\left(g_* - x_i^t\right) Else$.
15. Draw ε form a uniform distribution in [-1,1].
16. Do local pollination via $x_i^{t+1} = x_i^t + \varepsilon\left(x_j^t - x_k^t\right)$.
17. End if.
18. Build new solution at new location.
19. Estimate new solutions.
20. If evaluated solutions are better, update solutions in the population.
If
$X_j>X_i$ then
$x_i \leftarrow x_j$
$X_i \leftarrow X_j$
End if
End for
21. Find the current best solution g^*.
22. The FP retains on calculating the finest conceivable weight and bias at each epoch until the BPNN is converged as optimum solution.
End

4. SIMULATION ENVIRONMENT

For the performance, analysis purpose this research work emphases on two standards: (a) MSE and (b) classification average accuracy of testing data. For data collection machine learning UCI repository is used and the datasets organized into testing training. Proposed and standard algorithms trained on training datasets and its accuracy calculated on testing datasets.

Computer system, which used for this research work, has a 2.5-GHz CPU, RAM 4-GB whereas, OS used was Microsoft Window8.1. For simulation purpose, MATLAB used to run the proposed HFPBP and FPBP algorithms on three classification datasets Thyroid, Diabetes and Glass.

5. RESULTS AND DISCUSSION

In this portion the performance and precision of proposed algorithms are verified & authenticated. Proposed algorithms (i.e. HFPBP and FPBP) compared with the standard algorithms such as Artificial Bee Colony (ABCNN), Artificial Bee Colony Back Propagation (ABC-BP) and Back Propagation Neural

Network (BPNN). The performance evaluation of all algorithms carried out based on MSE and average accuracy on benchmark classification datasets.

Three selected benchmark classification datasets obtained from University California Irvine Machine Learning Repository (UCIMLR). The Datasets are Thyroid Disease (Quinlin, 1986), Glass (Evett & Spiehler, 1988) and Diabetes (Smith et al., 1988). The simulations performed on the proposed algorithms and their comparisons discussed in the next section.

Table 2 clearly expressed that the performance of the proposed HFPBP & FPBP algorithms is better than the conventional standard algorithms such as BPNN, ABCNN and ABC-BP in terms of MSE and Accuracy. According to table 1 the proposed algorithms have low MSE and achieved a high percentage of accuracy (HFPBP= 99.97283% and FPBP= 99.66667%). While the conventional standard algorithms (i.e. BPNN, ABCNN and ABC-BP) have MSE (0.291, 0.045, 0.044) and low accuracy of the percentage (94.64%, 99.09%, 95.58%) respectively. Figure 2 Comparison of average MSE, accuracy, epochs and timing for Glass classification.

Table 3 clearly expresses that the performance of the proposed HFPBP and FPBP algorithms is better than the conventional standard algorithms like BPNN, ABCNN and ABC-BP in terms of MSE and Accuracy. According to table 2 the proposed algorithms have low MSE and achieved a high percentage of accuracy (HFPBP= 99.89892% and FPBP=99.6873%). While the conventional standard algorithms (i.e. BPNN, ABCNN and ABC-BP) have MSE (0.262, 0.150 and 0.202), and low accuracy of the percentage (94.89%, 96.98%, 79.75%) respectively. Figure 3 Comparison of average MSE, accuracy, epochs and timing for Thyroid classification.

Table 4 displays performance of all the proposed and standard conventional algorithms. According to the table results, it concluded that the proposed algorithm's performance is better than the standard algorithms. For the glass, classification algorithms the proposed HFPBP and FPBP algorithms achieved small MSE and high accuracy of 99.95% and 99.86% percent. While the other algorithms like BPNN,

Table 2. Proposed algorithms performance of testing for thyroid classification problem

Algorithms	Epochs	Time/Sec	Accuracy%	MSE
BPNN	1000	32.41848	94.64329	0.291917
ABCNN	1000	11553.22	99.09981	0.04501
ABC-BP	1000	11845.33	95.58602	0.04414
FPBP	1000	230.883	99.66667	0.003333
HFPBP	1000	236.2508	99.97283	0.000543

Table 3. Performance of the proposed algorithms of testing for the diabetes classification problem

Algorithms	Epochs	Time/Sec	Accuracy%	MSE
BPNN	1000	35.60359	94.89875	0.262363
ABCNN	1000	7599.227	96.98078	0.150961
ABC-BP	1000	5718.069	79.75321	0.202468
FPBP	1000	106.2711	99.6873	0.003127
HFPBP	1000	107.9297	99.89892	0.002022

ABCNN and ABC-BP have large MSE of 0.360, 0.0068, 0.0331 and accuracy of 94.04%, 99.86% and 96.68% percent respectively. Figure 4 Comparison of average MSE, accuracy, epochs and timing for Diabetes classification.

The above Figure 2 the y-axis represents the total number of input values of the Thyroid dataset while x-axis represents the MSE, Timing, Epochs and accuracy of the proposed algorithms graphically, which are HFPBP and FPBP and also for the standard algorithms such as BPNN, ABCNN and ABC-BP. The dataset, which used for this purpose, was Thyroid. The simulation outcomes evidently illustrate that

Table 4. Performance of the proposed algorithms of testing for glass classification problem

Algorithms	Epochs	Time/Sec	Accuracy%	MSE
BPNN	1000	33.1664	94.04733	0.360404
ABCNN	1000	6308.108	99.86322	0.006839
ABC-BP	1000	5384.235	96.68856	0.033114
FPBP	1000	110.2479	99.86257	0.001374
HFPBP	1000	147.724	99.95363	0.000927

Figure 2. Comparison of average MSE, accuracy, epochs and timing for thyroid classification

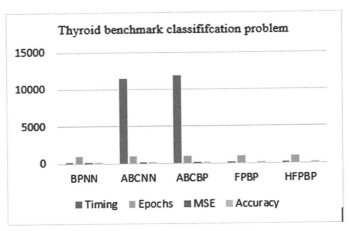

Figure 3. Comparison of average MSE, accuracy, epochs and timing for diabetes classification

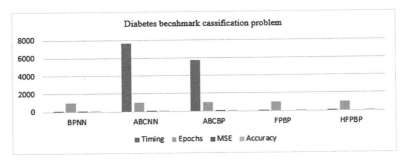

the proposed HFPBP and FPBP exhibit high accuracy and low MSE as compared to standard BPNN, ABCNN and ABC-BP algorithms.

Above Figure 3 the y-axis represents the total number of input values of the Diabetes dataset while x-axis represents the MSE, Timing, Epochs and accuracy of the proposed algorithms graphically, which are HFPBP and FPBP and also for the standard algorithms like BPNN, ABCNN and ABC-BP. The dataset, which used for this purpose, is Diabetes. The simulation outcomes evidently illustrate that the proposed HFPBP and FPBP exhibit high accuracy and low MSE as compared to standard BPNN, ABCNN and ABC-BP algorithms.

Above Figure 4 the y-axis represents the total number of input values of the Glass dataset while x-axis represents the MSE, Timing, Epochs and accuracy of the proposed algorithms graphically, which are HFPBP and FPBP and also for the standard algorithms such as BPNN, ABCNN and ABC-BP. The dataset, which used for this purpose, is Glass. The simulation outcomes evidently illustrate that the proposed HFPBP and FPBP exhibit high accuracy and low MSE as compared to standard BPNN, ABCNN and ABC-BP algorithms.

The above Figure 5 represents the MSE of proposed FPBP algorithm with log-sigmoid activation function. The dataset, which used in this graph, is Thyroid. The graph shows that initially the MSE is high, but when the epochs increases the value of MSE is decreased hence accuracy is also improved because with the passage of time the network becomes more intelligent and hence gives better results. The MSE, which achieved was 0.003, Accuracy is 99.66%, and the epochs (number of iterations) was 1000.

The above Figure 6 represents the MSE's of proposed Hybrid Flower Pollination based Back Propagation (HFPBP) algorithm with modified activation function. The dataset, which used in this graph, is Thyroid. The graph shows that initially the MSE is high, but when the epochs increases the value of MSE is decreased hence accuracy is also improved because with the passage of time the network becomes more intelligent and hence gives better results. The MSE, which achieved was 0.0005, Accuracy is 99.97%, and the epochs (number of iterations) was 1000.

The above Figure 7 denotes the MSE's of standard Back Propagation Neural Network (BPNN) algorithm with log-sigmoid activation function. The dataset, which used in this graph, is Thyroid. The graph shows that from start to end the oscillations is very high. The MSE, which achieved was 0.29, Accuracy is 94.64%, and the epochs (number of iterations) was 1000.

Figure 4. Comparison of average MSE, accuracy, epochs and timing for glass classification

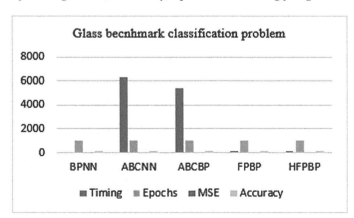

The above Figure 8 represents the MSE's of standard Artificial Bee Colony Neural Network (ABCNN) algorithm with log-sigmoid activation function. The dataset, which used in this graph, is Thyroid. The

Figure 5. MSE convergence performance of the proposed FPBP algorithm for thyroid classification

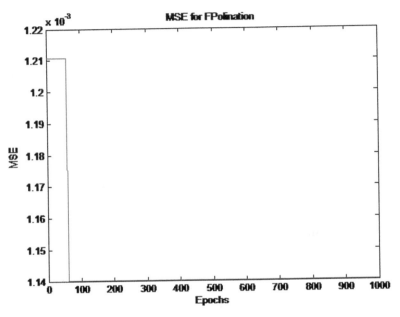

Figure 6. MSE convergence performance of the proposed HFPBP algorithm for thyroid classification

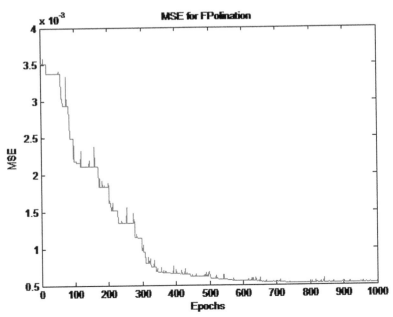

Figure 7. MSE convergence performance of BPNN algorithm for thyroid dataset

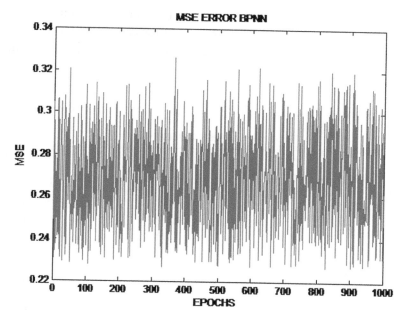

graph shows that from start to end the oscillations is very high. The MSE, which achieved was 0.04, Accuracy is 99.09%, and the epochs (number of iterations) was 1000.

The above Figure 9 represents the MSE's of the standard Artificial Bee Colony Back Propagation (ABC-BP) algorithm with log-sigmoid activation function. The dataset, which used in this graph, is

Figure 8. MSE convergence performance of ABCNN algorithm for thyroid dataset

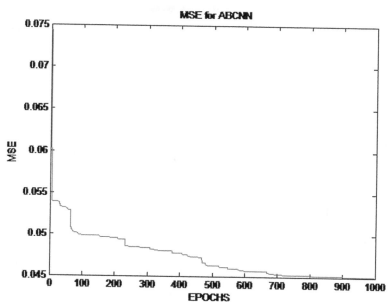

Thyroid. The graph shows that from start to finish the jumps in oscillations is very high. The MSE, which achieved was 0.04, Accuracy is 95.58%, and the epochs (number of iterations) was 1000.

The above Figure 10 represents the MSE's of proposed Flower Pollination Back Propagation (FPBP) algorithm with log-sigmoid activation function. The dataset, which used in this graph, is Diabetes. The

Figure 9. MSE convergence performance of ABC-BP algorithm for thyroid dataset

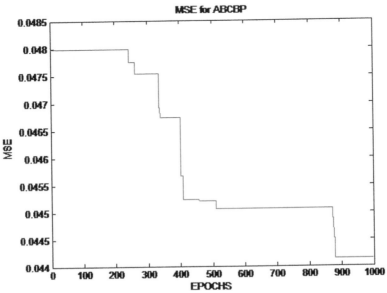

Figure 10. MSE convergence performance of proposed FPBP algorithm for diabetes dataset

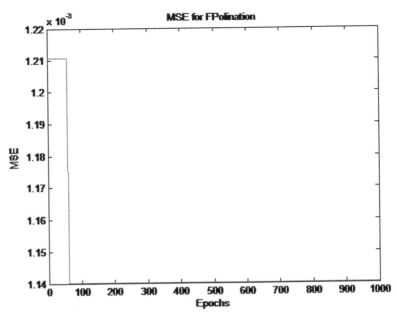

graph shows that initially the MSE is high, but when the epochs increases the value of MSE is decreased hence accuracy is also improved because with the passage of time the network become more intelligent and hence gives better results. The MSE, which achieved was 0.003, Accuracy is 99.68%, and the epochs (number of iterations) was 1000.

The above Figure 11 represents the MSE's of proposed Hybrid Flower Pollination based Back Propagation (HFPBP) algorithm with modified activation function. The dataset, which used in this graph, is Diabetes. The graph shows that initially the MSE is high, but when the epochs increases the value of MSE is decreased hence accuracy is also improved because with the passage of time the network becomes more intelligent and hence gives better results. The MSE, which achieved was 0.002, Accuracy is 99.89%, and the epochs (number of iterations) was 1000.

The above Figure 12 represents the MSE's of standard Back Propagation Neural Network (BPNN) algorithm with log-sigmoid activation function. The dataset, which used in this graph, is Diabetes. The graph shows that from start to end the oscillations is very high. The MSE, which achieved was 0.26, Accuracy is 94.89%, and the epochs (number of iterations) was 1000.

The above Figure 13 represents the MSE's of standard Artificial Bee Colony Neural Network (ABCNN) algorithm with log-sigmoid activation function. The dataset, which used in this graph, is Diabetes. The graph shows that from start to end the oscillations is very high. The MSE, which achieved was 0.15, Accuracy is 96.98%, and the epochs (number of iterations) was 1000.

The above Figure 14 represents the MSE's of the standard Artificial Bee Colony Back Propagation (ABC-BP) algorithm with log-sigmoid activation function. The dataset, which used in this graph, is Diabetes. The graph shows that from start to finish the jumps in oscillations is very high. The MSE, which achieved was 0.202, Accuracy is 79.75%, and the epochs (number of iterations) was 1000.

Figure 11. MSE convergence performance of the proposed HFPBP algorithm for diabetes dataset

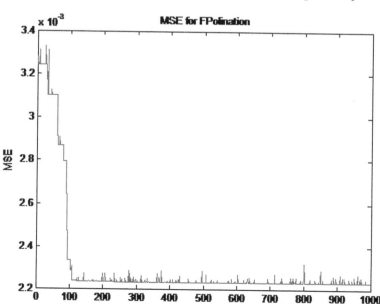

The above Figure 15 represents the MSE's of proposed Flower Pollination Back Propagation (FPBP) algorithm with log-sigmoid activation function. The dataset, which used in this graph, is Glass. The graph shows that initially the MSE is high, but when the epochs increases the value of MSE is decreased hence accuracy is also improved because with the passage of time the network becomes more intelligent and

Figure 12. MSE convergence performance of the standard BPNN algorithm for diabetes dataset

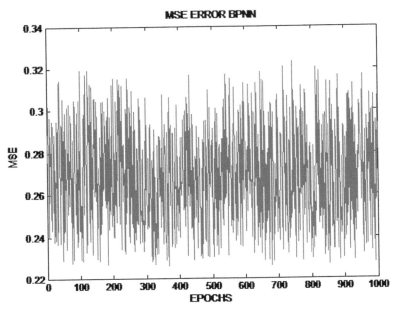

Figure 13. MSE convergence performance of the standard ABCNN algorithm for diabetes dataset

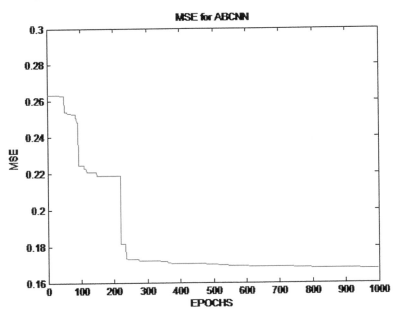

hence gives better results. The MSE, which achieved was 0.0013, Accuracy is 99.86%, and the epochs (number of iterations) was 1000.

The above Figure 16 represents the MSE's of proposed Hybrid Flower Pollination based Back Propagation (HFPBP) algorithm with modified activation function. The dataset, which used in this graph, is Glass. The graph shows that initially the MSE is high, but when the epochs increases the value of MSE is

Figure 14. MSE convergence performance of the standard ABC-BP algorithm for diabetes dataset

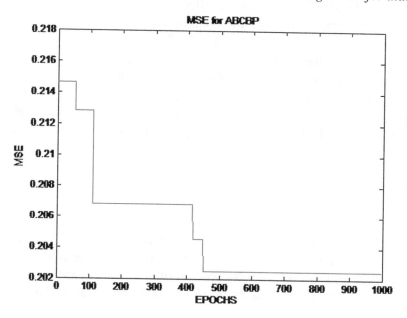

Figure 15. MSE Convergence performance of the proposed FPBP algorithm for glass dataset

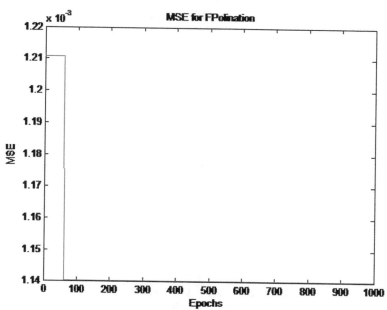

decreased hence accuracy is also improved because with the passage of time the network becomes more intelligent and hence gives better results. The MSE, which achieved was 0.0009, Accuracy is 99.95%, and the epochs (number of iterations) was 1000.

The above Figure 17 represents the MSE's of standard Back Propagation Neural Network (BPNN) algorithm with log-sigmoid activation function. The dataset, which used in this graph, is Glass. The graph shows that from start to end the oscillations is very high. The MSE, which achieved was 0.36, Accuracy is 94.04%, and the epochs (number of iterations) was 1000.

Figure 18 represents the MSE's of standard Artificial Bee Colony Neural Network (ABCNN) algorithm with log-sigmoid activation function. The dataset, which used in this graph, is Glass. The graph shows that from start to end the oscillations is very high. The MSE, which achieved was 0.15, Accuracy is 96.98%, and the epochs (number of iterations) was 1000.

The above Figure 19 represents the MSE's of the standard Artificial Bee Colony Back Propagation (ABC-BP) algorithm with log-sigmoid activation function. The dataset, which used in this graph, is Glass. The graph shows that from start to finish the jumps in oscillations is very high. The MSE, which achieved was 0.033, Accuracy is 96.68%, and the epochs (number of iterations) was 1000.

6. CONCLUSION AND FUTURE WORK

This research work proposed Hybrid Flower Pollination based Back Propagation (HFPBP) with modified activation function and Flower Pollination Back Propagation (FPBP) with log-sigmoid activation function. Several variants created in-order to improve the training of the ANN with respect to lowest MSE, high accuracy. The performance of proposed algorithms has been validated against the standard BPNN, ABCNN and ABC-BP algorithms by using different classification datasets such as Thyroid,

Figure 16. MSE Convergence performance of the proposed HFPBP algorithm for glass dataset

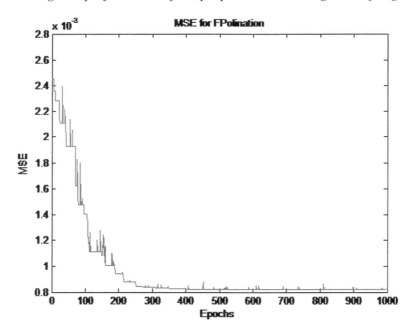

Figure 17. MSE convergence performance of the standard BPNN algorithm for glass dataset

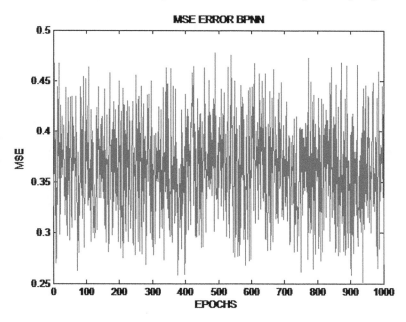

Figure 18. MSE convergence performance of the standard ABCNN algorithm for glass dataset

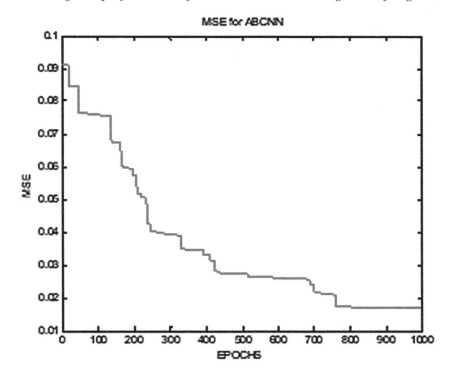

Figure 19. MSE convergence performance of the standard ABC-BP algorithm for glass dataset

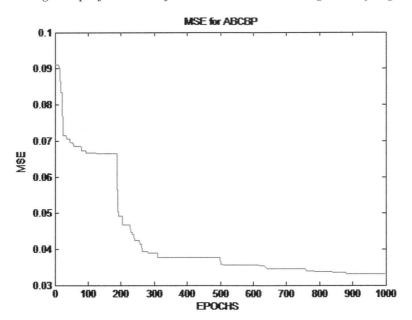

Diabetes and Glass. Based on simulations done the results shows that the proposed HFPBP and FPBP algorithms have high accuracy and low MSE.

In the future, we recommend the ABC algorithm the ABC is poor in the exploitation process to advance the exploitation and exploration ability of ABC the FP algorithms integrated with ABC algorithm.

ACKNOWLEDGMENT

The very first, I wish to utter my genuine thankfulness and appreciation to my respectable supervisor Dr. Abdullah for the nonstop backing of my MS research, for his serenity, motivation, and huge knowledge. The supervision of my respected advisor helped me a lot in all the phases of the research work and writing of this research paper as well. At the end, I would like to thank my family members and who supported me through all this process.

REFERENCES

Alsmadi, M. K. S., Omar, K. B., & Noah, S. A. (2009). Back propagation algorithm: The best algorithm among the multi-layer perceptron algorithm. *IJCSNS International Journal of Computer Science and Network Security*, *9*(4), 378–383.

Aydin, D., Ozyon, S., Yaşar, C., & Liao, T. (2014). Artificial bee colony algorithm with dynamic population size to combine economic and emission dispatch problem. *International Journal of Electrical Power & Energy Systems*, *54*, 144–153. doi:10.1016/j.ijepes.2013.06.020

Bi, J., Chk8en, Y., & Wang, J. Z. (2005, June). A sparse support vector machine approach to region-based image categorization. In *Proceedings of the 2005 IEEE Computer Society Conference on Computer Vision and Pattern Recognition (CVPR'05) (Vol. 1*, pp. 1121-1128). IEEE. 10.1109/CVPR.2005.48

Castellani, M., & Rowlands, H. (2009). Evolutionary artificial neural network design and training for wood veneer classification. *Engineering Applications of Artificial Intelligence, 22*(4), 732–741. doi:10.1016/j.engappai.2009.01.013

Celik, M., Koylu, F., & Karaboga, D. (2016). CoABC Miner: An algorithm for cooperative rule classification system based on artificial bee colony. *International Journal of Artificial Intelligence Tools, 25*(01), 1550028. doi:10.1142/S0218213015500281

Chakraborty, D., Saha, S., & Maity, S. (2015, February). Training feed forward neural networks using hybrid flower pollination-gravitational search algorithm. In *Proceedings of the 2015 International Conference on Futuristic Trends on Computational Analysis and Knowledge Management (ABLAZE)* (pp. 261-266). IEEE.

Chen, J., Huang, H., Tian, S., & Qu, Y. (2009). Feature selection for text classification with Naïve Bayes. *Expert Systems with Applications, 36*(3), 5432–5435. doi:10.1016/j.eswa.2008.06.054

Chiroma, H., Khan, A., Abubakar, A. I., Saadi, Y., Hamza, M. F., Shuib, L., & Herawan, T. (2016). A new approach for forecasting OPEC petroleum consumption based on neural network train by using flower pollination algorithm. *Applied Soft Computing, 48*, 50–58. doi:10.1016/j.asoc.2016.06.038

Chiroma, H., Shuib, N. L. M., Muaz, S. A., Abubakar, A. I., Ila, L. B., & Maitama, J. Z. (2015). A review of the applications of bio-inspired flower pollination algorithm. Procedia Coml2puter. *Science, 62*, 435–441.

Coppin, B. (2004). *Artificial intelligence illuminated*. Jones & Bartlett Learning.

Cunningham, P., & Delany, S. J. (2007). k-Nearest neighbour classifiers. *Multiple Classifier Systems, 34*(8), 1–17.

Dreiseitl, S., & Ohno-Machado, L. (2002). Logistic regression and artificial neural network classification models: A methodology review. *Journal of Biomedical Informatics, 35*(5), 352–359. doi:10.1016/S1532-0464(03)00034-0 PMID:12968784

Dunham, M. H. (2006). *Data mining: Introductory and advanced topics*. Pearson Education India.

Engelbrecht, A. P. (2007). *Computational intelligence: an introduction*. John Wiley & Sons. doi:10.1002/9780470512517

Eom, K., Jung, K., & Sirisena, H. (2003). Performance improvement of back propagation algorithm by automatic activation function gain tuning using fuzzy logic. *Neurocomputing, 50*, 439–460. doi:10.1016/S0925-2312(02)00576-3

Evett, I. W., & Spiehler, E. J. (1988). Knowledge based systems. In *Rule induction in forensic science*. Academic Press.

Hamid, N. A., Nawi, N. M., & Ghazali, R. (2011). The effect of adaptive gain and adaptive momentum in improving training time of gradient descent back propagation algorithm on classification problems. International Journal on Advanced Science. *Engineering and Information Technology, 1*(2), 178–184.

Hamid, N. A., Nawi, N. M., Ghazali, R., & Salleh, M. N. M. (2012). Solving Local Minima Problem in Back Propagation Algorithm Using Adaptive Gain, Adaptive Momentum and Adaptive Learning Rate on Classification Problems. *International Journal of Modern Physics: Conference Series, 9*, 448–455.

Haofei, Z., Guoping, X., Fangting, Y., & Han, Y. (2007). A neural network model based on the multi-stage optimization approach for short-term food price forecasting in China. *Expert Systems with Applications, 33*(2), 347–356. doi:10.1016/j.eswa.2006.05.021

Haykin, S. S., Haykin, S. S., Haykin, S. S., & Haykin, S. S. (2009). *Neural networks and learning machines* (Vol. 3). Upper Saddle River, NJ, USA: Pearson.

Hecht-Nielsen, R. (1990). On the algebraic structure of feed forward network weight spaces. Adval2nced. *Neural Computation*, 129–135.

Ho, Y. C., Bryson, A. E., & Baron, S. (1965). Differential games and optimal pursuit-evasion strategies. In *Proceedings of the Joint Automatic Control Conference* (No. 3, pp. 37-40). Academic Press. 10.1109/TAC.1965.1098197

Jayalakshmi, T., & Santhakumaran, A. (2010). Improved Gradient Descent Back Propagation Neural Networks for Diagnoses of Type II Diabetes Mellitus. *Global Journal of Computer Science and Technology, 9*(5).

Jung, K. K., Lim, J. K., Chung, S. B., & Eom, K. H. (2003). Performance Improvement of Back propagation Algorithm by Automatic Tuning of Learning Rate using Fuzzy Logic System. *Journal of information and communication convergence engineering, 1*(3), 157-162.

Karaboga, D. (2005). An idea based on honey bee swarm for numerical optimization (Vol. 200). Erciyes University.

Kathirvalavakumar, T., & Thangavel, P. (2006). A modified back propagation training algorithm for feed forward neural networks. *Neural Processing Letters, 23*(2), 111–119. doi:10.100711063-005-3501-2

Kim, H. C., Pang, S., Je, H. M., Kim, D., & Bang, S. Y. (2003). Constructing support vector machine ensemble. *Pattern Recognition, 36*(12), 2757–2767. doi:10.1016/S0031-3203(03)00175-4

Kim, J. W., Jung, K. K., & Eom, K. H. (2002). Auto-Tuning Method of Learning Rate for Performance Improvement of Back propagation Algorithm. *Journal of the Institute of Electronics Engineers of Korea CI, 39*(4), 19–27.

Kolen, J. F., & Pollack, J. B. (1991). Multi associative memory. In *Proceedings of the Thirteenth Annual Conference of the Cognitive Science Society* (pp. 785-789). Academic Press.

Kotsiantis, S. B., Kanellopoulos, D., & Pintelas, P. E. (2006). Data preprocessing for supervised leaning. *International Journal of Computational Science, 1*(2), 111–117.

Ku-Mahamud, K. R. (2015, August). Hybrid ant colony system and flower pollination algorithms for global optimization. In *Proceedings of the 2015 9th International Conference on IT in Asia (CITA)* (pp. 1-9). IEEE. 10.1109/CITA.2015.7349816

Lee, K., Booth, D., & Alam, P. (2005). A comparison of supervised and unsupervised neural networks in predicting bankruptcy of Korean firms. *Expert Systems with Applications, 29*(1), 1–16. doi:10.1016/j. eswa.2005.01.004

Li, J. B., & Chung, Y. K. (2005). A novel back-propagation neural network training algorithm designed by an ant colony optimization. In *Proceedings of the 2005 IEEE/PES Transmission & Distribution Conference & Exposition: Asia and Pacific* (pp. 1-5). IEEE.

Mushgil, H. M., Alani, H. A., & George, L. E. (2015). Comparison between Resilient and Standard Back Propagation Algorithms Efficiency in Pattern Recognition. *International Journal of Scientific & Engineering Research, 6*(3), 773–778.

Nandy, S., Sarkar, P. P., & Das, A. (2012). Training a feed-forward neural network with artificial bee colony based back propagation method.

Nawi, N. M., Ghazali, R., & Salleh, M. N. M. (2010, October). The development of improved back-propagation neural networks algorithm for predicting patients with heart disease. In *Proceedings of the International Conference on Information Computing and Applications* (pp. 317-324). Springer Berlin Heidelberg. 10.1007/978-3-642-16167-4_41

Nawi, N. M., Ransing, R. S., & Ransing, M. R. (2007). An improved conjugate gradient-based learning algorithm for back propagation neural networks. *International Journal of Computational Intelligence, 4*(1), 46–55.

Nawi, N. M., Ransing, R. S., Salleh, M. N. M., Ghazali, R., & Hamid, N. A. (2010). An improved back propagation neural network algorithm on classification problems. In Database Theory and Application, Bio-Science and Bio-Technology (pp. 177-188). Springer Berlin Heidelberg. doi:10.1007/978-3-642-17622-7_18

Nikam, S. S. (2015). A Comparative Study of Classification Techniques in Data Mining Algorithms. *Oriental Journal of Computer Science & Technology, 8*(1), 13–19.

Orosun, R. O., & Adamu, S. S. (2014). Neural Network Based Model of an Industrial Oil-fired Boiler System. *Nigerian Journal of Technology, 33*(3), 293–303. doi:10.4314/njt.v33i3.6

Otair, M. A., & Salameh, W. A. (2005, June). Speeding up back-propagation neural networks. In *Proceedings of the 2005 Informing Science and IT Education Joint Conference* (pp. 16-19). Academic Press.

Popescu, M. C., Balas, V. E., Perescu-Popescu, L., & Mastorakis, N. (2009). Multilayer perceptron and neural networks. *WSEAS Transactions on Circuits and Systems, 8*(7), 579–588.

Pop, C. B., Chifu, V. R., Salomie, I., Racz, D. S., & Bonta, R. M. (2017). Hybridization of the Flower Pollination Algorithm. A Case Study in the Problem of Generating Healthy Nutritional Meals for Older Adults. In *Nature-Inspired Computing and Optimization* (pp. 151–183). Springer International Publishing. doi:10.1007/978-3-319-50920-4_7

Quinlan, J. R. (1986). Induction of decision trees. *Machine Learning*, *1*(1), 81–106. doi:10.1007/BF00116251

Rehman, M. Z., Nawi, N. M., & Ghazali, M. I. (2011). Noise-Induced Hearing Loss (NIHL) prediction in humans using a modified back propagation neural network. International Journal on Advanced Science. *Engineering and Information Technology*, *1*(2), 185–189.

Ruggieri, S. (2002). Efficient C4. 5 [classification algorithm]. *IEEE Transactions on Knowledge and Data Engineering*, *14*(2), 438–444. doi:10.1109/69.991727

Rumelhart, D. E., Hinton, G. E., & Williams, R. J. (1988). Learning representations by back-propagating errors. *Cognitive modeling*, *5*(3), 1.

Schalkoff, R. J. (1997). *Artificial neural networks*. McGraw-Hill Higher Education.

Smith, J. W., Everhart, J. E., Dickson, W. C., Knowler, W. C., & Johannes, R. S. (1988, November). Using the ADAP learning algorithm to forecast the onset of diabetes mellitus. *In Proceedings of the Annual Symposium on Computer Application in Medical Care* (p. 261). American Medical Informatics Association.

Tong, S., & Koller, D. (2001). Support vector machine active learning with applications to text classification. *Journal of Machine Learning Research*, *2*(November), 45–66.

Umanol, M., Okamoto, H., Hatono, I., Tamura, H. I. R. O. Y. U. K. I., Kawachi, F., Umedzu, S., & Kinoshita, J. (1994, June). Fuzzy decision trees by fuzzy ID3 algorithm and its application to diagnosis systems. In *Proceedings of the Third IEEE Conference on Fuzzy Systems* (pp. 2113-2118). IEEE. 10.1109/FUZZY.1994.343539

Wang, L., Zeng, Y., & Chen, T. (2015). Back propagation neural network with adaptive differential evolution algorithm for time series forecasting. *Expert Systems with Applications*, *42*(2), 855-863.'2

Xiaoyuan, L., Bin, Q., & Lu, W. (2009, October). A new improved BP neural network algorithm. In *Proceedings of the Second International Conference on Intelligent Computation Technology and Automation ICICTA'09* (Vol. 1, pp. 19-22). IEEE. 10.1109/ICICTA.2009.12

Xu, Y., & Zhang, H. (2009, July). Study on the Improved BP Algorithm and Application. In *Proceedings of the Asia-Pacific Conference on Information Processing APCIP 2009* (Vol. 1, pp. 7-10). IEEE. 10.1109/APCIP.2009.9

Xu, S., & Wang, Y. (2017). Parameter estimation of photovoltaic modules using a hybrid flower pollination algorithm. *Energy Conversion and Management*, *144*, 53–68. doi:10.1016/j.enconman.2017.04.042

Yamany, W., Zawbaa, H. M., Emary, E., & Hassanien, A. E. (2015, August). Attribute reduction approach based on modified flower pollination algorithm. In *Proceedings of the 2015 IEEE International Conference on Fuzzy Systems (FUZZ-IEEE)* (pp. 1-7). IEEE. 10.1109/FUZZ-IEEE.2015.7338111

Yang, X. S. (2012, September). Flower pollination algorithm for global optimization. In *Proceedings of the International Conference on Unconventional Computing and Natural Computation* (pp. 240-249). Springer Berlin Heidelberg. 10.1007/978-3-642-32894-7_27

Zhang, J. R., Zhang, J., Lok, T. M., & Lyu, M. R. (2007). A hybrid particle swarm optimization–back-propagation algorithm for feed forward neural network training. *Applied Mathematics and Computation*, *185*(2), 1026–1037. doi:10.1016/j.amc.2006.07.025

Zweiri, Y. H., Whidborne, J. F., & Seneviratne, L. D. (2003). A three-term back propagation algorithm. *Neurocomputing*, *50*, 305–318. doi:10.1016/S0925-2312(02)00569-6

Additional Reading

Yazid, M. H. B. A., Talib, M. S., & Satria, M. H. (2019, August). Flower Pollination Neural Network for Heart Disease Classification. *IOP Conference Series. Materials Science and Engineering*, *551*(1), 012072. doi:10.1088/1757-899X/551/1/012072

Bangyal, W. H., Ahmad, J., & Rauf, H. T. (2019). Optimization of Neural Network Using Improved Bat Algorithm for Data Classification. *Journal of Medical Imaging and Health Informatics*, *9*(4), 670–681. doi:10.1166/jmihi.2019.2654

Alihodzic, A., Tuba, E., & Tuba, M. (2020). An Improved Extreme Learning Machine Tuning by Flower Pollination Algorithm. In *Nature-Inspired Computation in Data Mining and Machine Learning* (pp. 95–112). Cham: Springer. doi:10.1007/978-3-030-28553-1_5

Dhal, K. G., Gálvez, J., & Das, S. (2019). Toward the modification of flower pollination algorithm in clustering-based image segmentation. *Neural Computing & Applications*, 1–19.

Li, W., He, Z., Zheng, J., & Hu, Z. (2019). Improved Flower Pollination Algorithm and Its Application in User Identification Across Social Networks. *IEEE Access*, *7*, 44359–44371. doi:10.1109/ACCESS.2018.2889801

Sornam, M., & Prabhakaran, M. (2019). Logit-Based Artificial Bee Colony Optimization (LB-ABC) Approach for Dental Caries Classification Using a Back Propagation Neural Network. In *Integrated Intelligent Computing, Communication and Security* (pp. 79–91). Singapore: Springer. doi:10.1007/978-981-10-8797-4_9

Pandey, S. K., & Janghel, R. R. (2019). ECG Arrhythmia Classification Using Artificial Neural Networks. In *Proceedings of 2nd International Conference on Communication, Computing and Networking* (pp. 645-652). Springer Singapore. 10.1007/978-981-13-1217-5_63

Mohamed, S. T., Ebeid, H. M., Hassanien, A. E., & Tolba, M. F. (2019, March). Optimized Feed Forward Neural Network for Microscopic White Blood Cell Images Classification. In *Proceedings of the International Conference on Advanced Machine Learning Technologies and Applications* (pp. 758-767). Springer.

Desai, S. D., Giraddi, S., Narayankar, P., Pudakalakatti, N. R., & Sulegaon, S. (2019). Back-propagation neural network versus logistic regression in heart disease classification. In *Advanced Computing and Communication Technologies* (pp. 133–144). Springer Singapore. doi:10.1007/978-981-13-0680-8_13

KEY TERMS AND DEFINITIONS

Accuracy: Accuracy is the parameter for evaluating the performance of the machine or models which finds that how much the measured results are near to the actual value. Accuracy calculate all the correct prediction observation divided by the total observation number or actual number.

Ant Colony Optimization: In the field of computer sciences and operations research, the ant colony optimization algorithm (ACO) is a probabilistic method for resolving computational issues which can be decreased to resulting best routes via graphs. Artificial Ants stand for multi-agent technique which is inspired from the actual behavior of real ants.

Artificial Neural Network: Artificial Neural Network is actually modeled is a computational model which mimic the human brains works. There are units in the ANN called neurons these units are connected to other by link and every link is associated with a weight.

Back Propagation: BP is the utmost well-known supervised learning Artificial Neural Network algorithm presented by Rumelhart Hinton and Williams in 1986 mostly used to train Multi-Layer Perceptron. it is an algorithm which is used for optimization and applied to the Artificial Neural Network (ANN) to accelerate the network convergence to global optima throughout the training process. Like ANN BPNN also comprises of the input layer, one or more hidden layers and an output layer of neurons.

Classification: Classification is a technique in which the data are grouped into a given number of classes on the basis of some similarity and constraints. The main aim of the classification technique is to shrink the measure of the error.

Diabetes: It is a disease that happens when the glucose of your blood, also known as blood sugar, became too high. Blood glucose is the main source of energy for every human being and it comes from the food we and you eat. Insulin are, hormones which are made by the pancreas, it helps glucose from food get into your cells and will be utilizes for energy.

Flower pollination Algorithm: It is a bio-inspired algorithm which copies the pollination conduct of the flowering plants. Optimal plant reproduction policy includes the survival of the fittest as well as the optimal reproduction of plants in terms of numbers.

Local Minima: Local maxima are a point of a function with highest output (locally), while local minima are a point of a function with lowest output (also locally). Global maxima/minima, however, are different. They represent either the highest possible output of a function or the lowest possible output.

Mean Square Error: In statistics the mean square error initials are (MSE) of an estimator (it is a procedure for estimating an unobserved quantity) which has the ability to measure the average of all the square of errors. It is used to verify the accuracy in the classification results.

Optimization: It is the process in which there are various alternatives and the selection of best alternatives among them all is an optimization.

Swarm intelligence: It is the joint conduct of dispersed, self-organized scheme, natural or artificial. The concept is used in a work on artificial intelligence. The expression was introduced by Gerardo Beni and Jing Wang in 1989, in the context of cellular robotic systems.

Thyroid: It is a butterfly structure gland in the inner part of the neck. It produces hormones that control the speed of metabolism in the human body and also this system helps the body to use energy. The disorders of a thyroid gland can slow down the metabolism by disrupting the manufacturing of the thyroid hormones.

Chapter 14
The Effect of List–Liner–Based Interaction Technique in a 3D Interactive Virtual Biological Learning Environment

Numan Ali
University of Malakand, Pakistan

Sehat Ullah
University of Malakand, Pakistan

Zuhra Musa
University of Malakand, Pakistan

ABSTRACT

Various interaction techniques (such as direct, menu-based, etc.) are provided to allow users to interact with virtual learning environments. These interaction techniques improve their performance and learning but in a complex way. In this chapter, we investigated a simple list-liner based interface for gaining access to different modules within a 3D interactive Virtual Learning Environment (VLE). We have implemented a 3D interactive biological VLE for secondary school level students by using virtual mustard plant (VMP), where students interact by using 3D interactive device with the help of list-liner based interface. The aim of this work is to provide an easy interaction interface to use list-liner interaction technique by using 3D interactive device in an information-rich and complex 3D virtual environment. We compared list-liner interface with direct interface and evaluations reveal that the list-liner interface is very suitable and efficient for student learning enhancement and that the students can easily understand and use the system.

DOI: 10.4018/978-1-7998-2521-0.ch014

1. INTRODUCTION

The use of advance technology for teaching and training purposes is increasing day-by-day and many fields such as surgery, aeronautic assembly, architecture, businesses and education etc, are using digital technology applications to achieve efficiency in their work processes (Fung, 2002; Johansson & Wickman, 2018). These technologies are very helpful for the improvement of skill and independent learning (de Oliveira & Galembeck, 2016; Emvalotis & Koutsianou, 2018). As technological development are rapidly growing in science education, to develop new strategies and to enable teachers to develop pedagogical content knowledge around novel topics (Williams, Eames, Hume, & Lockley, 2012). According to Dalgarno and Lee, "technologies themselves do not directly cause learning to occur but can afford certain tasks that themselves may result in learning" (Dalgarno, Hedberg, & Harper, 2002). One of the advance technologies is the use of Virtual Reality (VR) technology that provides an efficient solution for problems where the physical alternative is not available, the cost of doing the actual work is high or the procedure of the task is very dangerous to perform, particularly in education because of their unique technological characteristics that differentiate them from the other Information and Communication Technologies (ICT) applications (Baggott la Velle, Wishart, McFarlane, Brawn, & John, 2007).

1.1 Virtual Reality (VR)

The recent advances in computer hardware and software have made VR technology capable to be used in many fields such as medical, military and education. According to Howard Rheingold VR is a three-dimensional computer-generated environment where user feels his/her presence. In the virtual environment user is able to navigate freely from one point to another, observe it from different sides, to get in touch with it, to seize it and manipulate it (Rheingold, 1991). VR can be described as a montage of technologies that support the creation of synthetic, highly interactive Three Dimensional (3D) spatial environments that represent real or non-real situations (Mikropoulos & Natsis, 2011). VR allows user to change the flow of occurrences in a virtual environment and hence to interact with virtual things. It uses many hardware components and software techniques for each application area. Virtual environment presents the 3D representation of the real or imaginary facts and provides to users a real time interaction (Hachet, 2010). Virtual reality can be classified into three basic schemes that are interaction, immersion and involvement (Pausch, Proffitt, & Williams, 1997). Interaction can be performed by pointing and gesturing, and by picking objects to manipulate them or examine them. The 3D interaction interfaces provide to users more realism and immersion in a virtual environment where users feel their presence. In virtual reality the 3D interaction is considered as a coercing component which allows the user to navigate, select, control and manipulate objects in a virtual environment (Ullah, 2011). Involvement is the user participation in a virtual world where he/she can navigate in a passive or active way (Pausch et al., 1997). Therefore, we must design the virtual environments in a way that is based on 3D interaction techniques where user feels more realism and immersion in it.

1.2 Virtual Reality in Education

In the teaching-learning process innovative approaches have been developed by using new technologies, in which VR is considered the essential one (Richard, Tijou, Richard, & Ferrier, 2006). VR is one of the most imperative contrivance that support students learning in different fields. Therefore, there are a lot of special virtual learning environments developed for different purposes in education such as Virtual Reality Physics Simulation (VRPS) (Kim, Park, Lee, Yuk, & Lee, 2001), Construct 3D for Mathematics Education (Sheridan, 2000), Virtual ChemLab Projects (Woodfield et al., 2004a) and biological education (Shim et al., 2003a) etc.

Virtual Learning Environment (VLE) is one of the most powerful tools that supports the learning process as ICT (Rajaei & Aldhalaan, 2011; Reis & Escudeiro, 2014). It is findings from the previous research that virtual learning environments are often more effective than traditional teaching tools (Clase et al., 2009). With the help of VR technology immersive and interactive virtual environments are created to facilitate or aid learning (Nonis, 2005; Richards & Kelaiah, 2012). These activities enable students to experience phenomena through their own eyes, ears and hands rather than through the eyes of a teacher or textbook writer (Ling & Rui, 2016; Totkov, 2003). Winn et al. suggested that interaction is more important facilitator for learning than immersion for some kinds of task (Winn et al., 1997). Therefore, the use of VR has become familiar technology in education for students learning improvement particularly in practical education.

Designing of virtual learning environment needs display hardware, tracking system, input device, environment model(s), rendering / display software and interaction software (Bowman et al., 2008; Wickens, 1992).

1.3 Virtual Reality in Biology Education

One of the solutions of the above problems and limitations is the use of VR technologies in biology education. Biology experiments are among the difficult tasks to be performed by students in laboratories (Mikropoulos, Katsikis, Nikolou, & Tsakalis, 2003a). Virtual biology laboratory curricula have been used efficiently as alternative or preliminary activities for hands-on experiments in high school and college level bi- ology courses, respectively. Virtual biology laboratories provide momentous benefits especially for the distance education, because it can be used anywhere and anytime for virtual experiments (Shim et al., 2003b). Virtual biology laboratories facilitate the students to perform the experiments many times without any costs and accidents. VR also enables students to explore very small (microscopic information), big or hazardous objects that cannot be accessed in normal situation in the real world (Bonser et al., 2013). The students' performance and learning capabilities can be enhanced by using visual, audio and haptic feedback in a virtual environment. Therefore, the use of VR has become familiar technology in biology education for students learning enhancement.

In this paper, we introduce a framework called virtual mustard plant (VMP), which uses a novel list-liner interaction technique, with a haptic interactive device. We invited, secondary school students for the evaluation of list-liner interaction technique in VMP. The students performed different tasks using list-liner as well as a direct interface. The experimental results reveal that the list-liner technique is efficient, more user friendly, easy in searching and exploration and has a higher user-satisfaction as compare to direct interface.

The rest of the paper is organized as follows. Section 2 elaborates some related studies in the field of virtual system for learning. Section 3 presents our proposed system. Section 4 is about the experiment and evaluation results of our proposed system. Finally, section 5 is related with conclusion and future work.

2. BACKGROUND

This section presents existing work in VR on biological education both in two-dimensional (2D) and Three Dimensional (3D) environments.

2.1 Virtual Biological Learning Environments

This subsection presents Virtual Biology Laboratories (VBLs) both in 2D and 3D environments.

Different Virtual Learning Environments (VLEs) have been developed for learning purposes by researchers that improve the learning capabilities of learners in biology education. Some of these learning environments are the following:

In 2005, Dede et al. developed an online graphical Multi-User Virtual Environments (MUVEs) in biology education to enhance middle school student motivation and learning about science and society (Dede, Clarke, Ketelhut, Nelson, & Bowman, 2005). Virtual environments for the structure of the plant cell and the process of photosynthesis were developed by Mikropoulos et al. In this VE exploration and interaction inside the virtual plant cell starts by navigation through the external plant tissue of the virtual cell. The internal cell structure is visible and the user can freely navigate, observe and study. The student can study about the organization of organelles in the 3D space inside the cell and the way they work together in order for the cell to function (Mikropoulos, Katsikis, Nikolou, & Tsakalis, 2003b). A typical cell environment was constructed at NDSU (North Dakota State University) by While et al. This VE contains 3D representations of all the components and organelles of a cell such as the nucleus, mitochondria, and chloroplasts. Students learn the structure and functions of a cell by interactively performing goal-oriented tasks in the 3D virtual cell (McClean, Slator, & White, 1999). Virtual environments for the structure of the plant cell and the process of photosynthesis were developed by Mikropoulos and Natsis (2011). Where the internal cell structure is visible and the user can freely navigate, observe and manipulate different objects. Here students can study about the organization of organelles in the 3D space inside the cell and the way they work together in order for the cell to function. This virtual environment is useful for teachers, but the user can lose orientation and navigation in this environment. Slator developed a Virtual Cell that provides an authentic problem-solving experience, engaging students in actively learning structures and functions of eukaryotic cells. The Virtual Cell simulation implements a series of cellular environments with a variety of assays, molecules, proteins, and tools providing an experimental context for the student. A virtual avatar acts as a guide and gives out assignments, and intelligent software tutor agents provide content and problem-solving advice. The Virtual Cell supports multi-user collaborations, where both students and teachers from remote sites can communicate with each other and work together on shared goals (Slator, 1999). VRBS (virtual Rety Biology Simulation) was developed to study the structure and function of human eye. Here the iris and pupil of the human eye have been visualized. While changing the viewpoint by repositioning some objects in the environment, the change in the iris and pupil have been visualized for understanding how these objects are seemed. In this system the interaction was based on number keys pressing in keyboard and it is difficult for students to memorize the functionality of each key to interact with different shapes (Shim et al., 2003c). Another approach was designed and implemented that is prototype web-based virtual 3D environment for teaching vertebrate biology for high school and middle school students. This 3D learning environment called Frog Island contains a Virtual Frog along with a rich array of related resources (images, sounds, data, and simulations) that students and teachers can use to study about information of frogs (Dev et al.,

1998). In 2012, Cheng and Annetta evaluated students' learning outcomes and their learning experiences through playing a Serious Educational Games (SEGs). They used different game based virtual learning environments (i.e. SEGs) to evaluate students learning interest. They found that students take more interest in learning by using actively immersing and enjoying the game worlds (Cheng & Annetta, 2012). In 2013, Bonser et al. developed a virtual microscopy for botany teaching. Virtual microscopy uses high-resolution digital 'virtual slides' that facilitate students to know about the using of actual microscope and glass slides. The framework is an effective tool for increasing student satisfaction in introductory botany courses (Bonser et al., 2013).

In a VLE it is necessary to provide some guidance where students take interest and perform their task more easily. However, most of the previously discussed techniques are providing a direct navigation to each individual part/object in the system. In addition, these techniques are complex and mostly useful for only expert users.

3. METHODS AND MATERIALS

The objective of this research work is to study the effect of list-liner and direct based interface in a complex 3D interactive VLE. We have developed a 3D interactive Virtual Mustard Plant (VMP) environment with simple list-liner and direct based interface. Our proposed system provides some advantages over previous:

- It provides 3D interaction interface with list-liner based technique for information rich and complex 3D virtual environment.
- It attracts the naive users by providing a direct simple 2D visual interface with each part of the plant in the virtual environment.
- It enhances students learning interest by hiding the irrelevant information and guessing the students learning.
- It provides detailed visual information about different parts of the plant.
- It provides two types of interaction techniques i.e. direct interaction and list-liner based interaction.

The proposed system is a 3D virtual environment like a real garden which contains a Virtual Mustard Plant (VMP) as shown in Figure 1. When the student selects any part of the plant then they get textual information about the selected part of the plant. This information is very useful for student learning enhancement where he/she comes to know about the properties of the plant.

3.1 Software Architecture

In this section we are going to discuss the principle components of the software architecture as shown in Figure 2, on which the VMP is based.

3.1.1 User Interaction

The first module of this architecture is the user interaction module. This provides an interface between the user and VMP enabling the user to navigate/move and select/manipulate virtual objects. User inter-

Figure 1. The inside scenario of VMP

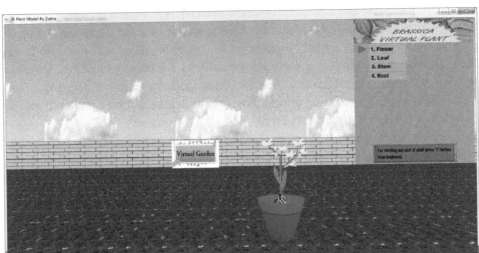

acts with VMP through both direct based and list-liner based interaction. We use Nintendo Wiimote as an input device. This subsection contains the following categories.

a. Nintendo Wiimote's Interface: There are many devices for 3D interaction like Microsoft Kinect (Microsoft Kinect, 2018), leap motion (Leap Motion Company, 2018), Nintendo Wiimote (Nintendo Wiimote, 2018), phantom (Phantom Company, 2018), joystick brand Joystick ("Joystick," 2018), etc. In VMP we have used Nintendo Wiimote for 3D interaction because it is a cost-effective device than other 3D interaction interfaces, it can also provide haptic sensation in the form of vibration. Wiimote is a 3D video game controller device which allows the user to interact with the virtual environment as shown in Figure 3.

Figure 2. Software architecture of VMP

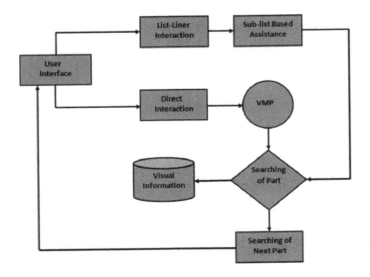

It senses every action of user and makes user feels less like a player and represents user's existence in the virtual environment Nintendo Wiimote (Wiimote, 2018). It contains 3- axis accelerometers, multiple buttons, a small speaker and a vibrator which support in game sound effects and user feedback. For connection with the system it uses Bluetooth technology. Its workspace is quite large and allows the interaction from a distance of 18 meters. The user in VMP is represented by a pointer which is controlled via Wiimote. Through Wiimote user can freely navigate and rotate any plant's object according to their hand's position and rotation and can feel them more immersion where he/she feels realism inside the virtual learning environment.

3.1.2 Direct Based Interaction

In this type of interaction, there is direct access to the plant by using Wiimote. The user can select different parts of the plant directly. When the student selects any part of the VMP textual information directly appears on the screen. The direct based interaction interface as shown in Figure 4.

a. Navigation in Direct based Interaction: The pointer representing the user can move (navigate) freely in all directions in the VMP. The navigation of pointer along X-axis is achieved through the rotation of Wiimote along its Y-axis as shown in part (b) of Figure 5. Similarly, the movement of pointer along Y-axis is controlled through the rotation of Wiimote along its X-axis as shown in part (a) of Figure 5. The Z-axis movement of pointer is controlled through the up and down buttons of Wiimote.

b. Selection and Manipulation in Direct based Interaction: Selection and manipulation are the important activities in any virtual environment. For the manipulation of a plant's object it needs to be selected first. In VMP an object becomes selectable when the pointer collides with it. After collision if the user presses the button "A" of the Wiimote, the object is selected the corresponding part of plant gets zoom- in on the screen. After selection the user is able to manipulate it i.e. to change its position or orientation and other attributes. For example he/she can zoom-in the selected plant's object and can explore it in depth and release it by just pressing the Wiimote "A" button again.

3.1.3 List-Liner Based Interaction

In this type of interaction there is given a list, in which information about the parts of the plant is displayed. When a student selects a list item by using Wiimote, the corresponding part of plant point-out

Figure 3. Wiimote's buttons and coordinates

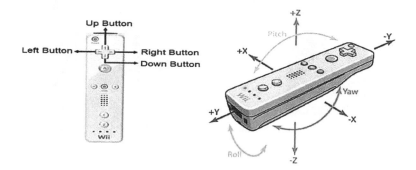

Figure 4. Direct based interaction interface

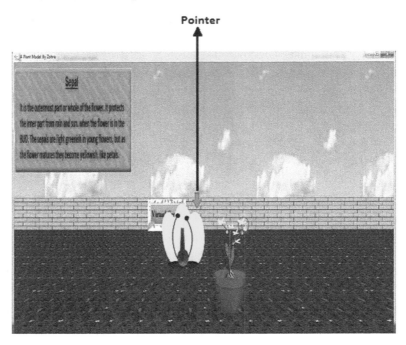

clearly by liner and can be zoom-in on the screen. Similarly, textual information is also displayed for the corresponding part of the plant.

a. Sub-List based Assistance: This is a very important module; it contains a list of all parts of the plant. First of all users select the name of a part of the plant from the list as shown in Figure 6 and then study its information. Navigate the pointer is representing the user can move from top to down freely

Figure 5. Wiimote's rotations

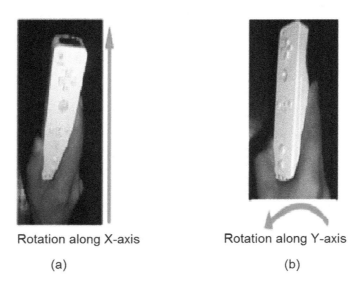

in the list. The movement of a pointer from top to down or down to top is achieved by pressing buttons "plus (+)" and "minus (-)". Similarly for sub-list the movement of a pointer from left to right or from right to left is controlled by pressing buttons "left" and "right."

b. Selection and Manipulation in List-Liner based Interaction: For the manipulation of a plant's object it needs to be selected first from the list through a pointer. If the user presses the button "A" of the Wiimote, the object is selected the corresponding part of plant gets zoom-in on the screen. After selection the user is able to manipulate it i.e. to change its position or orientation and other attributes. For example he/she can zoom-in the selected plant's object and can explore it in depth by pressing button "down" of the Wiimote.

3.1.4 Textual Information in VMP

Whenever a student selects any part of the plant, information about its name, proper ties and other details are provided in textual form which is shown in Figure 7, here student selects flower from the list and the sub-part i.e sepal of the flower zoom in and also its detailed information in textual form displayed. This information is very useful for students learning enhancement and improving their exam score.

4. METHODS

This section describes the experiment and evaluation of the 3D interactive VMP. We have implemented the 3D interactive VMP in MS Visual Studio 2012 using OpenGL on HP Corei3 Laptop having specication 2.4GHz processor, 2GB RAM and Intel(R) HD Graphics card. The Nintendo Wiimote was used as interfacing device. Similarly, an LED screen of 40 inches was used for display during experimentation.

4.1 Participants and Context

In order to evaluate the VMP, forty-five students participated in the evaluation. They were from secondary school level. They were from different institutes and had ages from 14 to 16 years. These students were

Figure 6. List-Liner based interaction interface

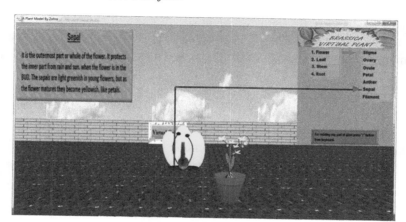

Figure 7. Textual information about plant's part in VMP.

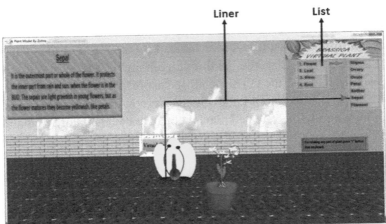

divided into two groups (i.e. G1, G2) containing equal numbers of students. There were eight females in G1 and nine in G2. As all the participants had no prior experience of VR systems or games, therefore, they were briefed with the help of a 25-minute demonstration about the use of the Nintendo Wiimote and VMP. For example, they were taught how they will navigate in the environment. Similarly, they were also guided about the selection and manipulation of different parts of the plant. Then each participant was asked to search different parts of the plant. The students in G1 tested the environment by using direct interaction with different parts of the plant. The students in G2 tested the same environment by using list-liner interaction with different parts of the plant. The students perform their tasks in VMP as shown in Figure 8. Here we recorded the search completion (plant's parts searching time) along with errors for each student. Each participant filled a questionnaire after getting experience in VMP. The subjective response of students was collected through a questionnaire.

The subjective responses of students regarding the easiness of the list-liner based interaction and its effect on the students' performance in VMP. The students answered each question on a scale of three to five options.

4.2 Data Sources and Data Analysis

This section describes analysis of the data accumulated during evaluation of the interaction techniques. Data was collected from the students of G1 (Group 1) and G2 (Group 2) through questionnaire, after evaluating both interaction techniques in VMP. The following aspects of the VMP were analyzed.

4.2.1 Questionnaire Interview

In first part of the analysis, data were gathered from the students of G1 and G2 using a questionnaire interview when they evaluated both interaction techniques in VMP with the help of direct and list-liner based interaction techniques. The questionnaire interview contained the following questions as shown in Table 1. During questionnaire interview the students answered each question on a scale of three to five options.

Figure 8. Task performing by participant in 3D interactive VMP

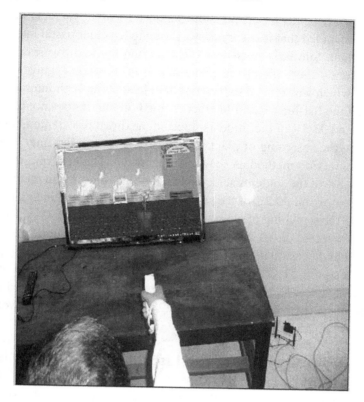

5. RESULTS

In this section we present the responses to the questions and also the analysis of the data recorded/ collected during the experiments. We used a statistical method Analysis of Variance (ANOVA) to find statistically significant difference between two groups.

Table 1. Questionnaire interview from students

S. No.	Questions
1	Which interaction method is easy?
2	Which interaction method is intuitive?
3	Which interaction method puts cognitive load on the user?
4	Which interaction method is easy to search/find a part(s) of the plant?
5	Which interaction method is more suitable for learning/education purpose?
6	Which interaction method is easy to find/search a known part of the plant?
7	Which interaction provides an easy and simple exploration method?
8	Overall, I am satisfied with virtual plant model.

For the first question, which is related to the easiness of list-liner and direct-based interaction, 65.7% of the students selected the list-liner based interaction and 34.3% of the students selected the direct-based interaction. It can be concluded that it is very easy to use the list-liner based interaction to evaluate the different parts of the plant. Similarly to answer Q2 regarding the intuitiveness, 59.2% chose list-liner based interaction and 40.8% chose direct based interaction as shown in Figure 9.

The third question, which was related to the cognitive load about both interaction interfaces, 66.5% of the students selected the list-liner based interaction method that it does not put more cognitive load on users' performance and 33.5% of the students selected the direct based interaction method. Similarly to answer Q4, regarding the searching of plant's parts, 70.3% choose list-liner interaction method and 29.7% choose direct interaction method as shown in Figure 10. The next question related to learning/education, for which 69.8% of the students selected that list-liner interaction method is more suitable for learning/education purposes and 30.2% of the students selected the based interaction method. Similarly to answer Q6, regarding the searching of already known parts of plant, 51.4% selected list-liner interaction method and 49.6% selected direct interaction method as shown in Figure 11.

The next question, which was related to the exploration that which interaction method is simple for exploration of the plant's part, 51.4% selected list-liner interaction method and 49.6% selected direct interaction method as shown in Figure 12. The last question, which was related to satisfaction about VMP, 54.3% students selected the higher level and 35.2% selected the highest level of satisfaction after using VMP as shown in Figure 13.

5.1 Performance Measure of Direct and List-Liner Interactions in VMP

The second part of the analysis was to check the performance of both groups (G1 and G2) in searching the same part of the plant in VMP using their respective interactional conditions. The conditions were the following for the groups:

G1: searched the plant's parts in VMP by using direct interaction.
G2: searched the plant's parts in VMP by using list-liner interaction.

Figure 9. Users' responses about the easiness and intuitiveness of interaction

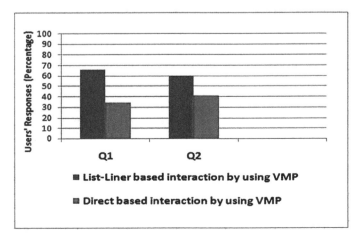

Figure 10. Cognitive load and ease of searching of plant's parts

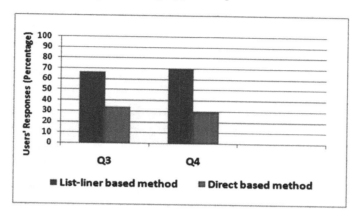

Figure 11. Learning and already known searching of plant's parts

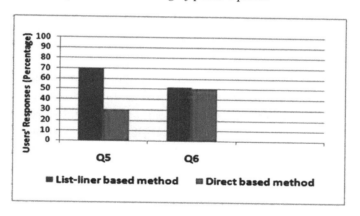

Figure 12. Exploration of plant's parts

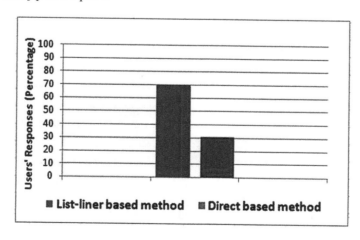

Figure 13. Satisfaction about VMP

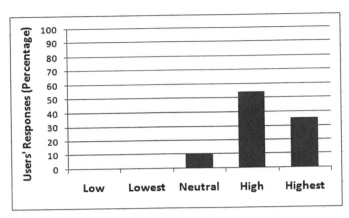

5.2 Task Assigning and Completion

For task assigning and completion we selected different main parts of the plant (i.e flower, leaf, stem and roots) to find their sub-parts and to read their textual information in detail. During searching of targeted plant's part and sub-part we counted students' searching time and errors of both groups i.e G1 and G2. After searching and reading of different sub-parts' textual information we asked different questions from both groups are given in Table 2. As stated earlier, textual information regarding each plant's part was equally avail- able to both groups (i.e. G1 and G2). The data recorded in this section consist of their search of parts completion times and the mean of errors that occurred during parts' searching.

5.3 Task Completion Time

The Analysis of Variance (ANOVA) for task completion time is significant (F (1, 47) = 22.24, P < 0.05). The average task completion time and standard deviation for each group are given in Table 3 and Figure

Table 2. Questionnaires from students about different parts of plant

S. No	Questions
1	What is a pollen grain in flower?
2	What is a filament?
3	What is a calyx and how many sepals it contains?
4	What is a sepal and role of sepal in flower?
5	What is a stele and how many types of stele?
6	What is the role of veins in leaf?
7	What is a midrib and the role of midrib in leaf?
8	What is a vascular bundle?
9	What is the role of pericycle in stele?
10	What is the role of pericycle in stele?

14. Comparing the task completion time of G1 with that of G2, we obtained a considerable difference, which means that students who used list-liner interaction method for searching of targeted plant's part in VMP were far better compared with those who used direct interaction method for searching of targeted plant's part in VMP.

5.4 Number of Errors during Searching of Plant's Parts

In this portion, we present a comprehensive analysis of errors occurred during searching of targeted plant's part which is shown in Table 4 and Figure 15. We counted the number of errors that has been done by a student during searching of targeted plant's part. These errors are the invalid/incorrect selection of plant's part.

5.5 Measuring Students' Learning in VMP

In order to find the individual learning of students, we asked different questions from the two groups such as identifying various parts of plant, information about parts and their functions in the plant. We used the following equation (1) for students' success rate.

$$SuccessRate = \frac{CorrectAnswer}{TotalQuestionsAsked} * 100 \qquad (1)$$

Table 3. Average task completion time and standard deviation for G1 and G2

Groups	Mean (Mints)	Standard Deviation (Mints)
G1	1.80	0.68
G2	0.67	0.40

Figure 14. Average task completion time of G1 and G2

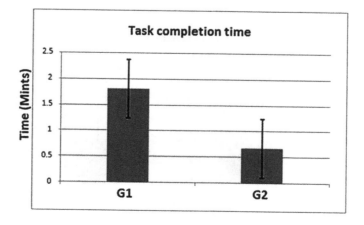

Here the mean success rate of G1 (Group 1) and G2 (Group 2) were 78.3% (SD= 10.2) and 82.7% (SD= 12.5) as shown in Figure 16. It was found that the learning capabilities of G2 to be slightly better than that of the G1, because both G1 and G2 guided by VMP by different interaction interfaces. However, on the bases of time and errors we observed a significant difference between the performance of G2 (students who used list-liner based interaction) and G1 (students who used direct-based interaction). We can say that students were overall satisfied with various aspects of the VMP such as textual information, direct and list-liner based interactions interfaces.

6. CONCLUSION

In this paper, we presented a 3D interactive VMP that we have developed for secondary school level students. Through evaluations of both groups (G1 and G2), we found that our proposed framework is very helpful for education institutions where students can simulate their biological tasks about plant like in a real world. Our proposed framework provides to students an advanced 3D interaction interface, visual information and list- liner interaction with different parts of the plant. We have combined the 3D interaction interface, visual information and list-liner interaction in VMP which show that it improves students' learning skills and they took more interest in biology learning. The visual information is very helpful for students' learning enhancement and also in improving their exam score.

The proposed framework is also suitable in the upgrading of education system. The introduction of this novel based interaction interface and 3D interactive advance technology explore and disclose new ways in the educational institutes for the upcoming students and also provide them with a sort of stimulus

Table 4. Average number of errors with standard deviation for G1 and G2

Groups	Mean (Errors)	Standard Deviation (Errors)
G1	3.91	1.05
G2	1.95	0.87

Figure 15. Average number of errors with standard deviation for G1 and G2

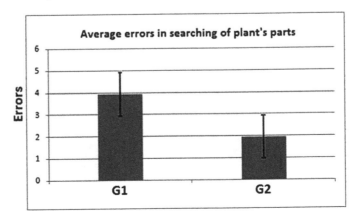

Figure 16. Mean success rate of G1 and G2 with standard deviations

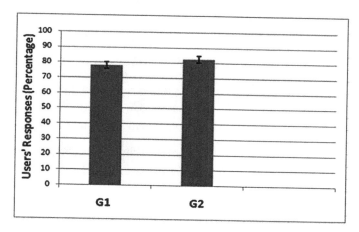

which are very useful for the encouragement of students and provoke them for further exploration and innovation in the field of education. Through this way the dignity and honor of the educational institutions can also be enhanced.

REFERENCES

Alam, A., Ullah, S., & Ali, N. (2016). A student-friendly framework for adaptive 3d-virtual learning environments. *Proceeding of Pakistan Academy of Sciences, 53*(3), 255–266.

Alam, A., Ullah, S., & Ali, N. (2018). The effect of learning-based adaptivity on students performance in 3d-virtual learning environments. *IEEE Access, 6*, 3400–3407. doi:10.1109/ACCESS.2017.2783951

Baggott la Velle, L., Wishart, J., McFarlane, A., Brawn, R., & John, P. (2007). Teaching and learning with ict within the subject culture of secondary school science. *Research in Science & Technological Education, 25*(3), 339–349. doi:10.1080/02635140701535158

Bonser, S. P., de Permentier, P., Green, J., Velan, G. M., Adam, P., & Kumar, R. K. (2013). Engaging students by emphasising botanical concepts over techniques: Innovative practical exercises using virtual microscopy. *Journal of Biological Education, 47*(2), 123–127. doi:10.1080/00219266.2013.764344

Bowman, D. A., Coquillart, S., Froehlich, B., Hirose, M., Kitamura, Y., Kiyokawa, K., & Stuerzlinger, W. (2008). 3d user interfaces: New directions and perspectives. *IEEE Computer Graphics and Applications, 28*(6), 20–36. doi:10.1109/MCG.2008.109 PMID:19004682

Cheng, M.-T., & Annetta, L. (2012). Students' learning outcomes and learning experiences through playing a serious educational game. *Journal of Biological Education, 46*(4), 203–213. doi:10.1080/00 219266.2012.688848

Clase, K. L., Adamo-Villani, N., Gooding, S. L., Yadav, A., Karpicke, J. D., & Gentry, M. (2009). Enhancing creativity in synthetic biology with interactive virtual environments. In Proceedings of the 39th IEEE Frontiers in education conference FIE '09 (pp. 1–6). doi:10.1109/FIE.2009.5350646 de Oliveira, M. L., & Galembeck, E. (2016). Mobile applications in cell biology present new approaches for cell modelling. *Journal of Biological Education*, *50*(3), 290–303. doi:10.1080/00219266.2015.1085428

Dede, C., Clarke, J., Ketelhut, D. J., Nelson, B., & Bowman, C. (2005). Students motivation and learning of science in a multi-user virtual environment. In *Proceedings of the American educational research association conference* (pp. 1–8). Academic Press.

Dev, P., Pichumani, R., Walker, D., Heinrichs, W., Karadi, C., & Lorie, W. (1998). Formative design of a virtual learning environment. *Studies in Health Technology and Informatics*, *50*, 392–398. PMID:10180582

Emvalotis, A., & Koutsianou, A. (2018). Greek primary school students images of scientists and their work: Has anything changed? *Research in Science & Technological Education*, *36*(1), 69–85. doi:10.1080/02635143.2017.1366899

Fung, Y. Y. H. (2002). A comparative study of primary and secondary school students' images of scientists. *Research in Science & Technological Education*, *20*(2), 199–213. doi:10.1080/0263514022000030453

Hachet, M. (2010). *3D User Interfaces, from Mobile Devices to Immersive Virtual Environments* [Habilitation `a diriger des recherches]. Universit'e Sciences et Technologies - Bordeaux I. Retrieved from https://tel.archives-ouvertes.fr/tel-00576663

Johansson, A.-M., & Wickman, P.-O. (2018). The use of organising purposes in science instruction as a scaffolding mechanism to support progressions: A study of talk in two primary science classrooms. *Research in Science & Technological Education*, *36*(1), 1–16. doi:10.1080/02635143.2017.1318272

Joysticks. (2018). Newegg. Retrieved From http://www.newegg.com/pc-game-controllers/subcategory/id-123

Kesner, M., Frailich, M., & Hofstein, A. (2013). Implementing the inter- net learning environment into the chemistry curriculum in high schools in Israel. In *Technology-rich learning environments* (p. 209-234). Retrieved from https://www.worldscientific.com/doi/abs/10.1142/97898125644120010

Kim, J.-H., Park, S., Lee, H., Yuk, K.-C., & Lee, H. (2001). Virtual reality simulations in physics education. *Interactive Multimedia Electronic* Additional Reading. *Journal of Computer-Enhanced Learning*, *3*(2).

Leap Motion Company. (n.d.). Retrieved from https://www.leapmotion.com/company

Ling, H., & Rui, L. (2016, Aug). Vr glasses and leap motion trends in education. In *Proceedings of the 2016 11th international conference on computer science education (ICCSE)* (p. 917-920). 10.1109/ICCSE.2016.7581705

McClean, P. E., Slator, B. M., & White, A. R. (1999). The virtual cell: An interactive, virtual environment for cell biology. In *Edmedia: World conference on educational media and technology* (pp. 1442–1443). Academic Press.

Mikropoulos, T. A., Katsikis, A., Nikolou, E., & Tsakalis, P. (2003a). Virtual environments in biology teaching. *Journal of Biological Education*, *37*(4), 176–181. doi:10.1080/00219266.2003.9655879

Mikropoulos, T. A., & Natsis, A. (2011). Educational virtual environments: A ten-year review of empirical research (1999–2009). *Computers & Education*, *56*(3), 769–780. doi:10.1016/j.compedu.2010.10.020

Nintendo Wiimote. (2018). Retrieved from https://store.nintendo.com

Nonis, D. (2005). *3d virtual learning environments (3d VLE)*. Singapore: Ministry of Education.

Pausch, R., Proffitt, D., & Williams, G. (1997). Quantifying immersion in virtual reality. In *Proceedings of the 24th annual conference on computer graphics and interactive techniques* (pp. 13–18). New York: ACM Press/Addison-Wesley Publishing Co. doi:10.1145/258734.258744

PCGamer. (2018). Microsoft Kinect. Retrieved from http://www.pcgamer.com/microsoft-ceases-production-of-kinect-for-windows

Phantom Company. P. C. (2018). Retrieved from http://www.immersion.fr/en/phantom-touch-x/

Rajaei, H., & Aldhalaan, A. (2011). Advances in virtual learning environments and class- rooms. In *Proceedings of the 14th communications and networking symposium* (pp. 133–142). San Diego, CA, USA: Society for Computer Simulation International. Retrieved From; http://dl.acm.org/citation.cfm?id=2048416.2048434

Reis, R., & Escudeiro, P. (2014). A model for implementing learning games on virtual world platforms. In *Proceedings of the XV international conference on human computer interaction* (pp. 98:1–98:2). New York: ACM. doi:10.1145/2662253.2662351

Rheingold, H. (1991). *Virtual reality*. New York: Simon & Schuster, Inc.

Richard, E., Tijou, A., Richard, P., & Ferrier, J.-L. (2006). Multi-modal virtual environments for education with haptic and olfactory feedback. *Virtual Reality (Waltham Cross)*, *10*(3), 207–225. doi:10.100710055-006-0040-8

Richards, D., & Kelaiah, I. (2012). Usability attributes in virtual learning environments. In *Proceedings of the 8th Australasian conference on interactive entertainment: Playing the system* (pp. 9:1–9:10). New York, NY, USA: ACM. doi:10.1145/2336727.2336736

Schofield, D., & Lester, E. (2010). Virtual chemical engineering: Guidelines for e-learning in engineering education.

Sheridan, T. B. (2000). Interaction, imagination and immersion some research needs. In *Proceedings of the ACM symposium on virtual reality software and technology* (pp. 1–7). ACM. 10.1145/502390.502392

Shim, K.-C., Park, J.-S., Kim, H.-S., Kim, J.-H., Park, Y.-C., & Ryu, H.-I. (2003a). Application of virtual reality technology in biology education. *Journal of Biological Education*, *37*(2), 71–74. doi:10.1080/00219266.2003.9655854

Slator, B. M. (1999). Intelligent tutors in virtual worlds. In *Proceedings of the 8th international conference on intelligent systems (ICIS-99)* (pp. 24–26). Academic Press.

Totkov, G. (2003). Virtual learning environments: Towards new generation. In *Proceedings of the 4th international conference on computer systems and technologies: E-learning* (pp. 8–16). New York: ACM. doi:10.1145/973620.973622

Ullah, S. (2011). *Multi-modal Interaction in Collaborative Virtual Environments: Study and analysis of performance in collaborative work* [Theses]. Universit'e d'Evry-Val d'Essonne. Retrieved From https://tel.archives-ouvertes.fr/tel-00562081

Wickens, C. D. (1992, October). Virtual reality and education. In *Proceedings of IEEE international conference on systems, man, and cybernetics* (Vol. 1, pp. 842-847). IEEE Press.

Williams, J., Eames, C., Hume, A., & Lockley, J. (2012). Promoting pedagogical content knowledge development for early career secondary teachers in science and technology using content representations. *Research in Science & Technological Education, 30*(3), 327–343.

Winn, W., Hoffman, H., Hollander, A., Osberg, K., Rose, H., & Char, P. (1997). The effect of student construction of virtual environments on the performance of high-and low-ability students. In *Proceedings of the Annual meeting of the American educational research association. Academic Press.*

Woodfield, B. F., Catlin, H. R., Waddoups, G. L., Moore, M. S., Swan, R., Allen, R., & Bodily, G. (2004a). The virtual chemlab project: A realistic and sophisticated simulation of inorganic qualitative analysis. *Journal of Chemical Education, 81*(11), 1672. doi:10.1021/ed081p1672

Yoon, S. A., Anderson, E., Park, M., Elinich, K., & Lin, J. (2018). How augmented reality, textual, and collaborative scaffolds work synergistically to improve learning in a science museum. *Research in Science & Technological Education*, 1–21.

ADDITIONAL READING

Alam, A., Ullah, S., & Ali, N. (2018). The Effect of Learning-Based Adaptivity on Students' Performance in 3D-Virtual Learning Environments. *IEEE, 6*(1), 3400–3407. doi:10.1109/ACCESS.2017.2783951

Eman, S., Florica, M., & Alin, M. (2012). A 3d virtual learning environment for teaching chemistry in high school. *Annals of DAAAM for 2012 & Proceedings of the 23rd International DAAAM Symposium, 23*, 2304–1382.

Katrina, B. S., Selcen, S. G., Richard, L., Michael, M., Christopher, D., Hazel, S. S., ... Janet, M. D. (2018). Learning neuroscience with technology: A scaffolded, active learning approach. *Journal of Science Education and Technology, Springer, 27*(6), 566–580. doi:10.100710956-018-9748-y PMID:31105416

Kihyun, R., Kristin, B., & Amanda, S. (2018). Promoting linguistically diverse students short-term and long-term understanding of chemical phenomena using visualizations. *Journal of Science Education and Technology, Springer, 27*(6), 508–522. doi:10.100710956-018-9739-z

Mehta, S., Bajaj, M., & Banati, H. (2019). An Intelligent Approach for Virtual Chemistry Laboratory. In Virtual Reality in Education: Breakthroughs in Research and Practice (pp 454-488). Academic Press. doi:10.4018/978-1-5225-8179-6.ch023

Tory, W., Jonathan, S., Jacqueline, K., Christopher, R., & Julia, R. (2019). Measuring Pedagogy and the Integration of Engineering Design in STEM Classrooms. *Journal of Science Education and Technology, 28*(3), 179–194. doi:10.100710956-018-9756-y

Ullah, S., Ali, N., & Rahman, S. (2016). The effect of procedural guidance on students' skill enhancement in a virtual chemistry laboratory. *Journal of Chemical Education, 93*(12), 2018–2025. doi:10.1021/acs.jchemed.5b00969

Winkelmann, K., Keeney-Kennicutt, W. L., Fowler, D., & Macik, M. (2017). Development, Implementation, and Assessment of General Chemistry Lab Experiments Performed in the Virtual World of Second Life. *Journal of Chemical Education, 94*(7), 849–858. doi:10.1021/acs.jchemed.6b00733

Wu, B., Wong, K., & Li, T. (2019). Virtual titration laboratory experiment with differentiated instruction. *Computer Animation and Virtual Worlds, 30*(3-4), e1882. doi:10.1002/cav.1882

KEY TERMS AND DEFINITIONS

3D Interaction: 3D interaction is a form of human-machine interaction where users are able to move and perform interaction in 3D space.

3D Interactive Virtual Environment: A virtual learning environment which is based on 3D interaction.

Biological Education: the study of structure, function, heredity, and evolution of all living organisms.

Cognitive Load: the used amount of working memory resources.

Computational Biology: is the science of using biological data to develop algorithms or models to understand biological systems and relationships.

Computer Animations: It is the process used for digitally generating animated images.

Computer-Based Learning: Computer-based learning (CBL) is the term used for any kind of learning with the help of computers.

Computer-Generated Environment: The application of computer graphics to create or contribute to images in art, printed media, video games, films, television programs, shorts, commercials, videos, and simulators.

Human Computer Interaction: It is a multidisciplinary field of study focusing on the design of computer technology and, in particular, the interaction between humans (the users) and computers.

Interactive Interface: It is the field of human–computer interaction, is the space where interactions between humans and machines occur.

Interactive Tutorials: media to allow students to interact with the content that they are learning.

Learning Technology: Technologies that can be used to support learning, teaching and assessment.

Virtual Learning Environment: a system for delivering learning materials to students via the web.

Virtual Reality: an artificial environment that is created with software and presented to the user in such a way that the user suspends belief and accepts it as a real environment.

Virtual Reality in Biology: using computer generated environment regarding structure, function, heredity, and evolution of all living organisms.

Compilation of References

Aalto, S., Haarala, C., Brück, A., Sipilä, H., Hämäläinen, H., & Rinne, J. O. (2006). Mobile phone affects cerebral blood flow in humans. *Journal of Cerebral Blood Flow and Metabolism*, *26*(7), 885–890. doi:10.1038j.jcbfm.9600279 PMID:16495939

Abhay, V. (2018). Why Mobile User Experience (UX) is Critical for iOS and Android Apps. Netsolutions. Retrieved from https://www.netsolutions.com/insights/7-reasons-to-customize-mobile-user-experience-for-ios-and-android/

Adetiba, E. (2015). Lung Cancer Prediction Using Neural Network Ensemble with Histogram of Oriented Gradient Genomic Features. *The Scientific World Journal*. doi:. doi:10.1155/2015/786013

Ahmed, M., Gagnon, M., Hamelin-Brabant, L., Mbemba, G., & Alami, H. (2017). A mixed methods systematic review of success factors of mhealth and telehealth for maternal health in Sub-Saharan Africa. *mHealth*, *3*(22), 1–10. PMID:28293618

Aimi Salihah, A. N., Mustafa, N., & Nashrul Fazli, M. N. (2009). Application of thresholding technique in determining ratio of blood cells for Leukemia detection.

Akter, S., Ray, P., & D'Ambra, J. (2013). Continuance of mHealth services at the bottom of the pyramid: The roles of service quality and trust. *Electronic Markets*, *23*(1), 29–47. doi:10.100712525-012-0091-5

Alam, A., Ullah, S., & Ali, N. (2016). A student-friendly framework for adaptive 3d-virtual learning environments. *Proceeding of Pakistan Academy of Sciences*, *53*(3), 255–266.

Alam, A., Ullah, S., & Ali, N. (2018). The effect of learning-based adaptivity on students performance in 3d-virtual learning environments. *IEEE Access*, *6*, 3400–3407. doi:10.1109/ACCESS.2017.2783951

Alamgir, K., Sami, U., & Salahuddin, K. (2018). Nutritional complications and its effects on human health. *J. Food Sci. Nutr.*, *1*(1), 17–20.

Albert, E. N., & Kerns, J. M. (1981). Reversible microwave effects on the blood-brain barrier. *Brain Research*, *230*(1-2), 153–164. doi:10.1016/0006-8993(81)90398-X PMID:7317776

Ali, A., Alrasheedi, M., Ouda, A., & Capretz, L. (2014). A study of the interface usability issues of mobile learning applications for smart phones from the user's perspective. *International Journal on Integrating Technology in Education*, *3*(4), 1–16. doi:10.5121/ijite.2014.3401

Ali, M. A., Tahir, N. M., & Ali, A. I. (2018). *Monitoring Healthcare System for Infants: A Review. Paper presented at the 2018 IEEE Conference on Systems, Process and Control* (pp. 44–47). IEEE Press. Retrieved from https://ieeexplore.ieee.org/abstract/document/8704143

Allen, H. C. (2002). *Keynotes and Characteristics with Comparisons of some of the Leading Remedies of the Materia Medica with Bowel Nosodes*. B. Jain Publishers.

Almeida, F., & Monteiro, J. (2017). Approaches and Principles for UX Web Experiences. *International Journal of Information Technology and Web Engineering, 12*(2), 49–65. doi:10.4018/IJITWE.2017040103

Almeida, F., Oliveira, J., & Cruz, J. (2010). Open Standards and Open Source: Enabling Interoperability. *International Journal of Software Engineering and Its Applications, 2*(1), 1–11. doi:10.5121/ijsea.2011.2101

Alotaibi, M., Albalawi, M., & Alwakeel, L. (2018). A Smart Mobile Pregnancy Management and Awareness System for Saudi Arabia. *International Journal of Interactive Mobile Technologies, 12*(5), 112–125. doi:10.3991/ijim.v12i5.9005

Alsmadi, M. K. S., Omar, K. B., & Noah, S. A. (2009). Back propagation algorithm: The best algorithm among the multilayer perceptron algorithm. *IJCSNS International Journal of Computer Science and Network Security, 9*(4), 378–383.

Al-Tarawneh, M. S. (2012). Lung Cancer Detection Using Image Processing Techniques. *Leonardo Electronic Journal of Practices and Technologies,* (20).

Altunkaynak, B. Z., Altun, G., Yahyazadeh, A., Kaplan, A. A., Deniz, O. G., Turkmen, A. P., ... Kaplan, S. (2016). Different methods for evaluating the effects of microwave radiation exposure on the nervous system. *Journal of Chemical Neuroanatomy, 75*, 62–69. doi:10.1016/j.jchemneu.2015.11.004 PMID:26686295

Amerah, Nurul Kassim1, a. D. A. A. (2017). Classification of DNA Sequences Using Convolutional Neural Network Approach. *Innovations in Computing Technology and Applications, 2*, 6.

Anand, S. V. (2010). Segmentation coupled textural feature classification for lung tumor prediction. In *Proceedings of the 2010 IEEE International Conference on Communication Control and Computing Technologies (ICCCCT)* (pp. 518-524). IEEE.

Anastasi, A., & Urbina, S. (1997). *Psychological testing.* Prentice Hall/Pearson Education.

Anisi, M. H., Abdullah, A. H., Razak, S. A., & Ngadi, M. (2012). Overview of data routing approaches for wireless sensor networks. *Sensors (Basel), 12*(4), 3964–3996. doi:10.3390120403964 PMID:23443040

Arber, S. L., & Lin, J. C. (1984). Microwave enhancement of membrane conductance: Effects of EDTA, caffeine, and tetracaine. *Physiological Chemistry and Physics and Medical NMR, 16*, 469–475. PMID:6443226

Arber, S. L., & Lin, J. C. (1985). Microwave-induced changes in nerve cells: Effects of modulation and temperature. *Bioelectromagnetics, 6*(3), 257–270. doi:10.1002/bem.2250060306 PMID:3836669

Arya, V. (2013, August). A quality of service analysis of energy aware routing protocols in mobile ad hoc networks. In *Proceedings of the 2013 Sixth International Conference on Contemporary Computing (IC3)* (pp. 439-444). IEEE.

Askarzadeh, A. (2016). A novel metaheuristic method for solving constrained engineering optimization problems: Crow search algorithm. *Computers & Structures, 169*, 1–12. doi:10.1016/j.compstruc.2016.03.001

Ater, T. (2017). *Building Progressive Web Apps: Bringing the Power of Native to the Browser.* Newton, MA: O'Reilly Media.

Athira Krishnan, S. K. (2014). A Survey on Image Segmentation and Feature Extraction Methods for Acute Myelogenous Leukemia Detection in Blood Microscopic Images. *International Journal of Computer Science and Information Technologies, 5*(6), 7877-7879.

Aydin, D., Ozyon, S., Yaşar, C., & Liao, T. (2014). Artificial bee colony algorithm with dynamic population size to combine economic and emission dispatch problem. *International Journal of Electrical Power & Energy Systems, 54*, 144–153. doi:10.1016/j.ijepes.2013.06.020

Babich, N. (2016). Designing UX Login Form and Process. UXPlanet. Retrieved from https://uxplanet.org/designing-ux-login-form-and-process-8b17167ed5b9

Babich, N. (2019). Using Red and Green in UI Design. UXPlanet. Retrieved from https://uxplanet.org/using-red-and-green-in-ui-design-66b39e13de91

Bag, A., & Bassiouni, M. A. (2008). Hotspot preventing routing algorithm for delay-sensitive applications of in vivo biomedical sensor networks. *Information Fusion*, *9*(3), 389–398. doi:10.1016/j.inffus.2007.02.001

Baggott la Velle, L., Wishart, J., McFarlane, A., Brawn, R., & John, P. (2007). Teaching and learning with ict within the subject culture of secondary school science. *Research in Science & Technological Education*, *25*(3), 339–349. doi:10.1080/02635140701535158

Bailey, N. T. J. (1952). A study of queues and appointment systems in hospital out-patient departments, with special reference to waiting-times. *Journal of the Royal Statistical Society. Series B. Methodological*, *14*(2), 185–199. doi:10.1111/j.2517-6161.1952.tb00112.x

Bangash, J. I., Abdullah, A. H., Anisi, M. H., & Khan, A. W. (2014a). A survey of routing protocols in wireless body sensor networks. *Sensors,* *14*(1), 1322-1357.

Bangash, J. I., Abdullah, A. H., Khan, A. W., Razzaque, M. A., & Yusof, R. (2015). Critical data routing (CDR) for intra wireless body sensor networks. *Telkomnika*, *13*(1), 181. doi:10.12928/telkomnika.v13i1.365

Bangash, J. I., Abdullah, A. H., Razzaque, M. A., & Khan, A. W. (2014b). Reliability aware routing for intra-wireless body sensor networks. *International Journal of Distributed Sensor Networks*, *10*(10), 786537. doi:10.1155/2014/786537

Bangash, J. I., Khan, A. W., & Abdullah, A. H. (2015). Data-centric routing for intra wireless body sensor networks. *Journal of Medical Systems*, *39*(9), 91. doi:10.100710916-015-0268-5 PMID:26242749

Barak, A. (2011). Internet-based psychological testing and assessment. In *Online Counseling* (pp. 225–255). Academic Press.

Baran, G. R., Kiani, M. F., & Samuel, S. P. (2014). *Science, Pseudoscience, and Not Science: How Do They Differ? In Healthcare and Biomedical Technology in the 21st Century* (pp. 19–57). Springer.

Barnes, P. M., Bloom, B., & Nahin, R. L. (2008). Complementary and alternative medicine use among adults and children; United States, 2007. CDC Stacks Public Health Publications.

Bas, O., Odaci, E., Mollaoglu, H., Ucok, K., & Kaplan, S. (2009). Chronic prenatal exposure to the 900 megahertz electromagnetic field induces pyramidal cell loss in the hippocampus of newborn rats. *Toxicology and Industrial Health*, *25*(6), 377–384. doi:10.1177/0748233709106442 PMID:19671630

Batista, M., & Gaglani, S. (2013). The Future of Smartphones in Health Care. *AMA Journal of Ethics*, *15*(11), 947–950. doi:10.1001/virtualmentor.2013.15.11.stas1-1311 PMID:24257085

Baukal, C. E., Ausburn, F. B., & Ausburn, L. J. (2013). A Proposed Multimedia Cone of Abstraction: Updating a Classic Instructional Design Theory. *Journal of Educational Technology*, *9*(4), 15–24.

Bawin, S. M., Kaczmarek, L. K., & Adey, W. R. (1975). Effects of modulated VHF fields on the central nervous system. *Annals of the New York Academy of Sciences*, *247*(1), 74–81. doi:10.1111/j.1749-6632.1975.tb35984.x PMID:1054258

Bawin, S. M., Satmary, W. M., Jones, R. A., Adey, W. R., & Zimmerman, G. (1996). Extremely-low-frequency magnetic fields disrupt rhythmic slow activity in rat hippocampal slices. *Bioelectromagnetics*, *17*(5), 388–395. doi:10.1002/(SICI)1521-186X(1996)17:5<388::AID-BEM6>3.0.CO;2-# PMID:8915548

Bawin, S. M., Sheppard, A. R., Mahoney, M. D., Abu-Assal, M., & Adey, W. R. (1986). Comparison between the effects of extracellular direct and sinusoidal currents on excitability in hippocampal slices. *Brain Research*, *362*(2), 350–354. doi:10.1016/0006-8993(86)90461-0 PMID:3942883

Bawin, S. M., Sheppard, A. R., Mahoney, M. D., & Adey, W. R. (1984). Influences of sinusoidal electric fields on excitability in the rat hippocampal slice. *Brain Research*, *323*(2), 227–237. doi:10.1016/0006-8993(84)90293-2 PMID:6098340

Ben-Othman, J., & Yahya, B. (2010). Energy efficient and QoS based routing protocol for wireless sensor networks. *Journal of Parallel and Distributed Computing*, *70*(8), 849–857. doi:10.1016/j.jpdc.2010.02.010

Benson, V. S., Pirie, K., Schüz, J., Reeves, G. K., Beral, V., & Green, J. (2017). Mobile phone use and risk of brain neoplasms and other cancers: Prospective study. *International Journal of Epidemiology*, *42*(3), 792–802. doi:10.1093/ije/dyt072 PMID:23657200

Bernier, R. H. (2017). What constitutes a public health problem? Epimonitor. Retrieved from http://epimonitor.net/List_of_Public_H ealth_Issues.htm

Berridge, M. J., & Irvine, R. F. (1984). Inositol triphosphate, a novel second messenger in cellular signal transduction. *Nature*, *312*(5992), 315–321. doi:10.1038/312315a0 PMID:6095092

Berwick, D. M. (2009). What 'patient-centered' should mean: confessions of an extremist: A seasoned clinician and expert fears the loss of his humanity if he should become a patient. *Health Affairs*, *28*(1), 555–565. doi:10.1377/hlthaff.28.4.w555

Beyerstein, B. L. (2001). Alternative medicine and common errors of reasoning. *Academic Medicine*, *76*(3), 230–237. doi:10.1097/00001888-200103000-00009 PMID:11242572

Bhartiya, S., Mehrotra, D., & Girdhar, A. (2016). Issues in Achieving Complete Interoperability while Sharing Electronic Health Records. *Procedia Computer Science*, *78*, 192–198. doi:10.1016/j.procs.2016.02.033

Bhaya, W. (2017). Review of Data Preprocessing Techniques in Data Mining. *Journal of Engineering and Applied Sciences (Asian Research Publishing Network)*, *12*, 4102–4107. doi:10.3923/jeasci.2017.4102.4107

Bhishagratna, K. L. (1911). *An English translation of The Sushruta Samhita: based on original Sanskrit text* (Vol. 2). author.

Bi, J., Chk8en, Y., & Wang, J. Z. (2005, June). A sparse support vector machine approach to region-based image categorization. In *Proceedings of the 2005 IEEE Computer Society Conference on Computer Vision and Pattern Recognition (CVPR'05)* (Vol. 1, pp. 1121-1128). IEEE. 10.1109/CVPR.2005.48

Binhi, V. N., Repiev, A. & Edelev. (2002). *Magnetobiology: underlying physical problems*. San Diego, CA: Academic Press.

Bin, Lv., Zhiye, C., Tongning, W., Qing, S., Duo, Y., Lin, M., ... Yi, X. (2013). The alteration of spontaneous low frequency oscillations caused by acute electromagnetic fields exposure. *Clinical Neurophysiology*. PMID:24012322

Blackman, C. F., Benane, S. G., Elliott, D. J., House, D. E., & Pollock, M. M. (1988). Influence of electromagnetic fields on the efflux of calcium ions from brain tissue in vitro: A three-model analysis consistent with the frequency response up to 510 Hz. *Bioelectromagnetics*, *9*(3), 215–227. doi:10.1002/bem.2250090303 PMID:3178897

Blackman, C. F., Elder, J. A., Weil, C. M., Benane, S. G., Eichinger, D. C., & House, D. E. (1979). Induction of calcium-ion efflux from brain tissue by radio-frequency radiation: Effects of modulation frequency and field strength. *Radiation Research*, *14*, 93–98.

Bloom, B. S. (1974). Time and learning. *The American Psychologist*, *29*(9), 682–688. doi:10.1037/h0037632

Bodeker, G., & Kronenberg, F. (2002). A public health agenda for traditional, complementary, and alternative medicine. *American Journal of Public Health*, *92*(10), 1582–1591. doi:10.2105/AJPH.92.10.1582 PMID:12356597

Bodeker, G., & Ong, C.-K. (2005). *WHO global atlas of traditional, complementary and alternative medicine* (Vol. 1). World Health Organization.

BodyFast UG. (2019, August 5). *BodyFast Intermittent Fasting: Coach, Diet Tracker*. Retrieved from https://play.google.com/store/apps/details?id=com.bodyfast&hl=en

Boericke, W. (2001). *New manual of homoeopathic materia medica and repertory*. B. Jain Publishers.

Boger, C. M. (1995). *Boenninghausen's Characteristics Materia Medica and Repertory. Indian Reprint Edition.* New Delhi: B. Jain Publishers.

Boger, C. M., & von der Lieth, B. (2004). *General Analysis*. Von der Lieth.

Bonser, S. P., de Permentier, P., Green, J., Velan, G. M., Adam, P., & Kumar, R. K. (2013). Engaging students by emphasising botanical concepts over techniques: Innovative practical exercises using virtual microscopy. *Journal of Biological Education, 47*(2), 123–127. doi:10.1080/00219266.2013.764344

Borbely, A. A., Huber, R., Graf, T., Fuchs, B., Gallmann, E., & Achermann, P. (1999). Pulsed high-frequency electromagnetic field affects human sleep and sleep electroencephalogram. *Neuroscience Letters, 275*(3), 207–210. doi:10.1016/S0304-3940(99)00770-3 PMID:10580711

Borisoft - Software development. (2019). *Zero Calories - fasting tracker for weight loss*. Retrieved from https://zero-caloriesfasting.com/index.html

Boulis, A., Smith, D., Miniutti, D., Libman, L., & Tselishchev, Y. (2012). Challenges in body area networks for healthcare: The MAC. *IEEE Communications Magazine, 50*(5), 100–106. doi:10.1109/MCOM.2012.6194389

Boushey, C. J., Spoden, M., Zhu, F. M., Delp, E. J., & Kerr, D. A. (2016). New mobile methods for dietary assessment: review of image-assisted and. *New technology in nutrition research and practice* (p. 12). Dublin: *Proceedings of the Nutrition Society*.

Boushey, C., Spoden, M., Zhu, F., Delp, E., & Kerr, D. (2017). New mobile methods for dietary assessment: Review of image-assisted and image-based dietary assessment methods. *The Proceedings of the Nutrition Society, 76*(3), 283–294. doi:10.1017/S0029665116002913 PMID:27938425

Bowman, D. A., Coquillart, S., Froehlich, B., Hirose, M., Kitamura, Y., Kiyokawa, K., & Stuerzlinger, W. (2008). 3d user interfaces: New directions and perspectives. *IEEE Computer Graphics and Applications, 28*(6), 20–36. doi:10.1109/MCG.2008.109 PMID:19004682

Bracq, M. S., Michinov, E., & Jannin, P. (2019). Virtual reality simulation in nontechnical skills training for healthcare professionals: A systematic review. *Simulation in Healthcare, 14*(3), 188–194. doi:10.1097/SIH.0000000000000347 PMID:30601464

Britannica, E. (1993). *Encyclopædia britannica*. Chicago: University of Chicago.

Bryman, A. (2016). *Social research methods*. United Kingdom: Oxford university press.

Bzhalava, Z., Tampuu, A., Bała, P., Vicente, R., & Dillner, J. (2018). Machine Learning for detection of viral sequences in human metagenomic datasets. *BMC Bioinformatics, 19*(1), 336. doi:10.118612859-018-2340-x PMID:30249176

Campbell, T., & Jacobson, H. (2014). *Whole: Rethinking the Science of Nutrition*. Dallas, TX: BenBella Books.

Can Yapan. (2017, November 25). *Diet Diary*. Retrieved from https://play.google.com/store/apps/details?id=com.canyapan.dietdiaryapp&hl=en

Carter, M. C., Burley, V. J., Nykjaer, C., & Cade, J. E. (2013). Adherence to a smartphone application for weight loss compared to website and paper diary: Pilot randomized controlled trial. *Journal of Medical Internet Research, 15*(4), e32. doi:10.2196/jmir.2283 PMID:23587561

Carter, M. C., Burley, V. J., Nykjaer, C., & Cade, J. E. (2013). Adherence to a Smartphone Application for Weight Loss. *Journal of Medical Internet Research, 15*(4). PMID:23587561

Castellani, M., & Rowlands, H. (2009). Evolutionary artificial neural network design and training for wood veneer classification. *Engineering Applications of Artificial Intelligence, 22*(4), 732–741. doi:10.1016/j.engappai.2009.01.013

Celik, M., Koylu, F., & Karaboga, D. (2016). CoABC Miner: An algorithm for cooperative rule classification system based on artificial bee colony. *International Journal of Artificial Intelligence Tools, 25*(01), 1550028. doi:10.1142/S0218213015500281

Chakraborty, D., Saha, S., & Maity, S. (2015, February). Training feed forward neural networks using hybrid flower pollination-gravitational search algorithm. In *Proceedings of the 2015 International Conference on Futuristic Trends on Computational Analysis and Knowledge Management (ABLAZE)* (pp. 261-266). IEEE.

Chakraborty, A., Baowaly, M., Arefin, A., & Bahar, A. (2012). The Role of Requirement Engineering in Software Development Life Cycle. *Journal of Emerging Trends in Computing and Information Sciences, 3*(5), 723–729.

Chandhok, C. (2012). A novel approach to image segmentation using artificial neural networks and k-means clustering. *International Journal of Engineering Research and Applications, 2*(3), 274–279.

Chao, K.-M. (2006). *Basic Concepts of DNA, Proteins, Genes and Genomes. Graduate Institute of Biomedical Electronics and Bioinformatics (Department of Computer Science and Information Engineering).* Taiwan: Graduate Institute of Networking and Multimedia National Taiwan University.

Chao, K.-M. (2006). *Basic Concepts of DNA, Proteins, Genes and Genomes.* Taiwan: National Taiwan University.

Chaudhary, A., & Singh, S. S. (2012). Lung cancer detection on CT images by using image processing. In *Proceedings of the 2012 International Conference on Computing Sciences (ICCS),* (pp. 142-146). IEEE. 10.1109/ICCS.2012.43

Chaurasiya, M., Chandulah, G. B., Misra, K., & Chaurasiya, V. K. (2010). Nearest-neighbor classifier as a tool for classification of protein families. *Bioinformation, 4*(9), 396–398. doi:10.6026/97320630004396 PMID:20975888

Cheng, M.-T., & Annetta, L. (2012). Students' learning outcomes and learning experiences through playing a serious educational game. *Journal of Biological Education, 46*(4), 203–213. doi:10.1080/00219266.2012.688848

Chen, J., Huang, H., Tian, S., & Qu, Y. (2009). Feature selection for text classification with Naïve Bayes. *Expert Systems with Applications, 36*(3), 5432–5435. doi:10.1016/j.eswa.2008.06.054

Cheruto, V. (2019, July 1). Rwanda and Ghana: Drones delivering medical supplies. *MSN News.* Retrieved from https://www.msn.com/en-za/news/other/rwanda-and-ghana-drones-delivering-medical-supplies/ar-AADJpCD

Chipara, O., He, Z., Xing, G., Chen, Q., Wang, X., Lu, C., ... Abdelzaher, T. (2006, June). Real-time power-aware routing in sensor networks. In *Proceedings of the 2006 14th IEEE International Workshop on Quality of Service* (pp. 83-92). IEEE. 10.1109/IWQOS.2006.250454

Chiroma, H., Khan, A., Abubakar, A. I., Saadi, Y., Hamza, M. F., Shuib, L., & Herawan, T. (2016). A new approach for forecasting OPEC petroleum consumption based on neural network train by using flower pollination algorithm. *Applied Soft Computing, 48*, 50–58. doi:10.1016/j.asoc.2016.06.038

Chiroma, H., Shuib, N. L. M., Muaz, S. A., Abubakar, A. I., Ila, L. B., & Maitama, J. Z. (2015). A review of the applications of bio-inspired flower pollination algorithm. Procedia Coml2puter. *Science, 62,* 435–441.

Christensen, H. C., Schüz, J., Kosteljanetz, M., Skovgaard, P. H., Boice, J. D., McLaughlin, J. K., & Johansen, C. (2004). Cellular Telephones and Risk for Acoustic Neuroma. *American Journal of Epidemiology, 159*(3), 277–283. doi:10.1093/aje/kwh032 PMID:14742288

Clarke, J. H. (1902). *A dictionary of pratical materia medica*: homoeopathic publishing Company.

Clarke, J. H. (1998). *The Prescriber: How to Practice Homoeopathy*: B. Jain Publishers. contributors, W. Alternative medicine. Retrieved from https://en.wikipedia.org/w/index.php?title=Alternative_medicine&oldid=906879807

Clase, K. L., Adamo-Villani, N., Gooding, S. L., Yadav, A., Karpicke, J. D., & Gentry, M. (2009). Enhancing creativity in synthetic biology with interactive virtual environments. In Proceedings of the 39th IEEE Frontiers in education conference FIE '09 (pp. 1–6). doi:10.1109/FIE.2009.5350646

Coello, C. A. (2000). An updated survey of GA-based multiobjective optimization techniques. *ACM Computing Surveys, 32*(2), 109–143. doi:10.1145/358923.358929

Collins, L., & Ellis, S. (2015). *Mobile Devices: Tools and Technologies*. Boca Raton, FL: Chapman and Hall/CRC. doi:10.1201/b18165

Coppin, B. (2004). *Artificial intelligence illuminated*. Jones & Bartlett Learning.

Craig, E. (1998). *Routledge encyclopedia of philosophy: questions to sociobiology* (Vol. 8). Taylor & Francis.

Crislip, M. (2010). Homeopathic Vaccines. *Science-Based Medicine.* Retrieved from https://sciencebasedmedicine.org/homeopathic-vaccines/

Croft, R. J., Chandler, J. S., Burgess, A. P., Barry, R. J., Williams, J. D., & Clarke, A. R. (2002). Acute mobile phone operation affects neural function in humans. *Clinical Neurophysiology, 113*(10), 1623–1632. doi:10.1016/S1388-2457(02)00215-8 PMID:12350439

Cronometer Software Inc. (2019, August 28). *Cronometer.* Retrieved from https://play.google.com/store/apps/details?id=com.cronometer.android.gold&hl=en

Cunningham, P., & Delany, S. J. (2007). k-Nearest neighbour classifiers. *Multiple Classifier Systems, 34*(8), 1–17.

Curcio, G., Ferrara, M., Moroni, F., D'Inzeo, G., Bertini, M., & De Gennaro, L. (2005). Is the brain influenced by a phone call? An EEG study of resting wakefulness. *Neuroscience Research, 53*(3), 265–270. doi:10.1016/j.neures.2005.07.003 PMID:16102863

Cylonblast Mobile Apps. (2019, August 31). *Best Boiled Egg Diet Plan.* Retrieved from https://play.google.com/store/apps/details?id=com.cylonblastmobileapps.bestboiledeggdiet&hl=en

D'Costa, H., Trueman, G., Tang, L., & … . (2003). Human brain wave activity during exposure to radiofrequency field emissions from mobile phones. *Australasian Physical & Engineering Sciences in Medicine, 26,* 162–167. doi:10.1007/BF03179176 PMID:14995060

Dagtas, S., Pekhteryev, G., Sahinoglu, Z., Cam, H., & Challa, N. (2008). Real-time and secure wireless health monitoring. *International Journal of Telemedicine and Applications, 2008,* 1–10. doi:10.1155/2008/135808 PMID:18497866

Daily Guide. (2017, November 17). Ghana ranks 6th on diabetes table in Africa. *Myjoyonline.* Retrieved from https://www.myjoyonline.com/lifestyle/2017/november-17th/ghana-ranks-6th-on-diabetes-table-in-africa.php

Dakhli, A., Bellil, W., & Amar, C. B. (2016). Wavelet Neural Networks for DNA Sequence Classification Using the Genetic Algorithms and the Least Trimmed Square. *Procedia Computer Science*, *96*, 418–427. doi:10.1016/j.procs.2016.08.088

Darwish, A., & Hassanien, A. E. (2011). Wearable and implantable wireless sensor network solutions for healthcare monitoring. *Sensors (Basel)*, *11*(6), 5561–5595. doi:10.3390110605561 PMID:22163914

Das, B. (1981). *Select your remedy*. Vishwamber Free Homeo Dispensary.

De Luca, R., Manuli, A., De Domenico, C., Voi, E. L., Buda, A., Maresca, G., ... Calabrò, R. S. (2019). Improving neuro-psychiatric symptoms following stroke using virtual reality. *Case Reports in Medicine*, *98*(19), e15236. PMID:31083155

de Oliveira, M. L., & Galembeck, E. (2016). Mobile applications in cell biology present new approaches for cell modelling. *Journal of Biological Education*, *50*(3), 290–303. doi:10.1080/00219266.2015.1085428

de Ribaupierre, S., Kapralos, B., Haji, F., Stroulia, E., Dubrowski, A., & Eagleson, R. (2014). Healthcare training enhancement through virtual reality and serious games. In *Virtual, Augmented Reality and Serious Games for Healthcare 1* (pp. 9–27). Berlin: Springer. doi:10.1007/978-3-642-54816-1_2

DeCastellarnau, A. (2018). A classification of response scale characteristics that affect data quality: A literature review. *Quality & Quantity*, *52*(4), 1523–1559. doi:10.100711135-017-0533-4 PMID:29937582

Dede, C., Clarke, J., Ketelhut, D. J., Nelson, B., & Bowman, C. (2005). Students motivation and learning of science in a multi-user virtual environment. In *Proceedings of the American educational research association conference* (pp. 1–8). Academic Press.

Delgado, J. M., Leal, J., Monteagudo, J. L., & Gracia, M. G. (1982). Embryological changes induced by weak, extremely low frequency electromagnetic fields. *Journal of Anatomy*, *134*(3), 533–551. PMID:7107514

Deniz, O. G., Kaplan, S., Selçuk, M. B., Terzi, M., Altun, G., Yurt, K. K., ... Davis, D. (2017). Effects of short and long term electromagnetic fields exposure on the human hippocampus. *Journal of microscopy and ultrastructure*, *5*(4), 191-197.

Dev, P., Pichumani, R., Walker, D., Heinrichs, W., Karadi, C., & Lorie, W. (1998). Formative design of a virtual learning environment. *Studies in Health Technology and Informatics*, *50*, 392–398. PMID:10180582

Dias, D., & Paulo Silva Cunha, J. (2018). Wearable health devices—Vital sign monitoring, systems and technologies. *Sensors (Basel)*, *18*(8), 12–18. doi:10.339018082414 PMID:30044415

Dimon, G. (2018). Password reset email design best practices. Postmarkapp. Retrieved from https://postmarkapp.com/guides/password-reset-email-best-practices

Djenouri, D., & Balasingham, I. (2009, September). New QoS and geographical routing in wireless biomedical sensor networks. In *Proceedings of the 2009 Sixth International Conference on Broadband Communications, Networks, and Systems* (pp. 1-8). IEEE. 10.4108/ICST.BROADNETS2009.7188

Dossey, A. (2019). A Guide to Mobile App Development: Web vs. Native vs. Hybrid [Infographic]. Clearbridgemobile. Retrieved from https://clearbridgemobile.com/mobile-app-development-native-vs-web-vs-hybrid/#What_are_Progressive_Web_Apps

Down to Earth. (2019). 5G: A dangerous generation.

Dreiseitl, S., & Ohno-Machado, L. (2002). Logistic regression and artificial neural network classification models: A methodology review. *Journal of Biomedical Informatics*, *35*(5), 352–359. doi:10.1016/S1532-0464(03)00034-0 PMID:12968784

Drummond, K. H., Houston, T., & Irvine, T. (2014). *The rise and fall and rise of virtual reality*. Vox Media.

Dubey, S. (1975). *Textbook of Materia Medica*. Dubey.

Dunaway, J., Searles, K., Sui, M., & Paul, N. (2018). News Attention in a Mobile Era. *Journal of Computer-Mediated Communication*, 23(2), 107–124. doi:10.1093/jcmc/zmy004

Dunham, M. H. (2006). *Data mining: Introductory and advanced topics*. Pearson Education India.

Durak, A., & Karaoglan Yilmaz, F. G. (2019). Artirilmiş gerçekliğin eğitsel uygulamalari üzerine ortaokul öğrencilerinin görüşleri [Opinions of secondary school students on educational practices of augmented reality]. *Abant İzzet Baysal Üniversitesi Eğitim Fakültesi Dergisi*, 19(2), 468–481. doi:10.17240/aibuefd.2019.19.46660-425148

Durant, J. R., Evans, G. A., & Thomas, G. P. (1989). The public understanding of science. *Nature*, 340(6228), 11–14. doi:10.1038/340011a0 PMID:2739718

Eames, S., Hoffmann, T., Worrall, L., & Read, S. (2010). Stroke patients' and carers' perception of barriers to accessing stroke information. *Topics in Stroke Rehabilitation*, 17(2), 69–78. doi:10.1310/tsr1702-69 PMID:20542850

Ehyaie, A., Hashemi, M., & Khadivi, P. (2009, June). Using relay network to increase life time in wireless body area sensor networks. In *Proceedings of the 2009 IEEE International Symposium on a World of Wireless, Mobile and Multimedia Networks & Workshops* (pp. 1-6). IEEE. 10.1109/WOWMOM.2009.5282405

Eickholt, J., & Cheng, J. (2013). DNdisorder: Predicting protein disorder using boosting and deep networks. *BMC Bioinformatics*, 14(1), 88.

El Beheiry, M., Doutreligne, S., Caporal, C., Ostertag, C., Dahan, M., & Masson, J. B. (2019). Virtual Reality: Beyond Visualization. *Journal of Molecular Biology*, 431(7), 315–321. doi:10.1016/j.jmb.2019.01.033 PMID:30738026

Elgamal, M. (2013). Automatic skin cancer images classification. *(IJACSA). International Journal of Advanced Computer Science and Applications*, 4(3), 287–294. doi:10.14569/IJACSA.2013.040342

Emvalotis, A., & Koutsianou, A. (2018). Greek primary school students images of scientists and their work: Has anything changed? *Research in Science & Technological Education*, 36(1), 69–85. doi:10.1080/02635143.2017.1366899

Engelbrecht, A. P. (2007). *Computational intelligence: an introduction*. John Wiley & Sons. doi:10.1002/9780470512517

Eom, K., Jung, K., & Sirisena, H. (2003). Performance improvement of back propagation algorithm by automatic activation function gain tuning using fuzzy logic. *Neurocomputing*, 50, 439–460. doi:10.1016/S0925-2312(02)00576-3

Eulitz, C., Ullsperger, P., Freude, G., & Elbert, T. (1998). Mobile phones modulate response patterns of human brain activity. *Neuroreport*, 9(14), 3229–3232. doi:10.1097/00001756-199810050-00018 PMID:9831456

Evett, I. W., & Spiehler, E. J. (1988). Knowledge based systems. In *Rule induction in forensic science*. Academic Press.

Fanguy, W. (2018). A comprehensive guide to designing UX buttons. Invisionapp. Retrieved from https://www.invisionapp.com/inside-design/comprehensive-guide-designing-ux-buttons/

Faridi, Z., Liberti, L., Shuval, K., Northrup, V., Ali, A., & Katz, D. L. (2008). Evaluating the impact of mobile telephone technology on type 2 diabetic patients' self-management: The NICHE pilot study. *Journal of Evaluation in Clinical Practice*, 14(3), 465–469. doi:10.1111/j.1365-2753.2007.00881.x PMID:18373577

FatSecret. (2019). *Play Store: Calorie Counter by FatSecret*. Retrieved from https://play.google.com/store/apps/details?id=com.fatsecret.android

Felemban, E., Lee, C. G., & Ekici, E. (2006). MMSPEED: Multipath Multi-SPEED protocol for QoS guarantee of reliability and. Timeliness in wireless sensor networks. *IEEE Transactions on Mobile Computing, 5*(6), 738–754. doi:10.1109/TMC.2006.79

Fenlander Software Solutions Ltd. (2019, August 30). *Ultimate Food Value Diary - Diet & Weight Tracker.* Retrieved from https://play.google.com/store/apps/details?id=com.fenlander.ultimatevaluediary&hl=en

Field, A. (2005). *Discovering statistics using SPSS.* London: Sage Publications.

Fields, G. P. (2014). *Religious therapeutics: Body and health in yoga, ayurveda, and tantra.* SUNY Press.

Fister, I., Yang, X.-S., Fong, S., & Zhuang, Y. (2014). Bat algorithm: Recent advances. *Paper presented at the 2014 IEEE 15th International Symposium on Computational Intelligence and Informatics (CINTI).* IEEE Press. 10.1109/CINTI.2014.7028669

Foley, T. (2017). Transforming the patient experience through "Smart Room" technologies: Tablets, flat-screen TVs and educational resources help engage patients in their healthcare during and after a hospital stay. *Health Tech Magazine.* Retrieved from https://healthtechmagazine.net/article/2017/01/transforming-patient-experience-through-smart-room-technologies

Free, C., Phillips, G., Watson, L., Galli, L., Felix, L., Edwards, P., ... Haines, A. (2013). The Effectiveness of Mobile-Health Technologies to Improve Health Care Service Delivery Processes: A Systematic Review and Meta-Analysis. *PLoS Medicine, 10*(1), 1–26. doi:10.1371/journal.pmed.1001363 PMID:23458994

Freude, G., Ullsperger, P., Eggert, S., & Ruppe, I. (1998). Effects of microwaves emitted by cellular phones on human slow brain potentials. *Bioelectromagnetics, 19*(6), 384–387. doi:10.1002/(SICI)1521-186X(1998)19:6<384::AID-BEM6>3.0.CO;2-Y PMID:9738529

Frey, A. H., Feld, S. R., & Frey, B. (1975). Neural function and behaviour: Defining the relationship. *Annals of the New York Academy of Sciences, 247*(1), 433–439. doi:10.1111/j.1749-6632.1975.tb36019.x PMID:46734

Fritze, K., Sommer, C., Schmitz, B., Mies, G., Hossmann, K. A., Kiessling, M., & Wiessner, C. (1997). Effect of GSM microwave exposure on blood-brain barrier. *Acta Neuropathologica, 94,* 465–470. doi:10.1007004010050734 PMID:9386779

Fung, Y. Y. H. (2002). A comparative study of primary and secondary school students' images of scientists. *Research in Science & Technological Education, 20*(2), 199–213. doi:10.1080/0263514022000030453

Gadelha, R. (2018). Revolutionizing Education: The promise of virtual reality. *Childhood Education, 94*(1), 40–43. doi:10.1080/00094056.2018.1420362

Gaggioli, A. (2017). An open research community for studying virtual reality experience. *Cyberpsychology, Behavior, and Social Networking, 20*(2), 138–139. doi:10.1089/cyber.2017.29063.csi

Gandhi, C. R., & Ross, D. H. (1989). Microwave induced stimulation of ^{32}Pi-incorporation into phosphoinositides of rat brain synaptosomes. *Radiation and Environmental Biophysics, 28*(3), 223–234. doi:10.1007/BF01211259 PMID:2552495

Gavalas, R. J., Walter, D. O., Hamer, J., & Rossadey, W. (1970). Effect of lowlevel, low-frequency electric fields on EEG and behavior in Macaca nemestrina. *Brain Research, 18*(3), 491–501. doi:10.1016/0006-8993(70)90132-0 PMID:4995199

Geetha, M. P., & Selvi, D. V. (2015). An impression of cancers and survey of techniques in image processing for detecting various cancers: A review. *International Research Journal of Engineering and Technology, 2.*

Genes, N., Violante, S., Cetrangol, C., Rogers, L., Schadt, E., Feng, Y., & Chan, Y. (2018). From smartphone to EHR: A case report on integrating patient-generated health data. *Digital Media, 23,* 1–6. PMID:31304305

Gerasimov, I., & Simon, R. (2002, April). A bandwidth-reservation mechanism for on-demand ad hoc path finding. In *Proceedings 35th Annual Simulation Symposium. SS 2002* (pp. 27-34). IEEE. 10.1109/SIMSYM.2002.1000079

Giang, N., Tran, V. A., Ngo, D. L., Phan, D., Lumbanraja, F., Faisal, M. R., ... Satou, K. (2016). DNA Sequence Classification by Convolutional Neural Network. *Journal of Biomedical Science and Engineering, 09*(05), 280–286. doi:10.4236/jbise.2016.95021

Gonzalez, H., Stakhanova, N., & Ghorbani, A. (2016). Measuring code reuse in Android apps. In *Proceedings of the 14th Annual Conference on Privacy, Security and Trust (PST)* (pp. 187-195). Academic Press. 10.1109/PST.2016.7906925

Goyal, A., Gopalakrishnan, M., Anantharaman, G., Chandrashekharan, D. P., Thachil, T., & Sharma, A. (2019). Smartphone guided wide-field imaging for retinopathy of prematurity in neonatal intensive care unit–a Smart ROP (SROP) initiative. *Indian Journal of Ophthalmology, 67*(6), 840. doi:10.4103/ijo.IJO_1177_18 PMID:31124499

Goyal, S., & Cafazzo, J. A. (2013). Mobile phone health apps for diabetes management: Current evidence and future developments, *QJM. International Journal of Medicine, 106*(1), 1067–1069. doi:10.1093/qjmed/hct203 PMID:24106313

Gropper, S., Smith, J., & Carr, T. (2017). *Advanced Nutrition and Human Metabolism*. London, UK: Cengage Learning.

Grym, K., Niela-Vilén, H., Ekholm, E., Hamari, L., Azimi, I., Rahmani, A, Liljeberg, P., Loyttyniemi, E. & Axelin, A. (2019). Feasibility of smart wristbands for continuous monitoring during pregnancy and one month after birth. *BMC pregnancy and childbirth, 19*(1), 34. doi:10.118612884-019-2187-9

Gunn, T., Jones, L., Bridge, P., Rowntree, P., & Nissen, L. (2018). The use of virtual reality simulation to improve technical skill in the undergraduate medical imaging student. *Interactive Learning Environments, 26*(5), 613–620. doi:10.1080/10494820.2017.1374981

Gupta, P., Sharma, V. K., & Sharma, S. (2014). *Healing traditions of the Northwestern Himalayas*. Springer. doi:10.1007/978-81-322-1925-5

Gyamfi, E. T. (2019). Metals and metalloids in traditional medicines (Ayurvedic medicines, nutraceuticals and traditional Chinese medicines). *Environmental Science and Pollution Research International*, 1–12. PMID:31004267

Haarala, C., Bjornberg, L., Ek, M., Laine, M., Revonsuo, A., Koivisto, M., & Hämäläinen, H. (2003). Effect of a 902 MHz electromagnetic field emitted by mobile phones on human cognitive function: A replication study. *Bioelectromagnetics, 24*(4), 283–288. doi:10.1002/bem.10105 PMID:12696088

Habash, R.W. (2011). *Non-Invasive microwave hyperthermia* [PhD Thesis]. ECE Deptt, IISc, Bangalore, India.

Hachet, M. (2010). *3D User Interfaces, from Mobile Devices to Immersive Virtual Environments* [Habilitation `a diriger des recherches]. Universit'e Sciences et Technologies - Bordeaux I. Retrieved from https://tel.archives-ouvertes.fr/tel-00576663

Hahnemann, S. (1996). Materia medica pura (Vol. 2). B. Jain Publishers.

Hahnemann, S. (1833). *The Homœopathic Medical Doctrine: Or," Organon of the Healing Art."* WF Wakeman.

Halvorsen, L. (2018). *Functional Web Development with Elixir, OTP, and Phoenix: Rethink the Modern Web App*. Raleigh, NC: Pragmatic Bookshelf.

Hamid, N. A., Nawi, N. M., & Ghazali, R. (2011). The effect of adaptive gain and adaptive momentum in improving training time of gradient descent back propagation algorithm on classification problems. International Journal on Advanced Science. *Engineering and Information Technology, 1*(2), 178–184.

Hamid, N. A., Nawi, N. M., Ghazali, R., & Salleh, M. N. M. (2012). Solving Local Minima Problem in Back Propagation Algorithm Using Adaptive Gain, Adaptive Momentum and Adaptive Learning Rate on Classification Problems. *International Journal of Modern Physics: Conference Series, 9*, 448–455.

Handayani, P., Meigasari, D., Pinem, A., Hidayanto, A., & Ayuningtyas, D. (2018). Critical success factors for mobile health implementation in Indonesia. *Heliyon (London), 4*(11), 1–26. doi:10.1016/j.heliyon.2018.e00981 PMID:30519665

Haofei, Z., Guoping, X., Fangting, Y., & Han, Y. (2007). A neural network model based on the multi-stage optimization approach for short-term food price forecasting in China. *Expert Systems with Applications, 33*(2), 347–356. doi:10.1016/j.eswa.2006.05.021

Harland, J. D., & Liburdy, R. P. (1997). Environmental magnetic fields inhibit the antiproliferative action of tamoxifen and melatonin in a human breast cancer cell line. *Bioelectromagnetics, 18*(8), 555–562. doi:10.1002/(SICI)1521-186X(1997)18:8<555::AID-BEM4>3.0.CO;2-1 PMID:9383244

Harrison, R., Flood, D., & Duce, D. (2013). Usability of mobile applications: Literature review and rationale for a new usability model. *Journal of Interaction Science, 1*(1), 1–16. doi:10.1186/2194-0827-1-1

Hartson, R., & Pyla, P. (2018). *The UX Book: Agile UX Design for a Quality User Experience.* Burlington, MA: Morgan Kaufmann.

Hashemi, A., Pilevar, A. H., & Rafeh, R. (2013). Mass detection in lung CT images using region growing segmentation and decision making based on fuzzy inference system and artificial neural network. *International Journal of Image. Graphics and Signal Processing, 5*(6), 16–24. doi:10.5815/ijigsp.2013.06.03

Hasic, H., Buza, E., & Akagic, A. (2017, May). A hybrid method for prediction of protein secondary structure based on multiple artificial neural networks. In *Proceedings of the 2017 40th International Convention on Information and Communication Technology, Electronics and Microelectronics (MIPRO)* (pp. 1195-1200). IEEE. doi:10.23919/MIPRO.2017.7973605

Haykin, S. S., Haykin, S. S., Haykin, S. S., & Haykin, S. S. (2009). *Neural networks and learning machines* (Vol. 3). Upper Saddle River, NJ, USA: Pearson.

HCD Team. (2017). Ayurveda. *Health Topics* Retrieved from https://www.healthlinkbc.ca/health-topics/aa116840spec

Hecht-Nielsen, R. (1990). On the algebraic structure of feed forward network weight spaces. Adval2nced. *Neural Computation*, 129–135.

Hemenway, H. B. (1894). Modern Homeopathy And Medical Science. *Journal of the American Medical Association, 22*(11), 367–377. doi:10.1001/jama.1894.02420900001001

Hietanen, M., Kovala, T., & Hamalainen, H. (2000). Human brain activity during exposure to radiofrequency fields emitted by cellular phones. *Scandinavian Journal of Work, Environment & Health, 26*(2), 87–92. doi:10.5271jweh.516 PMID:10817372

Hines, T. (1988). *Pseudoscience and the paranormal: A critical examination of the evidence.* Prometheus Books.

Hinrikus, H., Bachmann, M., Lass, J., Karai, D., & Tuulik, V. (2008a). Effect of low frequency modulated microwave exposure on human EEG: Individual sensitivity. *Bioelectromagnetics, 29*(7), 527–538. doi:10.1002/bem.20415 PMID:18452168

Hinrikus, H., Bachmann, M., Lass, J., Tomson, R., & Tuulik, V. (2008b). Effect of 7, 14 and 21 Hz modulated 450 MHz microwave radiation on human electroencephalographic rhythms. *International Journal of Radiation Biology, 84*(1), 69–79. doi:10.1080/09553000701691679 PMID:18058332

Ho, Y. C., Bryson, A. E., & Baron, S. (1965). Differential games and optimal pursuit-evasion strategies. In *Proceedings of the Joint Automatic Control Conference* (No. 3, pp. 37-40). Academic Press. 10.1109/TAC.1965.1098197

Hoernle, A. F. R. (1907). *Studies in the medicine of ancient India: Osteology, or the bones of the human body.* Clarendon Press.

Hoffmann, T., & McKenna, K. (2006). Analysis of stroke patients' and carers' reading ability and the content and design of written materials: Recommendations for improving written stroke information. *Patient Education and Counseling, 60*(3), 286–293. doi:10.1016/j.pec.2005.06.020 PMID:16098708

Holm, A., & Günzel-Jensen, F. (2017). Succeeding with freemium: Strategies for implementation. *The Journal of Business Strategy, 38*(2), 16–24. doi:10.1108/JBS-09-2016-0096

Honeine, P., Mourad, F., Kallas, M., Snoussi, H., Amoud, H., & Francis, C. (2011, May). Wireless sensor networks in biomedical: Body area networks. In *Proceedings of the International Workshop on Systems, Signal Processing and their Applications, WOSSPA* (pp. 388-391). IEEE. 10.1109/WOSSPA.2011.5931518

Hosseini-Sharifabad, M., Esfandiari, E., & Hosseini-Sharifabad, A. (2012). The effect of prenatal exposure to restraint stress on hippocampal granule neurons of adult rat offspring. *Iranian Journal of Basic Medical Sciences., 15*, 106–107. PMID:23493456

Huang, H. M., Liaw, S. S., & Lai, C. M. (2016). Exploring learner acceptance of the use of virtual reality in medical education: A case study of desktop and projection-based display systems. *Interactive Learning Environments, 24*(1), 3–19. doi:10.1080/10494820.2013.817436

Huber, R., Graf, T., Cote, K. A., Wittmann, L., Gallmann, E., Matter, D., ... Achermann, P. (2000). Exposure to pulsed high-frequency electromagnetic field during waking affects human sleep EEG. *Neuroreport, 11*(15), 3321–3325. doi:10.1097/00001756-200010200-00012 PMID:11059895

Huber, R., Treyer, V., Borbely, A. A., Schuderer, J., Gottselig, J. M., Landolt, H.-P., ... Achermann, P. (2002). Electromagnetic fields, such as those from mobile phones, alter regional cerebral blood flow and sleep and waking EEG. *Journal of Sleep Research, 11*(4), 289–295. doi:10.1046/j.1365-2869.2002.00314.x PMID:12464096

Hulkower, R. (2016). The history of the Hippocratic Oath: Outdated, inauthentic, and yet still relevant. *The Einstein Journal of Biology and Medicine; EJBM, 25*(1), 41–44. doi:10.23861/EJBM20102542

Hung, C. S., Anderson, C., Horne, J. A., & McEvoy, P. (2007). Mobile phone 'talk-mode' signal delays EEG-determined sleep onset. *Neuroscience Letters, 421*(1), 82–86. doi:10.1016/j.neulet.2007.05.027 PMID:17548154

Hussain, M., Al-Haiqi, A., Zaidan, A., Zaidan, B., Kiah, M., Anuar, N., & Abdulnabi, M. (2015). The landscape of research on smartphone medical apps: Coherent taxonomy, motivations, open challenges and recommendations. *Computer Methods and Programs in Biomedicine, 122*(3), 393–408. doi:10.1016/j.cmpb.2015.08.015 PMID:26412009

Hylton Iii, A., & Sankaranarayanan, S. (2012). Application of intelligent agents in hospital appointment scheduling system. *International Journal of Computer Theory and Engineering, 4*(4), 625.

Idrish, S., Rifat, A., Iqbal, M., & Nisha, N. (2017). Mobile Health Technology Evaluation: Innovativeness and Efficacy vs. Cost Effectiveness. *International Journal of Technology and Human Interaction, 13*(2), 1–21. doi:10.4018/IJTHI.2017040101

Iversen, J., & Eierman, M. (2013). *Learning Mobile App Development: A Hands-on Guide to Building Apps with iOS and Android.* Boston, MA: Addison-Wesley Professional.

Ja Kaun In. (2018). *Dining Note: Simple food diary*. Retrieved from https://apps.apple.com/us/app/dining-note-simple-food-diary/id1194971321

Jayalakshmi, T., & Santhakumaran, A. (2010). Improved Gradient Descent Back Propagation Neural Networks for Diagnoses of Type II Diabetes Mellitus. *Global Journal of Computer Science and Technology*, *9*(5).

Jenefer, B. M., & Cyrilraj, V. (2014). An efficient image processing methods for mammogram breast cancer detection. *Journal of Theoretical & Applied Information Technology*, *69*(1).

Johansson, A.-M., & Wickman, P.-O. (2018). The use of organising purposes in science instruction as a scaffolding mechanism to support progressions: A study of talk in two primary science classrooms. *Research in Science & Technological Education*, *36*(1), 1–16. doi:10.1080/02635143.2017.1318272

Johansson, D., & Andersson, K. (2015). Mobile e-Services: State of the Art, Focus Areas, and Future Directions. *International Journal of E-Services and Mobile Applications*, *7*(2), 1–24. doi:10.4018/ijesma.2015040101

Jonas, W. B. (2005). Dictionary of complementary and alternative medicine. *Journal of Alternative and Complementary Medicine*, *11*(4), 739–740. doi:10.1089/acm.2005.11.739

Joshi, M. D., Karode, A. H., & Suralkar, S. R. (2013). White blood cells segmentation and classification to detect acute leukemia. *International Journal of Emerging Trends and Technology in Computer Science*, *2*(3).

Jospe, M. R., Fairbairn, K. A., Green, P., & Perry, T. L. (2015). Diet app use by sports dietitians: A survey in five countries. *JMIR mHealth and uHealth*, *3*(1), e7. doi:10.2196/mhealth.3345 PMID:25616274

Joysticks. (2018). Newegg. Retrieved From http://www.newegg.com/pc-game-controllers/subcategory/id-123

Jung, K. K., Lim, J. K., Chung, S. B., & Eom, K. H. (2003). Performance Improvement of Back propagation Algorithm by Automatic Tuning of Learning Rate using Fuzzy Logic System. *Journal of information and communication convergence engineering*, *1*(3), 157-162.

Kahn, J. G., Yang, J. S., & Kahn, J. S. (2010). Mobile'health needs and opportunities in developing countries. *Health Affairs*, *29*(2), 252–258. doi:10.1377/hlthaff.2009.0965 PMID:20348069

Kale, S. D., Punwatkar, K. M., & Pusad, Y. (2013). Texture Analysis of Thyroid Ultrasound Images for Diagnosis of Benign and Malignant Nodule using Scaled Conjugate Gradient Backpropagation Training Neural Network. *IJCEM International Journal of Computational Engineering & Management*, *16*(6).

Kamble, V.B., & Deshmukh, S.N. (2017). Comparison Between Accuracy and MSE, RMSE by Using Proposed Method with Imputation Technique. *Orient. J. Comp. Sci. and Technol.*, *10*(4).

Kanakatte, A., Mani, N., Srinivasan, B., & Gubbi, J. (2008, May). Pulmonary tumor volume detection from positron emission tomography images. In *Proceedings of the International Conference on BioMedical Engineering and Informatics BMEI 2008* (Vol. 2, pp. 213-217). IEEE. 10.1109/BMEI.2008.354

Kandris, D., Tsagkaropoulos, M., Politis, I., Tzes, A., & Kotsopoulos, S. (2011). Energy efficient and perceived QoS aware video routing over wireless multimedia sensor networks. *Ad Hoc Networks*, *9*(4), 591–607. doi:10.1016/j.adhoc.2010.09.001

Kandris, D., Tsioumas, P., Tzes, A., Nikolakopoulos, G., & Vergados, D. (2009). Power conservation through energy efficient routing in wireless sensor networks. *Sensors (Basel)*, *9*(9), 7320–7342. doi:10.339090907320 PMID:22399998

Kan, P., Simonsen, S. E., Lyon, J. L., & Kestle, J. R. W. (2007). Cellular Phone Use and Brain Tumor: A Meta-Analysis. *Journal of Neuro-Oncology*, *86*(1), 71–78. doi:10.100711060-007-9432-1 PMID:17619826

Karaboga, D. (2005). An idea based on honey bee swarm for numerical optimization (Vol. 200). Erciyes University.

Karaoğlan Yılmaz, F. G., & Yılmaz, R. (2019). Examining the opinions of prospective teachers about the use of virtual reality applications in education [Sanal gerçeklik uygulamalarının eğitimde kullanımına ilişkin öğretmen adaylarının görüşlerinin incelenmesi]. In *Proceedings of the International Congress on Science and Education.* Academic Press.

Kartous, W., Layeb, A., & Chikhi, S. (2014). A new quantum cuckoo search algorithm for multiple sequence alignment. *Journal of Intelligent Systems, 23*(3), 261–275.

Kasinathan, V., Rahman, N., & Rani, M. (2014). Approaching Digital Natives with QR Code Technology in Edutainment. *International Journal of Education and Research, 2*(4), 169–178.

Kasmin, F., Prabuwono, A. S., & Abdullah, A. (2012). Detection of leukemia in human blood sample based on microscopic images: A study. *Journal of Theoretical & Applied Information Technology, 46*(2).

Kassim, N. A., & Abdullah, A. (2017). *Classification of DNA Sequences Using Convolutional Neural Network Approach.* Academic Press.

Kathirvalavakumar, T., & Thangavel, P. (2006). A modified back propagation training algorithm for feed forward neural networks. *Neural Processing Letters, 23*(2), 111–119. doi:10.100711063-005-3501-2

Kaufman, M. (1971). *Homeopathy in America: The rise and fall of a medical heresy.* The Johns Hopkins Press.

Kaur, A. R. (2013). Feature extraction and principal component analysis for lung cancer detection in CT scan images. *International Journal of Advanced Research in Computer Science and Software Engineering, 3*(3).

Kayne, S. B. (2006). *Homeopathic pharmacy: theory and practice.* Elsevier Health Sciences.

Kent, J. T. (1904). *Lectures on homeopathic materia medica with new remedies. New Dehli: B.* Jain Publishers.

Kent, J. T. (1992). *Repertory of the homoeopathic materia medica.* B. Jain Publishers.

Kesavaraj, G., & Sukumaran, S. (2013). A study on classification techniques in data mining. In *Proceedings of the 2013 Fourth International Conference on Computing, Communications and Networking Technologies (ICCCNT)* (pp. 1-7). IEEE. 10.1109/ICCCNT.2013.6726842

Kesner, M., Frailich, M., & Hofstein, A. (2013). Implementing the inter- net learning environment into the chemistry curriculum in high schools in Israel. In *Technology-rich learning environments* (p. 209-234). Retrieved from https://www.worldscientific.com/doi/abs/10.1142/97898125644120010

Khan, J. Y., Yuce, M. R., Bulger, G., & Harding, B. (2012). Wireless body area network (WBAN) design techniques and performance evaluation. *Journal of Medical Systems, 36*(3), 1441–1457. doi:10.100710916-010-9605-x PMID:20953680

Khan, Z. A., Sivakumar, S., Phillips, W., & Robertson, B. (2013). A QoS-aware routing protocol for reliability sensitive data in hospital body area networks. *Procedia Computer Science, 19*, 171–179. doi:10.1016/j.procs.2013.06.027

Khan, Z. A., Sivakumar, S., Phillips, W., & Robertson, B. (2014). ZEQoS: A new energy and QoS-aware routing protocol for communication of sensor devices in healthcare system. *International Journal of Distributed Sensor Networks, 10*(6), 627689. doi:10.1155/2014/627689

Khan, Z., Aslam, N., Sivakumar, S., & Phillips, W. (2012). Energy-aware peering routing protocol for indoor hospital body area network communication. *Procedia Computer Science, 10*, 188–196. doi:10.1016/j.procs.2012.06.027

Khan, Z., Sivakumar, S., Phillips, W., & Robertson, B. (2012, November). QPRD: QoS-aware peering routing protocol for delay sensitive data in hospital body area network communication. In *Proceedings of the 2012 Seventh International Conference on Broadband, Wireless Computing, Communication and Applications* (pp. 178-185). IEEE. 10.1109/BWCCA.2012.37

Khashman, A., & Al-Zgoul, E. (2010). Image segmentation of blood cells in leukemia patients. *Recent advances in computer engineering and applications, 2*(1), 104-109.

Kim, H. C., Pang, S., Je, H. M., Kim, D., & Bang, S. Y. (2003). Constructing support vector machine ensemble. *Pattern Recognition, 36*(12), 2757–2767. doi:10.1016/S0031-3203(03)00175-4

Kim, J. W., Jung, K. K., & Eom, K. H. (2002). Auto-Tuning Method of Learning Rate for Performance Improvement of Back propagation Algorithm. *Journal of the Institute of Electronics Engineers of Korea CI, 39*(4), 19–27.

Kim, J.-H., Park, S., Lee, H., Yuk, K.-C., & Lee, H. (2001). Virtual reality simulations in physics education. *Interactive Multimedia Electronic* Additional Reading. *Journal of Computer-Enhanced Learning, 3*(2).

King, D., Tee, S., Falconer, L., Angell, C., Holley, D., & Mills, A. (2018). Virtual health education: Scaling practice to transform student learning: Using virtual reality learning environments in healthcare education to bridge the theory/practice gap and improve patient safety. *Nurse Education Today, 71*, 7–9. doi:10.1016/j.nedt.2018.08.002 PMID:30205259

Kiran Chavan. (2019, September 8). *Smoothie Recipes: 500+ Healthy Smoothies.* Retrieved from https://play.google.com/store/apps/details?id=com.kiransmoothie.kiranchavan.juicerecipe&hl=en_US

Kleinlogel, H., Dierks, T., Koenig, T., Lehmann, H., Minder, A., & Berz, R. (2008). Effects of weak mobile phone - Electromagnetic fields (GSM, UMTS) on well-being and resting EEG. *Bioelectromagnetics, 29*(6), 479–487. doi:10.1002/bem.20419 PMID:18431738

Klopfer, E., & Squire, K. (2008). Environmental detectives: The development of an augmented reality platform for environmental simulations. *Educational Technology Research and Development, 56*(2), 203–228. doi:10.100711423-007-9037-6

Kohli, S., Miglani, S., & Rapariya, R. (2014). Basics of Artificial Neural Network. *International Journal of computing science and Mobile computing, 3*(9), 745-751.

Koivisto, M., Krause, C. M., Revonsuo, A., Laine, M., & Hamalainen, H. (2000b). The effects of electromagnetic field emitted by GSM phones on working memory. *Neuroreport, 11*(8), 1641–1643. doi:10.1097/00001756-200006050-00009 PMID:10852216

Koivisto, M., Revonsuo, A., Krause, C., Haarala, C., Sillanmaki, L., Laine, M., & Hamalainen, H. (2000a). Effects of 902 MHz electromagnetic field emitted by cellular telephones on response times in humans. *Neuroreport, 11*(2), 413–415. doi:10.1097/00001756-200002070-00038 PMID:10674497

Kolen, J. F., & Pollack, J. B. (1991). Multi associative memory. In *Proceedings of the Thirteenth Annual Conference of the Cognitive Science Society* (pp. 785-789). Academic Press.

Kotsiantis, S. B., Kanellopoulos, D., & Pintelas, P. E. (2006). Data preprocessing for supervised leaning. *International Journal of Computational Science, 1*(2), 111–117.

KP. (2018). 10 nutrition and diet apps for 2018. *Kaiser Permanente.* WA Health. Retrieved from https://wa-health.kaiserpermanente.org/best-diet-apps/

Kramarenko, A. V., & Tan, U. (2003). Effects of high-frequency electromagnetic fields on human EEG: A brain mapping study. *The International Journal of Neuroscience, 113*(7), 1007–1019. doi:10.1080/00207450390220330 PMID:12881192

Krause, C. M., Sillanmaki, L., Koivisto, M., Haggqvist, A., Saarela, C., Revonsuo, A., ... Hamalainen, H. (2000). Effects of electromagnetic field emitted by cellular phones on the EEG during a memory task. *Neuroreport, 11*(4), 761–764. doi:10.1097/00001756-200003200-00021 PMID:10757515

Krueger, M. W., & Wilson, S. (1985). VIDEOPLACE: A report from the artificial reality laboratory. *Leonardo, 18*(3), 145–151. doi:10.2307/1578043

Kukreja, H., Bharath, N., Siddesh, C. S., & Kuldeep, S. (2016). An introduction to artificial neural network. *International Journal Of Advance Research And Innovative Ideas In Education, 1*(5), 27–30.

Ku-Mahamud, K. R. (2015, August). Hybrid ant colony system and flower pollination algorithms for global optimization. In *Proceedings of the 2015 9th International Conference on IT in Asia (CITA)* (pp. 1-9). IEEE. 10.1109/CITA.2015.7349816

Kumar, P., & Lee, H. J. (2012). Security issues in healthcare applications using wireless medical sensor networks: A survey. *Sensors, 12*(1), 55-91.

Kumar, A. (2016). Artificial neural network model for effective cancer classification using microarray gene expression data. *Neural Computing & Applications*. doi:10.100700521-016-2701-1

Kumar, A. (2018). *Web Technology: Theory and Practice*. Boca Raton, FL: Chapman and Hall. doi:10.1201/9781351029902

Ladyman, J. (2013). Toward a demarcation of science from pseudoscience. In *Philosophy of pseudoscience: Reconsidering the demarcation problem* (pp. 45-59). Academic Press.

Lahkola, A., Tokola, K., & Auvinen, A. (2006). Meta-Analysis of Mobile Phone Use and Intracranial Tumors. *Scandinavian Journal of Work, Environment & Health, 32*(3), 171–177. doi:10.5271jweh.995 PMID:16804618

Lai, H. (1996). Single- and double-strand DNA breaks in rat brain cells after acute exposure to radiofrequency electromagnetic radiation. *International Journal of Radiation Biology, 69*(4), 513–521. doi:10.1080/095530096145814 PMID:8627134

Lai, H., & Singh, N. P. (1995). Acute low-intensity microwave exposure increases DNA single-strand breaks in rat brain cells. *Bioelectromagnetics, 16*(3), 207–210. doi:10.1002/bem.2250160309 PMID:7677797

Larson, R. (2018). A Path to Better-Quality mHealth Apps. *JMIR mHealth and uHealth, 6*(7), 1–6. doi:10.2196/10414 PMID:30061091

Lazzaro, V., Capone, F., Apollonio, F., Borea, P. A., & Cadossi, R. (2013). A consensus panel review of central nervous system effects of the exposure to low-intensity extremely low-frequency magnetic fields. *Brain Stimulation, 6*(4), 469–476. doi:10.1016/j.brs.2013.01.004 PMID:23428499

Le, K. (2011, January). Chest X-ray analysis for computer-aided diagnostic. In *Proceedings of the International Conference on Computer Science and Information Technology* (pp. 300-309). Springer Berlin Heidelberg.

Leap Motion Company. (n.d.). Retrieved from https://www.leapmotion.com/company

Lee, Y. S., Lee, H. J., & Alasaarela, E. (2013, July). Mutual authentication in wireless body sensor networks (WBSN) based on Physical Unclonable Function (PUF). In *Proceedings of the 2013 9th International Wireless Communications and Mobile Computing Conference (IWCMC)* (pp. 1314-1318). IEEE.

Lee, C., & Wong, G. K. C. (2019). Virtual reality and augmented reality in the management of intracranial tumors: A review. *Journal of Clinical Neuroscience, 62*, 14–20. doi:10.1016/j.jocn.2018.12.036 PMID:30642663

Lee, K., Booth, D., & Alam, P. (2005). A comparison of supervised and unsupervised neural networks in predicting bankruptcy of Korean firms. *Expert Systems with Applications, 29*(1), 1–16. doi:10.1016/j.eswa.2005.01.004

Leung, K., Lee, K., Wang, J., Ng, E. Y., Chan, H. L., Tsui, S. K., ... Sung, J. J. (2009). Data mining on dna sequences of hepatitis b virus. *IEEE/ACM Transactions on Computational Biology and Bioinformatics*, *8*(2), 428–440.

Liang, X., & Balasingham, I. (2007, October). A QoS-aware routing service framework for biomedical sensor networks. In *Proceedings of the 2007 4th International Symposium on Wireless Communication Systems* (pp. 342-345). IEEE. 10.1109/ISWCS.2007.4392358

Liang, X., Balasingham, I., & Byun, S. S. (2008, October). A reinforcement learning based routing protocol with QoS support for biomedical sensor networks. In *Proceedings of the 2008 First International Symposium on Applied Sciences on Biomedical and Communication Technologies* (pp. 1-5). IEEE.

Li, B. Y., & Chuang, P. J. (2013). Geographic energy-aware non-interfering multipath routing for multimedia transmission in wireless sensor networks. *Information Sciences*, *249*, 24–37. doi:10.1016/j.ins.2013.06.014

Libbrecht, M. W., & Noble, W. S. (2015). Machine learning applications in genetics and genomics. *Nature Reviews. Genetics*, *16*(6), 321–332. doi:10.1038/nrg3920 PMID:25948244

Li, J. B., & Chung, Y. K. (2005). A novel back-propagation neural network training algorithm designed by an ant colony optimization. In *Proceedings of the 2005 IEEE/PES Transmission & Distribution Conference & Exposition: Asia and Pacific* (pp. 1-5). IEEE.

Lin, L., Yang, C., Wong, K., Yan, H., Shen, J., & Phee, S. (2014). An energy efficient MAC protocol for multi-hop swallowable body sensor networks. *Sensors*, *14*(10), 19457-19476.

Linear Software LLC. (2012). *Body Tracker - body fat calc*. Retrieved from https://apps.apple.com/us/app/body-tracker-body-fat-calc/id581557588

Linet, M., & Inskip, P. (2010). Cellular Telephone Use and Cancer Risk. *Reviews on Environmental Health*, *25*(1), 51–55. doi:10.1515/REVEH.2010.25.1.51 PMID:20429159

Ling, H., & Rui, L. (2016, Aug). Vr glasses and leap motion trends in education. In *Proceedings of the 2016 11th international conference on computer science education (ICCSE)* (p. 917-920). 10.1109/ICCSE.2016.7581705

Lin, J. C., & Lin, M. F. (1982). Microwave hyperthermia-induced blood-brain barrier alterations. *Radiation Research*, *89*(1), 77–87. doi:10.2307/3575686 PMID:7063606

Lin, J. H., Chou, C. W., Yang, C. H., & Tsai, H. L. (2012). A chaotic Levy flight bat algorithm for parameter estimation in nonlinear dynamic biological systems. *Computer and Information Technology*, *2*(2), 56–63.

Lin-Lui, S., & Adey, W. R. (1982). Low frequency amplitude modulated microwave fields change calcium efflux rates from synaptosomes. *Biolectromagnetics*, *3*(3), 309–322. doi:10.1002/bem.2250030303 PMID:7126280

List of Sarcode and Nosode remedies in Homeopathy. (2016). Homeobook. Retrieved from https://www.homeobook.com/list-of-sarcode-and-nosode-remedies-in-homeopathy/

Loeb, S., Falchuk, B., & Panagos, T. (2009). *The Fabric of Mobile Services: Software Paradigms and Business Demands*. Hoboken, NJ: Wiley-Interscience. doi:10.1002/9780470478240

López, A., Detz, A., Ratanawongsa, N., & Sarkar, U. (2012). What patients say about their doctors online: A qualitative content analysis. *Journal of General Internal Medicine*, *27*(6), 685–692. doi:10.100711606-011-1958-4 PMID:22215270

Lui, J. H. L., Marcus, D. K., & Barry, C. T. (2017, February 20). Evidence-Based Apps? A Review of Mental Health Mobile Applications in a Psychotherapy Context. *Professional Psychology, Research and Practice*, *48*(3), 199–210; Advance online publication. doi:10.1037/pro0000122

Machado, J., Abelha, A., Santos, M., & Portela, F. (2017). *Next-Generation Mobile and Pervasive Healthcare Solutions.* Hershey, PA: IGI Global.

Madsen, R. (2019). Characteristics of Contemporary Methodologies of Classic Homeopathy. *Homœopathic Links, 32*(1), 18-22.

Malyapa, R. S., Ahern, E. W., Bi, C., Straube, W. L., La Regina, M., Pickard, W. F., & Roti, J. L. (1998). DNA damage in rat brain cells after in vivo exposure to 2450MHz electromagnetic radiation and various methods of euthanasia. *Radiation Research, 149*(6), 637–645. doi:10.2307/3579911 PMID:9611103

Malyapa, R. S., Ahern, E. W., Straube, W. L., Moros, E. G., Pickard, W. F., & Roti, J. L. (1997). Measurement of DNA damage after exposure to electromagnetic radiation in the cellular phone communication frequency band (835.62 and 847.74 MHz). *Radiation Research, 148*(6), 618–627. doi:10.2307/3579738 PMID:9399708

Mandala, M., Colletti, V., Sacchetto, L., Manganotti, P., Ramat, S., Marcocci, A., & Colletti, L. (2014). Effect of Bluetooth Headset and Mobile Phone Electromagnetic Fields on the Human Auditory Nerve. *Laryngoscope, 124*(1), 255–259. doi:10.1002/lary.24103 PMID:23619813

Mann, K., & Roschke, J. (1996). Effects of pulsed high-frequency electromagnetic fields on human sleep. *Neuropsychobiol, 33*(1), 41–47. doi:10.1159/000119247 PMID:8821374

MapMyFitness. (2019, September 7). *Map My Fitness Workout Trainer.* Retrieved from https://play.google.com/store/apps/details?id=com.mapmyfitness.android2&hl=en

Marotz, L. (2014). *Health, Safety, and Nutrition for the Young Child.* London, UK: Cengage Learning.

Masiliunas, R., & Vitkute, D. Stankevičius, E., Matijošaitis, V. & Petrikonis, K. (2018). Response inhibition set shifting and complex executive function in patients with chronic lower back pain. Medicina, 53, 26-33.

Matthew-Maich, N., Harris, L., Ploeg, J., Markle-Reid, M., Valaitis, R., Ibrahim, S., ... Isaacs, S. (2016). Designing, Implementing, and Evaluating Mobile Health Technologies for Managing Chronic Conditions in Older Adults: A Scoping Review. *JMIR mHealth and uHealth, 4*(2), 1–29. doi:10.2196/mhealth.5127 PMID:27282195

Mausset, A. L., de Seze, R., Montpeyroux, F., & Privat, A. (2001). Effects of radiofrequency exposure on the GABAergic system in the rat cerebellum: Clues from semiquantitative immunohistochemistry. *Brain Research, 912*(1), 33–46. doi:10.1016/S0006-8993(01)02599-9 PMID:11520491

Mayes, J., & White, A. (2016). How Smartphone Technology Is Changing Healthcare In Developing Countries. *The Journal of Global Health.* Retrieved from https://www.ghjournal.org/how-smartphone-technology-is-changing-healthcare-in-developing-countries/

McClean, P. E., Slator, B. M., & White, A. R. (1999). The virtual cell: An interactive, virtual environment for cell biology. In *Edmedia: World conference on educational media and technology* (pp. 1442–1443). Academic Press.

McRee, D. I., & Wachtel, H. (1980). The effects of microwave radiation on the vitality of isolated frog sciatic nerves. *Radiation Research, 82*(3), 536–546. doi:10.2307/3575320 PMID:7384419

McRee, D. I., & Wachtel, H. (1986). Elimination of microwave effects on the vitality of nerves after blockage of active transport. *Radiation Research, 108*(3), 260–268. doi:10.2307/3576914 PMID:3492008

Mehmood, M. (2014). Use of Bioinformatics Tools in Different Spheres of Life Sciences. *Journal of Data Mining in Genomics & Proteomics, 5.* doi:10.4172/2153-0602.1000158

Meier, R., & Lake, I. (2018). *Professional Android.* Hoboken, New Jersey: Wrox. doi:10.1002/9781119419389

Merritt, J. H., Chamness, A. P., & Allen, S. J. (1978). Studies on blood-brain barrier permeability after microwave radiation. *Radiation and Environmental Biophysics, 15*(4), 367–377. doi:10.1007/BF01323461 PMID:756056

Meulenbeld, G. J. (1999). *A history of Indian medical literature* (Vol. 3). E. Forsten Groningen.

Michrowski, A. (2018). What you should know about the coming 5G – and what to do about it. Whole Life Expo 2019.

Mikropoulos, T. A., Katsikis, A., Nikolou, E., & Tsakalis, P. (2003a). Virtual environments in biology teaching. *Journal of Biological Education, 37*(4), 176–181. doi:10.1080/00219266.2003.9655879

Mikropoulos, T. A., & Natsis, A. (2011). Educational virtual environments: A ten-year review of empirical research (1999–2009). *Computers & Education, 56*(3), 769–780. doi:10.1016/j.compedu.2010.10.020

Mishra, L.-c., Singh, B. B., & Dagenais, S. (2001). Healthcare and disease management in Ayurveda. *Alternative Therapies in Health and Medicine, 7*(2), 44–51. PMID:11253416

Monowar, M. M., Mehedi Hassan, M., Bajaber, F., Hamid, M. A., & Alamri, A. (2014). Thermal-aware multiconstrained intrabody QoS routing for wireless body area networks. *International Journal of Distributed Sensor Networks, 10*(3), 676312. doi:10.1155/2014/676312

Morel, M., Bideau, B., Lardy, J., & Kulpa, R. (2015). Advantages and limitations of virtual reality for balance assessment and rehabilitation. *Neurophysiologie Clinique [Clinical Neurophysiology], 45*(4-5), 315–326. doi:10.1016/j.neucli.2015.09.007 PMID:26527045

Movassaghi, S., Abolhasan, M., & Lipman, J. (2013). A review of routing protocols in wireless body area networks. *Journal of Networks, 8*(3), 559–575. doi:10.4304/jnw.8.3.559-575

Movassaghi, S., Abolhasan, M., Lipman, J., Smith, D., & Jamalipour, A. (2014). Wireless body area networks: A survey. *IEEE Communications Surveys and Tutorials, 16*(3), 1658–1686. doi:10.1109/SURV.2013.121313.00064

Movvahedi, M. M., Tavakkoli-Golpayegani, A., Mortazavi, S. A., Haghani, M., Razi, Z., & Shojaie-Fard, M. B. (2014). Does exposure to GSM 900 MHz mobile phone radiation affect short-term memory of elementary school students. *Journal of Pediatric Neurosciences, 9*(2), 121–124. doi:10.4103/1817-1745.139300 PMID:25250064

Mukkamala, S. R., & Madhusudhanan, M. (2016). *U.S. Patent Application No. 14/478,277.*

Muoio, D. (2017). New technologies are transforming health, but culture lags behind. Mobile Health News. Retrieved from https://www.mobihealthnews.com/content/new-technologies-are-transforming-health-culture-lags-behind

Murthi, S., & Varshney, A. (2018). How Augmented Reality Will Make Surgery Safer. *Harvard Business Review*. Retrieved from https://hbr.org/2018/03/how-augmented-reality-will-make-surgery-safer

Murugesan, S. (2013). Mobile apps in Africa. *IT Professional, 15*(5), 8–11. doi:10.1109/MITP.2013.83

Mushgil, H. M., Alani, H. A., & George, L. E. (2015). Comparison between Resilient and Standard Back Propagation Algorithms Efficiency in Pattern Recognition. *International Journal of Scientific & Engineering Research, 6*(3), 773–778.

MyNetDiary Inc. (2019). *Calorie Counter PRO MyNetDiary*. Retrieved from https://apps.apple.com/us/app/calorie-counter-pro-mynetdiary/id352247139

Nandy, S., Sarkar, P. P., & Das, A. (2012). Training a feed-forward neural network with artificial bee colony based back propagation method.

Narayanaswamy, V. (1981). Origin and development of ayurveda:(a brief history). *Ancient Science of Life, 1*(1), 1. PMID:22556454

Naresh, P., & Shettar, R. (2014). Image Processing and Classification Techniques for Early Detection of Lung Cancer for Preventive Health Care: A Survey. *Int. J. of Recent Trends in Engineering & Technology, 11.*

Nasi, G., Cucciniello, M., & Guerrazzi, C. (2015). The role of mobile technologies in health care processes: the case of cancer supportive care. *Journal of medical Internet research, 17*(2), e26. doi:10.2196/jmir.3757

Nawi, N. M., Ghazali, R., & Salleh, M. N. M. (2010, October). The development of improved back-propagation neural networks algorithm for predicting patients with heart disease. In *Proceedings of the International Conference on Information Computing and Applications* (pp. 317-324). Springer Berlin Heidelberg. 10.1007/978-3-642-16167-4_41

Nawi, N. M., Ransing, R. S., Salleh, M. N. M., Ghazali, R., & Hamid, N. A. (2010). An improved back propagation neural network algorithm on classification problems. In Database Theory and Application, Bio-Science and Bio-Technology (pp. 177-188). Springer Berlin Heidelberg. doi:10.1007/978-3-642-17622-7_18

Nawi, N. M., Ransing, R. S., & Ransing, M. R. (2007). An improved conjugate gradient based learning algorithm for back propagation neural networks. *International Journal of Computational Intelligence, 4*(1), 46–55.

Nawi, N. M., Ransing, R. S., & Ransing, M. R. (2007). An improved conjugate gradient-based learning algorithm for back propagation neural networks. *International Journal of Computational Intelligence, 4*(1), 46–55.

Nazia, S., & Ekta, S. (2014). Online appointment scheduling system for hospitals–an analytical study. *Int J Innov Res Sci Eng Technol, 4*(1), 21–27.

Nazir, B., & Hasbullah, H. (2013). Energy efficient and QoS aware routing protocol for clustered wireless sensor network. *Computers & Electrical Engineering, 39*(8), 2425–2441. doi:10.1016/j.compeleceng.2013.06.011

Ng, H. P., Ong, S. H., Foong, K. W. C., Goh, P. S., & Nowinski, W. L. (2006, March). Medical image segmentation using k-means clustering and improved watershed algorithm. In *Proceedings of the 2006 IEEE Southwest Symposium on Image Analysis and Interpretation* (pp. 61-65). IEEE. 10.1109/SSIAI.2006.1633722

Ngai, E., Zhou, Y., Lyu, M. R., & Liu, J. (2010). A delay-aware reliable event reporting framework for wireless sensor–actuator networks. *Ad Hoc Networks, 8*(7), 694–707. doi:10.1016/j.adhoc.2010.01.004

Nikam, S. S. (2015). A Comparative Study of Classification Techniques in Data Mining Algorithms. *Oriental Journal of Computer Science & Technology, 8*(1), 13–19.

Nintendo Wiimote. (2018). Retrieved from https://store.nintendo.com

Nisha, N., Iqbal, M., Rifat, A., & Idrish, S. (2015). Mobile Health Services: A New Paradigm for Health Care Systems. *International Journal of Asian Business and Information Management, 6*(1), 1–17. doi:10.4018/IJABIM.2015010101

Nonis, D. (2005). *3d virtual learning environments (3d VLE).* Singapore: Ministry of Education.

NoomInc. (2017). *Noom.* Retrieved from https://apps.apple.com/us/app/noom/id634598719

Norris, M. W., Spicer, K., & Byrd, T. (2019). Virtual Reality: The New Pathway for Effective Safety Training. *Professional Safety, 64*(06), 36–39.

Nunes, F., Andersen, T., & Fitzpatrick, G. (2019). The agency of patients and carers in medical care and self-care technologies for interacting with doctors. *Health Informatics Journal, 25*(2), 330–349. doi:10.1177/1460458217712054 PMID:28653552

Nutritionix. (2019, June 7). *Track - Calorie Counter.* Retrieved from https://play.google.com/store/apps/details?id=com. nutritionix.nixtrack&hl=en

Online Psychology Degree Guide. (n.d.). What Technology Advances Are Affecting Psychology Studies? Retrieved From https://www.onlinepsychologydegree.info/faq/what-technology-advances-are-affecting-psychology-studies/

Organic Facts. (2018, January 16). *Health, Nutrition & Diet Guide*. Retrieved from https://play.google.com/store/apps/details?id=com.organicfacts.app&hl=en

Orosun, R. O., & Adamu, S. S. (2014). Neural Network Based Model of an Industrial Oil-fired Boiler System. *Nigerian Journal of Technology*, *33*(3), 293–303. doi:10.4314/njt.v33i3.6

Oscar, K. J., & Hawkins, T. D. (1977). Microwave alteration of the blood– brain barrier system of rats. *Brain Research*, *126*(2), 281–293. doi:10.1016/0006-8993(77)90726-0 PMID:861720

Otair, M. A., & Salameh, W. A. (2005, June). Speeding up back-propagation neural networks. In *Proceedings of the 2005 Informing Science and IT Education Joint Conference* (pp. 16-19). Academic Press.

Outlier. (2015, July 22). *Nutritionist-Dieting made easy*. Retrieved from https://play.google.com/store/apps/details?id=com.nutritionist.development&hl=en

Owusu, E., & Chakraborty, J. (2019). User requirements gathering in mHealth: Perspective from Ghanaian end users. In *Proceedings of the International Conference on Human-Computer Interaction* (pp. 386-396). Springer. 10.1007/978-3-030-22577-3_28

Page, R. L. (2000). Brief history of flight simulation. In *SimTecT 2000 Proceedings* (pp. 11-17). Academic Press.

Pankomera, R., & Greunen, D. (2018). A model for implementing sustainable mHealth applications in a resource-constrained setting: A case of Malawi. *The Electronic Journal on Information Systems in Developing Countries*, *84*(2), 1–12. doi:10.1002/isd2.12019

Pasche, B., Erman, M., Hayduk, R., Mitler, M. M., Reite, M., Higgs, L., ... Lebet, J. P. (1996). Effects of low energy emission therapy in chronic psychophysiological insomnia. *Sleep*, *19*(4), 327–336. doi:10.1093leep/19.4.327 PMID:8776791

Patel, M., Mehta, D., Patterson, P., & Rawal, R. (2016). Applying Back Propagation Algorithm for classification of fragile genome sequence. *IOSR Journal of Computer Engineering*, *18*(5), 1–10. doi:10.9790/0661-1805010110

Patil, A. D., Chinche, A. D., Singh, A. K., Peerzada, S. P., Barkund, S. A., Shah, J. N., & Jadhav, A. B. (2019). Ultra high dilutions: A review on in vitro studies against pathogens.

Patil, B. G., & Jain, S. N. (2014). Cancer cells detection using digital image processing methods. *International Journal of Latest Trends in Engineering and Technology*.

Patwardhan, B., Warude, D., Pushpangadan, P., & Bhatt, N. (2005). Ayurveda and traditional Chinese medicine: A comparative overview. *Evidence-Based Complementary and Alternative Medicine*, *2*(4), 465–473. doi:10.1093/ecam/neh140 PMID:16322803

Pausch, R., Proffitt, D., & Williams, G. (1997). Quantifying immersion in virtual reality. In *Proceedings of the 24th annual conference on computer graphics and interactive techniques* (pp. 13–18). New York: ACM Press/Addison-Wesley Publishing Co. doi:10.1145/258734.258744

PCGamer. (2018). Microsoft Kinect. Retrieved from http://www.pcgamer.com/microsoft-ceases-production-of-kinect-for-windows

Pelargos, P. E., Nagasawa, D. T., Lagman, C., Tenn, S., Demos, J. V., Lee, S. J., ... Bari, A. (2017). Utilizing virtual and augmented reality for educational and clinical enhancements in neurosurgery. *Journal of Clinical Neuroscience*, *35*, 1–4. doi:10.1016/j.jocn.2016.09.002 PMID:28137372

Phantom Company. P. C. (2018). Retrieved from http://www.immersion.fr/en/phantom-touch-x/

Philippe, R. (2017). The importance of psychology. Owlcation. Retrieved From https://owlcation.com/social-sciences/Psychology-and-its-Importance

Philippe, R. (n.d.). The Importance of Psychology. Owlcation. Retrieved from https://owlcation.com/social-sciences/Psychology-and-its-Importance?

Piane, G. M., & Eggleston, B. M. (2016). Complementary, Alternative, And Integrative Health Approaches Among West Asian American Communities. *Complementary, Alternative, and Integrative Health, Multicultural Perspectives*, 305.

Pollak, J., Gay, G., Byrne, S., Wagner, E., Retelny, D., & Humphreys, L. (2010). It's time to eat! Using mobile games to promote healthy eating. *IEEE Pervasive Computing*, *9*(3), 21–27. doi:10.1109/MPRV.2010.41

Pop, C. B., Chifu, V. R., Salomie, I., Racz, D. S., & Bonta, R. M. (2017). Hybridization of the Flower Pollination Algorithm. A Case Study in the Problem of Generating Healthy Nutritional Meals for Older Adults. In *Nature-Inspired Computing and Optimization* (pp. 151–183). Springer International Publishing. doi:10.1007/978-3-319-50920-4_7

Popescu, M.-C., Balas, V. E., Perescu-Popescu, L., & Mastorakis, N. (2009). Multilayer perceptron and neural networks. *WSEAS Transactions on Circuits and Systems*, *8*(7), 579–588.

Powers, D. M. W. (2008). Evaluation: From precision, recall and f-factor to roc, informedness, markedness and correlation. *J Mach Learn Technol*, *2*, 2229–3981.

Prasad, R. (2007). Homoeopathy booming in India. *Lancet*, *370*(9600), 1679–1680. doi:10.1016/S0140-6736(07)61709-7 PMID:18035598

Pray, W. S., & Worthen, D. B. (2003). *A history of nonprescription product regulation*. CRC Press.

Preece, A. W., Iwi, G., Davies-Smith, A., Wesnes, K., Butler, S., Lim, E., & Varey, A. (1999). Effect of a 915-MHz simulated mobile phone signal on cognitive function in man. *International Journal of Radiation Biology*, *75*(4), 447–456. doi:10.1080/095530099140375 PMID:10331850

Premier Inc. (2019, September 06). How health systems are prioritizing maternal and infant health. [Blog post]. Retrieved from https://www.premierinc.com/newsroom/blog/how-health-systems-are-prioritizing-maternal-and-infant-health

Preston, E., Vavasour, E. J., & Assenheim, H. M. (1979). Permeability of the blood-brain barrier to mannitol in the rat following 2,450 MHz microwave irradiation. *Brain Research*, *174*(1), 109–117. doi:10.1016/0006-8993(79)90807-2 PMID:487114

Psychological testing. (n.d.). Retrieved from https://psycnet.apa.org/record/1998-07223-000

Quinlan, J. R. (1986). Induction of decision trees. *Machine Learning*, *1*(1), 81–106. doi:10.1007/BF00116251

Quwaider, M., & Biswas, S. (2009, October). Probabilistic routing in on-body sensor networks with postural disconnections. In *Proceedings of the 7th ACM international symposium on Mobility management and wireless access* (pp. 149-158). ACM. 10.1145/1641776.1641803

Quwaider, M., Rao, J., & Biswas, S. (2010). Body-posture-based dynamic link power control in wearable sensor networks. *IEEE Communications Magazine*, *48*(7), 134–142. doi:10.1109/MCOM.2010.5496890

Rajaei, H., & Aldhalaan, A. (2011). Advances in virtual learning environments and class- rooms. In *Proceedings of the 14th communications and networking symposium* (pp. 133–142). San Diego, CA, USA: Society for Computer Simulation International. Retrieved From; http://dl.acm.org/citation.cfm?id=2048416.2048434

Raju, V. (2003). Susruta of ancient India. *Indian Journal of Ophthalmology, 51*(2), 119. PMID:12831140

Rashidi, P., & Mihailidis, A. (2012). A survey on ambient-assisted living tools for older adults. *IEEE Journal of Biomedical and Health Informatics, 17*(3), 579–590. doi:10.1109/JBHI.2012.2234129 PMID:24592460

Rau, P. L., Plocher, T., & Choong, Y. Y. (2012). *Cross-cultural design for IT products and services.* CRC Press. doi:10.1201/b12679

Ravi, D. K., Kumar, N., & Singhi, P. (2017). Effectiveness of virtual reality rehabilitation for children and adolescents with cerebral palsy: An updated evidence-based systematic review. *Physiotherapy, 103*(3), 245–258. doi:10.1016/j.physio.2016.08.004 PMID:28109566

Razzaque, M. A., Alam, M. M., Mamun-Or-Rashid, M., & Hong, C. S. (2008). Multi-constrained QoS geographic routing for heterogeneous traffic in sensor networks. *IEICE Transactions on Communications, 91*(8), 2589–2601. doi:10.1093/ietcom/e91-b.8.2589

Razzaque, M., Hong, C. S., & Lee, S. (2011). Data-centric multiobjective QoS-aware routing protocol for body sensor networks. *Sensors (Basel), 11*(1), 917–937. doi:10.3390110100917 PMID:22346611

RecoveryBull.com. (2019, May 4). *Health Diet Foods Fitness Help.* Retrieved from https://play.google.com/store/apps/details?id=com.medical.guide_health.diet.tips&hl=en

Rehman, M. Z., Nawi, N. M., & Ghazali, M. I. (2011). Noise-Induced Hearing Loss (NIHL) prediction in humans using a modified back propagation neural network. *International Journal on Advanced Science. Engineering and Information Technology, 1*(2), 185–189.

Rehman, M. Z., Nawi, N. M., & Ghazali, M. I. (2011). Noise-Induced Hearing Loss (NIHL) Prediction in Humans Using a Modified Back Propagation Neural Network. International Journal on Advanced Science. *Engineering and Information Technology., 1*, 185–189. doi:10.18517/ijaseit.1.2.39

Reiser, H., Dimpfel, W., & Schober, F. (1995). The influence of electromagnetic fields on human brain activity. *European Journal of Medical Research, 1*, 27–32. PMID:9392690

Reis, R., & Escudeiro, P. (2014). A model for implementing learning games on virtual world platforms. In *Proceedings of the XV international conference on human computer interaction* (pp. 98:1–98:2). New York: ACM. doi:10.1145/2662253.2662351

Reite, M., Higgs, L., Lebet, J. P., Barbault, A., Rossel, C., Kuster, N., ... Amato, D. B. P. (1994). Sleep inducing effect of low energy emission therapy. *Bioelectromagnetics, 15*(1), 67–75. doi:10.1002/bem.2250150110 PMID:8155071

Rheingold, H. (1991). *Virtual reality.* New York: Simon & Schuster, Inc.

Richard, E., Tijou, A., Richard, P., & Ferrier, J.-L. (2006). Multi-modal virtual environments for education with haptic and olfactory feedback. *Virtual Reality (Waltham Cross), 10*(3), 207–225. doi:10.100710055-006-0040-8

Richards, D., & Kelaiah, I. (2012). Usability attributes in virtual learning environments. In *Proceedings of the 8th Australasian conference on interactive entertainment: Playing the system* (pp. 9:1–9:10). New York, NY, USA: ACM. doi:10.1145/2336727.2336736

Riener, R., & Harders, M. (2012). *Virtual reality in medicine.* Springer Science & Business Media. doi:10.1007/978-1-4471-4011-5

Riva, G. (2005). Virtual reality in psychotherapy [review]. *Cyberpsychology & Behavior, 8*(3), 220–240. doi:10.1089/cpb.2005.8.220 PMID:15971972

Robert, L., Lee, F., Keinrath, C., Scherer, R., & Bisch, H. (2007). Brain-Compute Communication: Motivation, Aim, and Impact of Exploring a Virtual Apartment. *IEEE Transactions on Neural Systems and Rehabilitation Engineering*, *15*(4), 473–482. doi:10.1109/TNSRE.2007.906956 PMID:18198704

Roschke, J., & Mann, K. (1997). No Short-Term Effects of Digital Mobile Radio Telephone on the Awake Human Electroencephalogram. *Bioelectromagnetics*, *18*(2), 172–176. doi:10.1002/(SICI)1521-186X(1997)18:2<172::AID-BEM10>3.0.CO;2-T PMID:9084868

Rosenthal, F. (2015). *The physician in medieval Muslim society. In Man versus Society in Medieval Islam* (pp. 1026–1042). BRILL.

Rose, T., Nam, C. S., & Chen, K. B. (2018). Immersion of virtual reality for rehabilitation-Review. *Applied Ergonomics*, *69*, 153–161. doi:10.1016/j.apergo.2018.01.009 PMID:29477323

Rowe, T. (1998). *Homeopathic Methodology: Repertory, Case Taking, and Case Analysis: an Introductory Homeopathic Workbook*. North Atlantic Books.

Roy, E., Bakr, M. M., & George, R. (2017). The need for virtual reality simulators in dental education: A review. *The Saudi Dental Journal*, *29*(2), 41–47. doi:10.1016/j.sdentj.2017.02.001 PMID:28490842

Ruggieri, S. (2002). Efficient C4. 5 [classification algorithm]. *IEEE Transactions on Knowledge and Data Engineering*, *14*(2), 438–444. doi:10.1109/69.991727

Rumelhart, D. E., Hinton, G. E., & Williams, R. J. (1988). Learning representations by back-propagating errors. *Cognitive modeling*, *5*(3), 1.

Russo, J. E., McCool, R. R., & Davies, L. (2016). VA telemedicine: An analysis of cost and time savings. *Telemedicine Journal and e-Health*, *22*(3), 209–215. doi:10.1089/tmj.2015.0055 PMID:26305666

Ruthenbeck, G. S., & Reynolds, K. J. (2015). Virtual reality for medical training: The state-of-the-art. *Journal of Simulation*, *9*(1), 16–26. doi:10.1057/jos.2014.14

Sacks, R., Perlman, A., & Barak, R. (2013). Construction safety training using immersive virtual reality. *Construction Management and Economics*, *31*(9), 1005–1017. doi:10.1080/01446193.2013.828844

Sadeghian, F., Seman, Z., Ramli, A. R., Kahar, B. H. A., & Saripan, M. I. (2009). A framework for white blood cell segmentation in microscopic blood images using digital image processing. *Biological Procedures Online*, *11*(1), 196–206. doi:10.100712575-009-9011-2 PMID:19517206

Saikumar, T., Anoop, B. K., Murthy, P. S., & Meghanathan, N. (2012). Robust adaptive threshold algorithm based on kernel fuzzy clustering on image segmentation. *Computer Science & Information Technology (CS & IT)*, 99-103.

Saleh, A. B., Sibley, M. J., & Mather, P. (2015, March). QoS Aware Inter-Cluster Routing Protocol for IEEE 802.15. 4 Networks. In *Proceedings of the 2015 17th UKSim-AMSS International Conference on Modelling and Simulation (UKSim)* (pp. 538-543). IEEE.

Salford, L. G., Brun, A. E., Eberhardt, J. L., Malmgren, L., & Persson, B. R. (2003). Nerve cell damage in mammalian brain after exposure to microwaves from GSM mobile phones. *Environmental Health Perspectives*, *111*(7), 881–883. doi:10.1289/ehp.6039 PMID:12782486

Sampson, W. (1995). Antiscience Trends In The Rise of The "Alternative Medicine' movement. *Annals of the New York Academy of Sciences*, *775*(1), 188–197. doi:10.1111/j.1749-6632.1996.tb23138.x PMID:8678416

Sánchez-Cabrero, R., Costa-Román, Ó., Pericacho-Gómez, F. J., Novillo-López, M. Á., Arigita-García, A., & Barrientos-Fernández, A. (2019). Early virtual reality adopters in Spain: Sociodemographic profile and interest in the use of virtual reality as a learning tool. *Heliyon (London)*, *5*(3), e01338. doi:10.1016/j.heliyon.2019.e01338 PMID:30923768

Saper, R. B., Phillips, R. S., Sehgal, A., Khouri, N., Davis, R. B., Paquin, J., ... Kales, S. N. (2008). Lead, mercury, and arsenic in US-and Indian-manufactured Ayurvedic medicines sold via the Internet. *Journal of the American Medical Association*, *300*(8), 915–923. doi:10.1001/jama.300.8.915 PMID:18728265

Sarhan, A. M. (2009). Cancer classification based on microarray gene expression data using DCT and ANN. *Journal of Theoretical & Applied Information Technology*, *6*(2).

Sarwar, M., & Soomro, T. (2013). Impact of Smartphone's on Society. *European Journal of Scientific Research*, *98*(2), 216–226.

Sayrafian-Pour, K., Yang, W. B., Hagedorn, J., Terrill, J., & Yazdandoost, K. Y. (2009, September). A statistical path loss model for medical implant communication channels. In *Proceedings of the 2009 IEEE 20th International Symposium on Personal, Indoor and Mobile Radio Communications* (pp. 2995-2999). IEEE. 10.1109/PIMRC.2009.5449869

Scarella, O. C., Lanteri, S., Beaume, G., Oudot, S., & Piperno, S. (2006). Realistic numerical modeling of human head tissue exposure to electromagnetic waves from cellular phones. *Comptes Rendus Physique*, *7*(5), 501–508. doi:10.1016/j.crhy.2006.03.002

Schalkoff, R. J. (1997). *Artificial neural networks*. McGraw-Hill Higher Education.

Schirmacher, A., Winters, S., Fischer, S., Goeke, J., Galla, H. J., Kullnick, U., ... Stogbauer, F. (2000). Electromagnetic fields (1.8 GHz) increase the permeability to sucrose of the blood-brain barrier in vitro. *Bioelectromagnetics*, *21*, 338–345. doi:10.1002/1521-186X(200007)21:5<338::AID-BEM2>3.0.CO;2-Q PMID:10899769

Schoeni, A., Roser, K., & Roosli, M. (2015). Symptoms and cognitive functions in adolescents in relation to mobile phone use during night. *PLoS One*, *10*(7), 0133528. doi:10.1371/journal.pone.0133528 PMID:26222312

Schofield, D., & Lester, E. (2010). Virtual chemical engineering: Guidelines for e-learning in engineering education.

Scott Kruse, C., Karem, P., Shifflett, K., Vegi, L., Ravi, K., & Brooks, M. (2018). Evaluating barriers to adopting telemedicine worldwide: A systematic review. *Journal of Telemedicine and Telecare*, *24*(1), 4–12. doi:10.1177/1357633X16674087 PMID:29320966

Seaman, R. L., & Wachtel, H. (1978). Slow and rapid responses to CW and pulsed microwave radiation by individual Aplysia pacemakers. *The Journal of Microwave Power*, *13*(1), 77–86. doi:10.1080/16070658.1978.11689079 PMID:213605

Seguin, R., Aggarwal, A., Vermeylen, F., & Drewnowski, A. (2016). Consumption frequency of foods away from home linked with higher body mass index and lower fruit and vegetable intake among adults: A cross-sectional study. *Journal of Environmental and Public Health*, *2016*, 1–12. doi:10.1155/2016/3074241 PMID:26925111

Sekar, S. (2007). Traditional alcoholic beverages from Ayurveda and their role on human health.

Selin, H. (2002). A History of Indian Medical Literature.

Selin, H. (2013). *Encyclopaedia of the history of science, technology, and medicine in non-westen cultures*. Springer Science & Business Media.

Seo, K. S. (2005, May). Improved fully automatic liver segmentation using histogram tail threshold algorithms. In *Proceedings of the International Conference on Computational Science* (pp. 822-825). Springer Berlin Heidelberg. 10.1007/11428862_115

Seymour, N. (2008). VR to OR: A review of the evidence that virtual reality simulation improves operating room performance. *World Journal of Surgery*, *32*(2), 182–188. doi:10.100700268-007-9307-9 PMID:18060453

Sezer, B., & Yilmaz, R. (2019). Learning management system acceptance scale (LMSAS): A validity and reliability study. *Australasian Journal of Educational Technology*, *35*(3), 15–30. doi:10.14742/ajet.3959

Sezer, B., Yilmaz, R., & Karaoglan Yilmaz, F. G. (2013). Integrating technology into classroom: The learner-centered instructional design. *International Journal on New Trends in Education and Their Implications*, *4*(4), 134–144.

Shahid, M., & Tasneem, K. (2017). Impact of Avoiding Non-functional Requirements in Software Development Stage. *American Journal of Information Science and Computer Engineering*, *3*(4), 52–55.

Shapiro, H. (2006). *Medicine across cultures: history and practice of medicine in non-western cultures* (Vol. 3). Springer Science & Business Media.

Sharif, M., Ansari, G. J., Yasmin, M., & Fernandes, S. L. (2018). Reviews of the Implications of VR/AR Health Care Applications in Terms of Organizational and Societal Change. *Emerging Technologies for Health and Medicine: Virtual Reality, Augmented Reality, Artificial Intelligence, Internet of Things, Robotics Industry*, *4*(0), 1–19.

Shen, H., Bai, G., Tang, Z., & Zhao, L. (2014). QMOR: QoS-aware multi-sink opportunistic routing for wireless multimedia sensor networks. *Wireless Personal Communications*, *75*(2), 1307–1330. doi:10.100711277-013-1425-0

Sheridan, T. B. (2000). Interaction, imagination and immersion some research needs. In *Proceedings of the ACM symposium on virtual reality software and technology* (pp. 1–7). ACM. 10.1145/502390.502392

Shim, K.-C., Park, J.-S., Kim, H.-S., Kim, J.-H., Park, Y.-C., & Ryu, H.-I. (2003a). Application of virtual reality technology in biology education. *Journal of Biological Education*, *37*(2), 71–74. doi:10.1080/00219266.2003.9655854

Shorofi, S. A., & Arbon, P. (2017). Complementary and alternative medicine (CAM) among Australian hospital-based nurses: Knowledge, attitude, personal and professional use, reasons for use, CAM referrals, and socio-demographic predictors of CAM users. *Complementary Therapies in Clinical Practice*, *27*, 37–45. doi:10.1016/j.ctcp.2017.03.001 PMID:28438278

Siddiquee, M.A. & Tasnim, H. (2018). A Comprehensive Study of Decision Tre es to Classify DNA Sequences. *University of New Mexico*.

Silva, B., Rodrigues, J., de la Torre Díez, I., López-Coronado, M., & Saleem, K. (2015). Mobile-health: A review of current state in 2015. *Journal of Biomedical Informatics*, *56*, 265–272. doi:10.1016/j.jbi.2015.06.003 PMID:26071682

Singh, S. (2012). Cancer cells detection and classification in biopsy image. *International Journal of Engineering Science and Technology*.

Singh, S., & Ernst, E. (2008). *Trick or treatment: The undeniable facts about alternative medicine*. WW Norton & Company.

Slator, B. M. (1999). Intelligent tutors in virtual worlds. In *Proceedings of the 8th international conference on intelligent systems (ICIS-99)* (pp. 24–26). Academic Press.

Smith, J. W., Everhart, J. E., Dickson, W. C., Knowler, W. C., & Johannes, R. S. (1988, November). Using the ADAP learning algorithm to forecast the onset of diabetes mellitus. *In Proceedings of the Annual Symposium on Computer Application in Medical Care* (p. 261). American Medical Informatics Association.

Smith, K. (2012). Homeopathy is unscientific and unethical. *Bioethics*, *26*(9), 508–512. doi:10.1111/j.1467-8519.2011.01956.x PMID:22506737

Soegaard, M. (2019). Consistency: More than what you think. Interaction Design. Retrieved from https://www.interaction-design.org/literature/article/consistency-more-than-what-you-think

Sommerville, I. (2018). *Software Engineering*. New Delhi: Pearson India.

SparkPeople. (2013, January 30). *Perfect Produce*. Retrieved from https://play.google.com/store/apps/details?id=com.sparkpeople.android.produce&hl=en

SparkPeople. (2016, August 24). *Nutrition Lookup - SparkPeople*. Retrieved from https://play.google.com/store/apps/details?id=com.sparkpeople.foodLookup&hl=en

SparkPeople. (2016, August 26). *Healthy Slow Cooker Recipes*. Retrieved from https://play.google.com/store/apps/details?id=com.sparkpeople.SlowCookerRecipes&hl=en_US

SparkPeople. (2016, November 8). *Pregnancy Health & Fitness*. Retrieved from https://play.google.com/store/apps/details?id=com.SparkPeople.pregnancyHealth&hl=en_US

SparkPeople. (2017, August 13). *Healthy Recipes & Calculator*. Retrieved from https://play.google.com/store/apps/details?id=com.sparkpeople.android.cookbook&hl=en

Srinivasan, P., & Kamalakkannan, P. (2012, December). REAQ-AODV: Route stability and energy aware QoS routing in mobile Ad Hoc networks. In *Proceedings of the 2012 Fourth International Conference on Advanced Computing (ICoAC)* (pp. 1-5). IEEE. 10.1109/ICoAC.2012.6416845

StayWell. (2019). *My Diet Diary Calorie Counter*. Retrieved from https://play.google.com/store/apps/details?id=org.medhelp.mydiet&hl=en

Stone, M. (2019, February 8). *Simple Diet Diary*. Retrieved from https://play.google.com/store/apps/details?id=com.rarepebble.dietdiary&hl=en

Stremetska, D. (2016). Why mobile development is so expensive. STFalcon. Retrieved from https://stfalcon.com/en/blog/post/why-mobile-development-is-so-expensive

Sudha, V., & Jayashree, P. (2012). Lung nodule detection in CT images using thresholding and morphological operations. *International Journal of Emerging Science and Engineering, 1*(2), 17–21.

Sundararajan, R., Xu, H., Annangi, P., Tao, X., Sun, X., & Mao, L. (2010, April). A multiresolution support vector machine based algorithm for pneumoconiosis detection from chest radiographs. In *Proceedings of the 2010 IEEE International Symposium on Biomedical Imaging: From Nano to Macro* (pp. 1317-1320). IEEE. 10.1109/ISBI.2010.5490239

Su, S., Yu, H., & Wu, Z. (2013). An efficient multi–objective evolutionary algorithm for energy–aware QoS routing in wireless sensor network. *International Journal of Sensor Networks, 13*(4), 208–218. doi:10.1504/IJSNET.2013.055583

Susruta, S. (1963). *An English translation of the Sushruta samhita, based on original Sanskrit text* (Vol. 30). Рипол Классик.

Sutton, C. H., & Carrol, F. B. (1979). Effects of microwave-induced hyperthermia on the blood-brain barrier of the rat. *Radiat Sci, 14*(6S), 329–334. doi:10.1029/RS014i06Sp00329

Svoboda, R. (1992). *Ayurveda: Life, health and longevity*. Penguin Books India.

Takahashi, D., Xiao, Y., Hu, F., Chen, J., & Sun, Y. (2008). Temperature-aware routing for telemedicine applications in embedded biomedical sensor networks. *EURASIP Journal on Wireless Communications and Networking, 2008*, 26.

Talukdar, N. A., Deb, D., & Roy, S. (2014, August). Automated Blood Cancer Detection Using Image Processing Based on Fuzzy System. *International Journal of Advanced Research in Computer Science and Software Engineering, 4*(8), 1–6.

Tandel, S., & Jamadar, A. (2018). Impact of Progressive Web Apps on Web App Development. *International Journal of Innovative Research in Science, Engineering and Technology, 7*(9), 9349–9444.

Tang, Q., Tummala, N., Gupta, S. K., & Schwiebert, L. (2005, June). TARA: thermal-aware routing algorithm for implanted sensor networks. In *Proceedings of the International Conference on Distributed Computing in Sensor Systems* (pp. 206-217). Springer. 10.1007/11502593_17

Taniar, D. (2008). *Mobile Computing: Concepts, Methodologies, Tools, and Applications*. Hershey, PA: IGI Global.

Tan, K. K., Le, N. Q. K., Yeh, H. Y., & Chua, M. C. H. (2019). Ensemble of Deep Recurrent Neural Networks for Identifying Enhancers via Dinucleotide Physicochemical Properties. *Cells, 8*(7), 767. doi:10.3390/cells8070767 PMID:31340596

Tasteaholics. (2019, August 4). *Total Keto Diet: Low Carb Recipes & Keto Meals*. Retrieved from https://play.google.com/store/apps/details?id=com.totalketodiet.ketodiet&hl=en

Teke, A., Londh, S., Oswal, P., & Malwade, S. S. (2019). Online Clinic Management System. *International Journal (Toronto, Ont.), 4*(2).

Thompson-Butel, A. G., Shiner, C. T., McGhee, J., Bailey, B. J., Bou-Haidar, P., McCorriston, M., & Faux, S. G. (2019). The Role of Personalized Virtual Reality in Education for Patients Post Stroke— A Qualitative Case Series. *Journal of Stroke and Cerebrovascular Diseases, 28*(2), 450–457. doi:10.1016/j.jstrokecerebrovasdis.2018.10.018 PMID:30415917

Thompson, E. A., Mathie, R. T., Baitson, E. S., Barron, S. J., Berkovitz, S. R., Brands, M., ... Mercer, S. W. (2008). Towards standard setting for patient-reported outcomes in the NHS homeopathic hospitals. *Homeopathy, 97*(03), 114–121. doi:10.1016/j.homp.2008.06.005 PMID:18657769

Tocci, P. G. (2019). *Wireless Technology: Ultra Convenient. Endlessly Entertaining. Criminally Instigated*. Terminally Pathological.

Tong, S., & Koller, D. (2001). Support vector machine active learning with applications to text classification. *Journal of Machine Learning Research, 2*(November), 45–66.

Totkov, G. (2003). Virtual learning environments: Towards new generation. In *Proceedings of the 4th international conference on computer systems and technologies: E-learning* (pp. 8–16). New York: ACM. doi:10.1145/973620.973622

Trower, B. (2013). Wi-Fi- A thalidomide in the making. Who cares?

Tuomela, R. (1987). *Science, protoscience, and pseudoscience. In Rational Changes in Science* (pp. 83–101). Springer.

Tyagi, A., Jain, V., Bhatia, D., & Duhan, M. (2010). Review of Effect of Electromagnetic Radiations of Mobile Phone on Human Health. In *Proceeding of Control Instrumentation System Conference*. Academic Press.

Tyagi, A., Duhan, M., & Bhatia, D. (2011). *Effect of Mobile Phone Radiation on Brain Activity GSM Vs CDMA*. IJSTM.

Ullah, S. (2011). *Multi-modal Interaction in Collaborative Virtual Environments: Study and analysis of performance in collaborative work* [Theses]. Universit'e d'Evry-Val d'Essonne. Retrieved From https://tel.archives-ouvertes.fr/tel-00562081

Ullah, S., Higgins, H., Braem, B., Latre, B., Blondia, C., Moerman, I., ... Kwak, K. S. (2012). A comprehensive survey of wireless body area networks. *Journal of Medical Systems, 36*(3), 1065–1094. doi:10.100710916-010-9571-3 PMID:20721685

Ullah, S., Shen, B., Riazul Islam, S. M., Khan, P., Saleem, S., & Sup Kwak, K. (2010). A study of MAC protocols for WBANs. *Sensors (Basel)*, *10*(1), 128–145. doi:10.3390100100128 PMID:22315531

Umanol, M., Okamoto, H., Hatono, I., Tamura, H. I. R. O. Y. U. K. I., Kawachi, F., Umedzu, S., & Kinoshita, J. (1994, June). Fuzzy decision trees by fuzzy ID3 algorithm and its application to diagnosis systems. In *Proceedings of the Third IEEE Conference on Fuzzy Systems* (pp. 2113-2118). IEEE. 10.1109/FUZZY.1994.343539

Under Armour, Inc. (2019). *MyFitnessPal*. Retrieved from https://apps.apple.com/us/app/myfitnesspal/id341232718

Underwood, E., & Rhodes, P. (2008). History of medicine. In *Encyclopaedia Brittanica*. Chicago, IL: Encyclopaedia Brittanica.

Van Velthoven, M., & Cordon, C. (2019). Sustainable Adoption of Digital Health Innovations Perspectives From a Stakeholder Workshop. *Journal of Medical Internet Research*, *21*(3), 1–8. doi:10.2196/11922 PMID:30907734

Vaughan, N., Dubey, V. N., Wainwright, T. W., & Middleton, R. G. (2016). A review of virtual reality based training simulators for orthopaedic surgery. *Medical Engineering & Physics*, *38*(2), 59–71. doi:10.1016/j.medengphy.2015.11.021 PMID:26751581

Venkatesh, V., Morris, M. G., Davis, G. B., & Davis, F. D. (2003). User acceptance of information technology: Toward a unified view. *Management Information Systems Quarterly*, *27*(3), 425–478. doi:10.2307/30036540

Ventola, C. (2014). Mobile Devices and Apps for Health Care Professionals: Uses and Benefits. *P&T*, *39*(5), 356–364. PMID:24883008

Verma, S. C., Tejaswini, T. M., & Pradhan, D. (2019). Harmful effects of 5G radiations: review. In *Proceedings of IRAJ International Conference* (pp. 71-75). Academic Press.

Verma, N., Kansal, S., & Malvi, H. (2018). Development of Native Mobile Application Using Android Studio for Cabs and Some Glimpse of Cross Platform Apps. *International Journal of Applied Engineering Research*, *13*(16), 12527–12530.

Vijayakar, P. (1999). *Predictive Homoeopathy*. Preeti Publishers.

Viswanathan, P. (2019). Native Apps vs. Web Apps: What Is the Better Choice? Lifewire. Retrieved from https://www.lifewire.com/native-apps-vs-web-apps-2373133

Wachtel, H., Seaman, R., & Joines, W. (1975). Effects of low-intensity microwaves on isolated neurons. *Annals of the New York Academy of Sciences*, *247*(1), 46–62. doi:10.1111/j.1749-6632.1975.tb35982.x PMID:1054247

Wagner, P., Roschke, J., Mann, K., Fell, J., Hiller, W., Frank, C., & Grozinger, M. (2000). Human sleep EEG under the influence of pulsed radiofrequency electromagnetic fields. Results from polysomnographies using submaximal high power flux densities. *Neuropsychobiol*, *42*, 207–212. doi:10.1159/000026695 PMID:11096337

Wagner, P., Roschke, J., Mann, K., Hiller, W., & Frank, C. (1998). Human sleep under the influence of pulsed radiofrequency electromagnetic fields: A polysomnographic study using standardized conditions. *Bioelectromagnetics*, *19*(3), 199–202. doi:10.1002/(SICI)1521-186X(1998)19:3<199::AID-BEM8>3.0.CO;2-X PMID:9554698

Wainstein, L. (2018). Why You Should Use Responsive Images. Lab21. Retrieved from https://www.lab21.gr/blog/use-responsive-images

Wang, L., Zeng, Y., & Chen, T. (2015). Back propagation neural network with adaptive differential evolution algorithm for time series forecasting. *Expert Systems with Applications*, *42*(2), 855-863.'2

Wang, Y., Zou, Z., Song, H., Xu, X., Wang, H., d'Oleire Uquillas, F., & Huang, X. (2016). Altered grey matter volume and white matter integrity in college students with mobile phone dependence. *Frontiers in Psychology*, *7*, 597. PMID:27199831

Warburton, S. (2009). Second Life in higher education: Assessing the potential for and the barriers to deploying virtual worlds in learning and teaching. *British Journal of Educational Technology*, *40*(3), 414–426. doi:10.1111/j.1467-8535.2009.00952.x

Watchers, W. International, Inc. (2019, September 9). *WW (formerly Weight Watchers)*. Retrieved from https://play.google.com/store/apps/details?id=com.weightwatchers.mobile&hl=en

We Will Bring The Health Care Where It's Convenient For You. (2019). UberGP. Retrieved from http://www.ubergp.co.uk/

Wen, J., Liu, Y., Shi, Y., Huang, H., Deng, B., & Xiao, X. (2019). A classification model for lncRNA and mRNA based on k-mers and a convolutional neural network. *BMC Bioinformatics*, *20*(1), 469. doi:10.118612859-019-3039-3 PMID:31519146

What is homeopathy? (2019). *Homeopathy*. Retrieved from https://www.britishhomeopathic.org/homeopathy/what-is-homeopathy/

Wickens, C. D. (1992, October). Virtual reality and education. In *Proceedings of IEEE international conference on systems, man, and cybernetics* (Vol. 1, pp. 842-847). IEEE Press.

Wikipedia. (2019b). History of medicine. Retrieved from https://en.wikipedia.org/w/index.php?title=History_of_medicine&oldid=905929535

Wikipedia. (n.d.). Mobile Phone. Retrieved From http://en.wikipedia.org/wiki/Mobile_phone

Wikipedia. (n.d.a). Ayurveda.

Williams, J., Eames, C., Hume, A., & Lockley, J. (2012). Promoting pedagogical content knowledge development for early career secondary teachers in science and technology using content representations. *Research in Science & Technological Education*, *30*(3), 327–343.

Winn, W., Hoffman, H., Hollander, A., Osberg, K., Rose, H., & Char, P. (1997). The effect of student construction of virtual environments on the performance of high-and low-ability students. In *Proceedings of the Annual meeting of the American educational research association. Academic Press*.

Wong, E. (2019). Principle of Consistency and Standards in User Interface Design. Interaction Design. Retrieved from https://www.interaction-design.org/literature/article/principle-of-consistency-and-standards-in-user-interface-design

Woodfield, B. F., Catlin, H. R., Waddoups, G. L., Moore, M. S., Swan, R., Allen, R., & Bodily, G. (2004a). The virtual chemlab project: A realistic and sophisticated simulation of inorganic qualitative analysis. *Journal of Chemical Education*, *81*(11), 1672. doi:10.1021/ed081p1672

World Health Organisation. (2018). Maternal mortality: Key facts. Retrieved from https://www.who.int/news-room/fact-sheets/detail/maternal-mortality

World Health Organization (WHO). (2018). Ageing and Health. Rederived from https://www.who.int/news-room/fact-sheets/detail/ageing-and-health

World Health Organization (WHO). (2018). World Health Statistics 2018. Rederived from https://www.who.int/gho/publications/world_health_statistics/2018/en/

World Health Organization. (2000). Nutrition for health and development: a global agenda for combating malnutrition.

World Health Organization. (2016). Disease burden and mortality estimates. Retrieved from https://www.who.int/healthinfo/global_burden_disease/estimates/en/index1.html

World Population Aging. (2017). "Population Division", Department of Economic and Social Affairs, United Nations, 2018. Rederived From https://www.un.org/en/development/desa/population/publications/pdf/ageing/WPA2017_Highlights.pdf

Wu, C. H., & McLarty, J. W. (Eds.). (2012). *Neural networks and genome informatics*. Elsevier.

Wu, C., Berry, M., Shivakumar, S., & McLarty, J. (1995). Neural networks for full-scale protein sequence classification: Sequence encoding with singular value decomposition. *Machine Learning, 21*(1-2), 177–193. doi:10.1007/BF00993384

Wujastyk, D. (2012). *Well-mannered medicine: Medical ethics and etiquette in classical ayurveda*. Oxford University Press. doi:10.1093/acprof:oso/9780199856268.001.0001

Wujastyk, D., & Smith, F. M. (2013). *Modern and global Ayurveda: pluralism and paradigms*. Suny Press.

Xiao, Y., Shen, X., Sun, B. O., & Cai, L. (2006). Security and privacy in RFID and applications in telemedicine. *IEEE Communications Magazine, 44*(4), 64–72. doi:10.1109/MCOM.2006.1632651

Xiaoyuan, L., Bin, Q., & Lu, W. (2009, October). A new improved BP neural network algorithm. In *Proceedings of the Second International Conference on Intelligent Computation Technology and Automation ICICTA'09* (Vol. 1, pp. 19-22). IEEE. 10.1109/ICICTA.2009.12

Xing, Z., Pei, J., & Keogh, E. (2010). A brief survey on sequence classification. *ACM Sigkdd Explorations Newsletter, 12*(1), 40–48. doi:10.1145/1882471.1882478

Xu, Y., & Zhang, H. (2009, July). Study on the Improved BP Algorithm and Application. In *Proceedings of the Asia-Pacific Conference on Information Processing APCIP 2009* (Vol. 1, pp. 7-10). IEEE. 10.1109/APCIP.2009.9

Xu, S., & Wang, Y. (2017). Parameter estimation of photovoltaic modules using a hybrid flower pollination algorithm. *Energy Conversion and Management, 144*, 53–68. doi:10.1016/j.enconman.2017.04.042

Xyris Software (Australia) Pty Ltd. (2019). *Easy Diet Diary*. Retrieved from https://apps.apple.com/au/app/easy-diet-diary/id436104108

Yamany, W., Zawbaa, H. M., Emary, E., & Hassanien, A. E. (2015, August). Attribute reduction approach based on modified flower pollination algorithm. In *Proceedings of the 2015 IEEE International Conference on Fuzzy Systems (FUZZ-IEEE)* (pp. 1-7). IEEE. 10.1109/FUZZ-IEEE.2015.7338111

Yang, X. S. (2012, September). Flower pollination algorithm for global optimization. In *Proceedings of the International Conference on Unconventional Computing and Natural Computation* (pp. 240-249). Springer Berlin Heidelberg. 10.1007/978-3-642-32894-7_27

Yang, G. Z. (2014). *Body Sensor Networks* (1st ed.). London, UK: Springer Berlin Heidelberg, London. doi:10.1007/978-1-4471-6374-9

Yao, S., Swetha, P., & Zhu, Y. (2018). Nanomaterial-Enabled wearable sensors for healthcare. *Advanced Healthcare Materials, 7*(1), 1–27. doi:10.1002/adhm.201700889 PMID:29193793

YAZIO GmbH. (2018). *YAZIO — Diet & Food Tracker*. Retrieved from https://apps.apple.com/us/app/yazio-diet-food-tracker/id946099227

Yilmaz, R., Karaoglan Yilmaz, F. G., & Ezin, C. C. (2018). Self-directed learning with technology and academic motivation as predictors of tablet PC acceptance. In Handbook of Research on Mobile Devices and Smart Gadgets in K-12 Education (pp. 87-102). Hershey, PA: IGI Global. doi:10.4018/978-1-5225-2706-0.ch007

Yin, L., Zhang, A., Ye, X., & Xie, X. (2019). Security-Aware Department Matching and Doctor Searching for Online Appointment Registration System. *IEEE Access: Practical Innovations, Open Solutions*, 7, 41296–41308. doi:10.1109/ACCESS.2019.2904724

Yoon, S. A., Anderson, E., Park, M., Elinich, K., & Lin, J. (2018). How augmented reality, textual, and collaborative scaffolds work synergistically to improve learning in a science museum. *Research in Science & Technological Education*, 1–21.

Zadeh, H. G., Janianpour, S., & Haddadnia, J. (2013). Recognition and Classification of the Cancer Cells by Using Image Processing and LabVIEW. *International Journal of computer theory and engineering, 5*(1).

Zadeh, H. G., Janianpour, S., & Haddadnia, J. (2013). Recognition and Classification of the Cancer Cells by using Image Processing and Lab VIEW. *International Journal of Computer Theory and Engineering, 5*(1), 104–107. doi:10.7763/IJCTE.2013.V5.656

Zaman, S., & Toufiq, R. (2017). Codon based back propagation neural network approach to classify hypertension gene sequences. In *Proceedings of the 2017 International Conference on Electrical, Computer and Communication Engineering (ECCE)* (pp. 443-446). Academic Press. 10.1109/ECACE.2017.7912945

zeronica.com. (2015, May 16). *Weight Tracker "Weigh My Diet"*. Retrieved from https://play.google.com/store/apps/details?id=com.zeronica.weighmydiet&hl=en_GB

Zhang, J. R., Zhang, J., Lok, T. M., & Lyu, M. R. (2007). A hybrid particle swarm optimization–back-propagation algorithm for feed forward neural network training. *Applied Mathematics and Computation, 185*(2), 1026–1037. doi:10.1016/j.amc.2006.07.025

Zhang, M., Zhang, Z., Chang, Y., Aziz, E. S., Esche, S., & Chassapis, C. (2018). Recent developments in game-based virtual reality educational laboratories using the Microsoft Kinect. *International Journal of Emerging Technologies in Learning, 13*(1), 138–159. doi:10.3991/ijet.v13i01.7773

Zheng, X., Xu, S., Zhang, Y., & Huang, X. (2019). Nucleotide-level Convolutional Neural Networks for Pre-miRNA Classification. *Scientific Reports, 9*(1), 628. doi:10.103841598-018-36946-4 PMID:30679648

Zweiri, Y. H., Whidborne, J. F., & Seneviratne, L. D. (2003). A three-term back propagation algorithm. *Neurocomputing*, 50, 305–318. doi:10.1016/S0925-2312(02)00569-6

Zykina, A. V. (2004). A lexicographic optimization algorithm. *Automation and Remote Control, 65*(3), 363–368. doi:10.1023/B:AURC.0000019366.84601.8e

About the Contributors

Sajid Umair is a Lecturer in Computer Science at the Institute of Computer Science and Information Technology (ICS&IT), The University of Agriculture Peshawar, Pakistan. He was born in Nowshera KPK, Pakistan in 1992. He received his M.S. degree in computer science from School of Electrical Engineering and Computer Science (SEECS), National University of Sciences and Technology (NUST), Islamabad Pakistan in 2016 under the supervision of Professor Dr. Asad Anwar Butt. He completed his B.S. degree in computer science from The University of Agriculture Peshawar, Pakistan, in 2014 with a distinction of Silver Medal. His areas of interest include android/desktop applications development, mobile cloud computing, mobile devices and smart gadgets, mobile technologies and electronic media, and mobile journalism. His research papers have been published in different journals, conferences and also as book chapters. His recently published book, "Handbook of Research on Mobile Devices and Smart Gadgets in K-12 Education" by IGI Global USA 2017, was indexed by SCOPUS. He is also the Editor-in-chief of the book, "Mobile Devices and Smart Gadgets in Human Rights" which is published by IGI Global USA 2018. He is a former member of High Performance Computing (HPC) Lab and Excellence for Mobile Computing (EMC) Lab at School of Electrical Engineering and Computer Science (SEECS), National University of Sciences and Technology (NUST), Islamabad Pakistan. He achieved many awards as an outstanding boy scout, most important among them being: Chief Commissioner Award from Pakistan Boy Scouts Association.

* * *

Syed Bakhtawar Shah Abid was born on May 05, 1978, in Dir (Lower), KPK Province, Pakistan. He did his BSc degree in Computer Science from the University of Peshawar from 1997-1999. In 2000, he joined the Department of Computer Science, University of Peshawar, KPK Province, Pakistan for MSc in Computer Science. He later enrolled in the Department of Computer Science, University of Peshawar, KPK Province, Pakistan to continue his Master of Science (MS) degree in 2013. He enrolled in Ph.D. at the Department of Computer Science, University of Peshawar, KPK Province, Pakistan in spring 2018. His main research interests include privacy-preserving data publishing and cloud computing. He joined Abdul Wali Khan University Timergara campus as a lecturer in computer science in 2011. Now he is a lecturer in the Institute of Computer Science and Information Technology (ICSIT), Faculty of Management and Computer Sciences (FMCS), The University of Agriculture, Peshawar since 2017. He has 17 years of national and international teaching experience.

Theodora Dame Adjin-Tettey is a lecturer at the University of Professional Studies, Accra, Ghana. She holds a bachelor's degree in Linguistics and Information Studies and a Master of Philosophy degree in Communication Studies both from the University of Ghana. Theodora also obtained her PhD in Communication degree from the University of South Africa, Pretoria, South Africa. She has published in the areas of new media usage and appropriation, body image and influence of media, climate change communication, among others. She has a special interest in how media technologies are used and adapted into socio-cultural practices. Apart from her academic work, Theodora is also passionate about sharing informative and inspiring stories through her articles widely published by www.myjoyonline.com, one of Ghana's leading media outlets. Through Theodora's stories, you will find one who is capable of sharing her thoughts through writing and one who is not afraid to share her story to inspire others.

Muzamil Ahmad is currently pursuing BS Computer Science from The University of Agriculture Peshawar, Pakistan. He is amongst top ten position holders at his department. He belongs to Lakki Marwat, Khyberpakhtukhwah (KPK), and Pakistan. His native language is Pashto. Urdu and English are his second languages. He received his degree of intermediate in Computer Science from Government Post Graduate Collage Bannu, KPK. During second year of F.Sc, he also secured Certificate of Information and Technology from Micro-Tech Computer Institute Bannu. Earlier on, he completed matriculation at Government High School Tabbi Murad Lakki Marwat, KPK. He won distinctions in Naat competition, and Cricket Tournament at Government Centennial Model High School No. 1 Lakki Marwat, KPK. He is Interested in Programming, Graphic Designing, development, Innovation and Business Planning. He has published "An Efficient System for Human Detection Using PIR Sensor and Mobile Technology", (in Handbook of Research on Mobile Devices and Smart Gadgets in Human Rights, with Muhammad Shoaib and Aizaz ul Haq). In order to hone up these skills, he developed a number of projects, including hostel management system, library management system, hospital management system, student report card, tic tac toe game, digital watch, GPA calculator, and pc controller through commands, water level detector, sensor security system, and passive infrared radial (PIR) sensor security system connected with mobile technology.

Maria Ali was born on February 2, 1991, in KPK Province, Pakistan. She did her BS degree in Computer Science from the Institute of Computer Science and Information Technology (ICSIT), Faculty of Management and Computer Sciences (FMCS), The University of Agriculture, Peshawar, during 2010-2014. Later in 2015, she joined the Institute of Computer Science and Information Technology (ICSIT), Faculty of Management and Computer Sciences (FMCS), The University of Agriculture, Peshawar, KPK Province, Pakistan, to continue her Master of Science (MS) degree. During her MS in Computer Science at the Institute of Computer Science and Information Technology (ICSIT), Faculty of Management and Computer Sciences (FMCS), The University of Agriculture, Peshawar, she started her research journey under professional guidance and the supervision of Assistant Professor Dr. Abdullah. Her main research interests include neural networks, data mining, hybrid neural networks, knowledge-based systems, and data mining, deep learning, and web mining.

Numan Ali was born in Pakistan, in 1988. He received the B.S. (CS) degree (Hons.) and the M.S. (CS) degree with a specialization in virtual reality and intelligent systems from the University of Malakand, Pakistan, in 2011 and 2015, respectively, where he is currently pursuing the Ph.D. degree. He is also a Lecturer with the Institute of Computer Science and IT, ICS/IT, The University of Agriculture Peshawar, Pakistan. His current research interests include 3-D graphics, virtual reality, and human computer interaction and intelligent systems.

Fernando Luís Almeida has a PhD in Computer Science Engineering from Faculty of Engineering of University of Porto (FEUP). He also holds an MSc in Innovation and Entrepreneurship and an MSc in Informatics Engineering from FEUP. He has around 10 years of teaching experience at higher education levels in the field of computer science and management. He has also worked for 15 years in several positions as software engineer and project manager for large organizations and research centers like Critical Software, CICA/SEF, INESC TEC and ISR Porto. His current research areas include innovation policies, entrepreneurship, software development and decision support systems.

Abu Baker has received his Bachelor of Science in Information Technology and Master of Science in Information Technology from The University of Agriculture Peshawar, Pakistan. Currently working at The Bank of Khyber, Pakistan as a Senior Software Developer. He is also the founder and CEO at KHYBERCODED software solution and research center Peshawar, Pakistan. He ihas a four-year experience in development and designing applications in JAVA, ANDROID, and ASP.net. He developed many government applications like E-Gov mobile application for Khyber Pakhtoon Khwa E-Governance department, JPSC KP for Joint Public Safety Cell, MIS for Directorate of IT, Account System for The University of Agriculture and MIS for Peoples Primary Health Care Initiative. His research interest is Android Security, Machine Learning, Data Mining, and Artificial Inelegance.

Javed Iqbal Bangash received his Ph.D. degree from the University of Technology Malaysia (UTM), M.Sc. degree (with Distinction) from London Metropolitan University, London, UK, and B.E. degree from University of Engineering and Technology, Peshawar, Pakistan. He is currently an Assistant Professor at the Department of Computer Science and Information Technology, The Agriculture University, Peshawar, Pakistan. His research areas include communication protocols for IoT, WSNs, WBANs, & Adhoc Networks, and Digital Image Processing & Multimedia Processing.

Mairaj Bibi was born in Quetta Balochistan, Pakistan in 1994. She did her Matriculation from Govt. Girls High school Kasi Road Quetta in 2008 and F.S.C in Pre-Medical in Islamia Girls College Quetta in 2010. She got MBBS seat in Bolan Medical college Quetta in 2012 and completed her MBBS in 2017. She done her Internship in Medicine and Allied and surgery and allied in Bolan Medical complex in 2018. She cleared FCPS part 1 in Gynae Obs in 2019 and has started her FCPS part 2 training in gynae obs in Bolan Medical Complex Quetta from July 2019. She is also a member of Royel College Obs gynae(UK). She loves her patients and works hard to save life of patients.

Ines Carvalho has a B.E. in Computer Systems and Network. Throughout her academic and professional career she has developed projects for the information technology sector and led development teams using agile methodologies and waterfall methodologies. She has been involved in the development of several projects for mobile platforms. She has also worked together on international projects under the Erasmus+ initiative with an industrial impact on the definition of new production processes and technologies. She has experience in the field of networks security, information systems and software development. In the future, she intends to continue to carry out research and business work in these areas.

Bukhtawar Elahi received the Bachelor of Engineering in Information Technology (BEIT) degree from the University of Engineering and Technology (UET), Taxila, Pakistan and Master of Science in Information Technology (MSIT) degree from the National University of Sciences and Technology (NUST), Islamabad, Pakistan. Her research interests include cloud computing, distributed systems, internet of things, machine learning and deep learning.

Sana Elahi has been working as a lecturer at Dr. A. Q. Khan Institute of Computer Sciences and Information Technology Kahuta, Pakistan, since September 2018. She is a computer engineer with research interests in MRI, Medical image and Signal processing. She received her MS degree from COMSATS University Islamabad. She has her research publications in the field of MRI.

Furqan Iqbal is appointed senior software developer and researcher at Khyber Coded Software's, Games & Research Lab specializing in java and research papers. He completed his Bachelor Degree in Computer Science from Pakistan and currently enrolled in a Master in Software Technology at the University of Stuttgart, Germany. His current research interest falls into two main areas: the BIG Data, Data analysis and storage, and secondly, Medical Science.

Maria Kanwal is doing her Masters of Science in Information Technology from National University of Sciences and Technology (NUST), Islamabad, Pakistan. Her research interests include distributed simulation and IoT.

Abdul Waheed Khan is Assistant Professor at Military College of Signals, National University of Science and Technology (NUST), Pakistan. He completed his Ph.D. in Computer Science at University Technology Malaysia in 2015. He did his MSc in Digital Communication Networks (Distinction) from London Metropolitan University in 2008. Prior to his MSc, he graduated from the Department of Computer Science, the University of Peshawar in 2005. In recognition of his academic and research achievements, he was awarded Best Postgraduate Student award for session 2014/15 at University Technology Malaysia. His research interests include communication protocols for Wireless Sensor Networks, Mobile Ad-Hoc Networks, and Internet of Things.

Abdullah Khan was born on February 06, 1985, in Dir (Lower), KPK Province, Pakistan. He did his BSc degree from Malakand University during 2004-2006. In 2006, he joined University to Science and Technology, Bannu, KPK Province, Pakistan for MSc in Computer Science. He later enrolled in the Universiti Tun Hussein Onn Malaysia to continue his Ph.D. at the end of 2010. During his Doctor of Philosophy (Ph.D.) in Information Technology at Universiti Tun Hussein Onn Malaysia (UTHM), he started his research journey under the professional guidance of the supervision of Associate Professor Dr. Nazri Mohd. Nawi. He is currently an Assistant Professor at the institute of computer science and information technology faculty of Management and computer sciences The University of Agriculture, Peshawar, Pakistan. He has published several research articles in the field of optimization and meta-heuristics, neural network, data mining, prediction etc. His main research interests include hybrid neural networks, knowledge-based systems, and data mining, deep learning, and web mining.

Asfandyar Khan received his MSc degree from University of Peshawar, Pakistan in 2003 and his PhD Degree from Department of Computer and Information Sciences, University Technology PETRO-

NAS, Malaysia in 2011. During his PhD, he was working as Graduate Assistant in University Technology Petronas, Malaysia. He is currently working as a faculty member with ICS & IT, The University of Agriculture, Peshawar. His research interest includes wireless sensor networks, green computing, bio informatics, and medical imaging systems.

Muhammad Abbas Khan was born in Quetta Balochistan, Pakistan in 1998. He did Matriculation from Tameer-I-Nau Public School, Quetta in 2013 and F.Sc. in Pre-Engineering from Tameer-I-Nau Public College Quetta, in 2015. He is student of B.Sc. (Hons) Agriculture at University of Agriculture Peshawar KP, Pakistan. He is currently Coordinator of Pakistan International Human Rights Organization (PIHRO) District Killa Saifullah, Balochistan, for a 2 year period, member of Breeding & Genetics Society of Pakistan (BGSP) and member of Society for Horticulture Development. He remained member of Pakistan International Human Rights Organization Youth Wing Khyber Pakhtunkhwa for 2 years. He also remained as Organizer of 1st KP Women Super League, Peshawar and 1st National Tourism Conference at Gilgit Baltistan, Pakistan and many more. He always focused on Promotion and Protection of Human Rights.

Rafiullah Khan received the B.S. degree in Computer Science from University of Peshawar, Peshawar, Pakistan, in 2007 and the M.S. degree in Internetworking and Digital Communication from Institute of Management Sciences, Peshawar, Pakistan in 2010. He received Ph.D. degree in Computer Science from Capital University of Science and Technology, Islamabad, Pakistan. He worked as Lecturer as Preston University and Iqra National University Peshawar, Pakistan from 2007 to 2011 and currently he is working as Senior Lecturer at the Institute of Computer Science and Information Technology, the University of Agriculture Peshawar since 2011. He also conducted different projects related to Distance learning, Online marketing, android app for rescue, behavioral analysis of search engine users, sentiment-based product rating, user privacy, private information retrieval, and effects of moringa plant on diabetic patients. His research interests include data mining, machine learning, web user privacy, sentiment analysis, computer networks, gender studies, history, and Islamic mysticism.

Siyab Khan was born on February 20, 1992, in Batkhela Totakaan, KPK Province, Pakistan. He did his BS degree in Computer Science from the Department of Computer Science, Islamia College University, Peshawar during 2011-2015. He later enrolled in the Institute of Computer Science and Information Technology (ICSIT), Faculty of Management and Computer Sciences (FMCS), The University of Agriculture, Peshawar to continue his Master of Science (MS) degree at the start of 2017. During his MS in Computer Science at the Institute of Computer Science and Information Technology (ICSIT), Faculty of Management and Computer Sciences (FMCS), The University of Agriculture, Peshawar, he started his research journey under professional guidance and the supervision of Assistant Professor Dr. Abdullah. His main research interests include neural networks, data mining, hybrid neural networks, knowledge-based systems, and data mining, deep learning, and web mining. He is working as a lecturer in CECOS university Hayatabad phase 6 since October 2019.

Mahnoor Laila is a Psychologist. She did her MPhil from University of Peshawar. Currently doing Ph.D. from Pakistan. She in International certified Hypnotherapist. Took session with drug addict with collaboration if Dost Welfare Foundation. Worked with UNICEF as a District Consultant and has training and educational experience in different departments.

Junaid Ahmad Malik completed his PhD in Zoology (Wildlife) in 2015. He is working as a Lecturer in Zoology at Govt. Degree College, Bijbehara, Anantnag. Dr. Malik has published many research articles and technical papers in many international and nationally reputed journals. He has also authored several books and book chapters of reputed publishers. He is in the editorial board and a regular reviewer of several journals of reasonable reputation.

Zuhra Musa is a primary school teacher and graduated from University of Malakand Pakistan.

Urooj Beenish Orakzai received a M.S. degree in Information Technology from Institute of Business and Management Sciences, Peshawar, Pakistan, in 2011. She is currently working as an Assistant Professor at Government Girls Degree College Hayatabad No. 1 Peshawar, Pakistan, since 2008. Her research interests include networks, security, and wireless networks.

Muhammad Roman is a Lecturer at Elementary and Secondary Education, Department Khyber Pakhtunkhwa, Government of Pakistan.

Lala Rukh received the MS-IT Degree from Institute of Computer Sciences/Information Technology University of Agriculture. She is now working as Senior Lecturer at Institute of Computer Sciences/ Information Technology University; she joined university as a lecturer in 2009. She has remained a member of the board of studies of MS Degree. Her research interest includes Networking, Information Privacy and Android Programming. She has published different research papers in the field of networking.

Bushra Shafi received the Ph.D. degree in Social Work from University of Peshawar in 2010 and she is currently perusing Post Doctorate from University of Dundee, Scotland. She is working as Assistant Professor at the Department of Rural Sociology, The University of Agriculture Peshawar since 2010. She also conducted different projects for the uplift and empowerment of Rural women in northern area of Pakistan. Her research interests include social work, sociology, gender studies, gender development, and community welfare.

Seema Shafi is a homeopathic doctor, she received her Diploma in Homeopathic medical Sciences(DHMS) from National council for Homeopathy Pakistan in 1993, and Diploma in Health technician/educator from UNICEF. She also received a Doctor of Homeopathic Medicines (HMD) Degree from British Council for Homeopathy UK in 1996 and received Master's degree in Urdu Literature from University of Peshawar in 1997 and Master's Degree in Education from Allama Iqbal Open University Islamabad in 2012. She is running a Homeopathic Medical College, a Technical College, two Private Secondary level schools, and a Homeopathic Hospital and Research center in Charsadda, Pakistan since 1997. She also conducted a project on effects of moringa plant on diabetic patients. Her research interests include homeopathy, naturopathy, home remedies, and education.

Said Khalid Shah received his Master of Science degree in computer science (1999) from the Department of Computer Science, University of Peshawar, KPK, Pakistan. From 2000 to 2004, he worked as a lecturer at the Department of Computer Science, University of Peshawar, KPK, Pakistan. In 2004, he joined the University of Science and Technology, Bannu, KPK, Pakistan as a lecturer and then has been promoted to assistant professor in 2012. He received his Doctor of Philosophy (Ph.D.) degree from the University of East Anglia, UK, with a thesis on the topic of non-rigid medical image registration in the year 2011. After completing his Ph.D., he joined the University of Science and Technology, Bannu, KPK, Pakistan and where he was responsible for teaching various computer science subjects and as well as supervising academic/industrial research projects in the area of medical image processing and analysis such as segmentation, visualization, and registration.

Syed Tanveer Shah was born in Mardan, Pakistan, in 1987. He received the B.Sc (Hons), M.Sc (Hons) and Ph.D Degree in Agriculture with Major Horticulture from the Department of Horticulture, The University of Agriculture, Peshawar, Pakistan, in 2009, 2011 and 2017, respectively. In 2012, he joined the Department of Horticulture, The University of Agriculture, Peshawar, as a lecturer and still serving Horticulture Dept. His current research interests include general horticulture, fruit production, post harvest horticulture, and nursery management, etc. Dr. Shah is involved in various types of academic and administrative activities of the University. He is a member of various horticultural society namely Society for Horticulture Development, Pakistan Society for Horticulture Sciences, etc. He is practically involved in Horticultural related activities in planning and solving various problems for the growers also for their livelihood uplift. He has not only participated in various trainings, workshops and conferences but also organized trainings and conferences as well. He remained as Judge in "Annual Winter and Spring Flower Show" arranged by Cantonment Board Peshawar. He has published more than 30 research articles. He is a reviewer for so many national as well as international journals. His contribution in the field of agriculture especially horticulture is outstanding.

Adil Sheraz graduated from Abasyn University Peshawar, Pakistan in February 2018 with a Master's of Science (MS) in Telecommunication and Networks. Prior to his MS, he has done his Bachelor of Science (BS) in Telecommunication from Preston Institute of Management Sciences and Technology, Karachi, Pakistan in 2013. He has a research background in Wireless Sensor Networks (WSN), Wireless Body Area Networks (WBAN) and holds a keen interest in Artificial Intelligence (AI) and Software Defined Networks (SDN).

Mohib Ullah received the M.Sc. degree in Computer Science from University of Peshawar, Peshawar, Pakistan, in 2003 and the M.S. degree in Data Network and Security from Birmingham City University, Birmingham, UK in 2009. He received Ph.D. degree in Computer Science from Capital University of Science and Technology, Islamabad, Pakistan. Currently he is working as Senior Lecturer at the Institute of Computer Science and Information Technology, the University of Agriculture Peshawar since 2011. His research interests include Networks, Security & wireless Network and Web User Privacy.

Rahat Ullah is working as lecturer of Computer science in the University of Malakand KP, Pakistan. He received MS degree in Information Technology from the University of Agriculture Peshawar. Currently he is the research member of NSSRG (Network System and Security Research Group) at University of Malakand. His areas of interest include Vehicular Networks, IoT in Education, SDN, WSN and Smart traffic light.

Rehan Ullah was born on February 2, 1991, in Dir (Lower), KPK Province, Pakistan. He did his BSc degree in Computer Science from the University of Peshawar during 2010-2012. In 2013, he joined the Department of Computer Science, University of Peshawar, KPK Province, Pakistan for MSc in Computer

Science. He later enrolled in the Institute of Computer Science and Information Technology (ICSIT), Faculty of Management and Computer Sciences (FMCS), The University of Agriculture, Peshawar to continue his Master of Science (MS) degree at the start of 2017. During his MS in Computer Science at the Institute of Computer Science and Information Technology (ICSIT), Faculty of Management and Computer Sciences (FMCS), The University of Agriculture, Peshawar, he started his research journey under professional guidance and the supervision of Assistant Professor Dr. Abdullah. His main research interests include neural networks, data mining, hybrid neural networks, knowledge-based systems, and data mining, deep learning, and web mining.

Sehat Ullah was born in Pakistan, in 1977. He received the M.Sc. degree in computer science from the University of Peshawar, Pakistan, in 2001, and the M.S. degree in virtual reality and intelligent systems and the Ph.D. degree in robotics from the University of Evry, France, in 2007 and 2011, respectively. He is currently an Associate Professor with the Department of Computer Science and IT, University of Malakand, Pakistan, where he is also a Provost.

Zia Ullah is currently a lecturer at the University of Agriculture Peshawar-Pakistan. He has completed his MS in Finance from Gandhara University Peshawar Pakistan in the year 2012. Prior to this he has obtained his MBA Degree with a specialization in Finance from the University of Peshawar in the year 2007. He has a very strong background in Finance and Accounting along with a very handsome blend of Information Technology like Accounting Information Systems and Management Information Systems as his basic courses at his bachelor level (B.com). He remained very outstanding during his studies. In the year 2007, he has completed his two months training in State Bank of Pakistan Karachi which was a part of a merit internship during his MBA and submitted a report on the Management of Risks in Banks to State Bank of Pakistan Karachi. He also worked as an internee in the Excise and Taxation Department, Government of Pakistan for one-year time duration. During his MBA he also worked as an internee in Bank Al-Falah main branch Peshawar Pakistan and submitted a thesis report on the Credit Policy of Bank Al-Falah to the concerned University. He obtained years of experience in different renowned Universities like FAST University of Science and Information Technology, Qurtuba University of Management Sciences, Sarhad University and currently Agriculture University Peshawar (Computer Sciences & Information Technology Department) and through the years he taught many hard subjects, like finance, accounting, cost accounting, management accounting, business communications, production and operations management, professional practices in information technology and financial management for information technology. He also worked as an Account Officer in the Department of Reclamation and Probation for 2 years which is a constituent body of the Home Department working in collaboration with the prison and judiciary. His research area includes the management of risks in banks, corporate ownership, credit policy and the impact of artificial intelligence on professional practices of accounting in multinational corporations.

Ahmet Berk Üstün is a lecturer in the Department of Computer Technology & Information Systems at Bartin University in Turkey. He received his M.A. degree in Computer Education & Instructional Technology from Gazi University in 2011. He obtained his Ph.D. in Learning Design and Technology (LDT) at Wayne State University, Detroit, Michigan in 2018. While studying for a Ph.D., he worked as a graduate research assistant for three years in LDT. He is also certified in College and University Teaching and Online Teaching by obtaining graduate certificates from Wayne State University. His research interests focus on instructional design and technology, mobile learning, blended learning, online learning, virtual reality and emerging technologies such as augmented reality and the internet of things.

Annas Waheed is an Android Developer. He did his BCS (Hons) from the University of Peshawar, Pakistan. He has never lost his enthusiasm for developing great things with attention to detail. He has over three years of experience with Java, including two years on Android by developing software for high-profile companies. He brings a passion for perfect user experience and UI into every Android project.

Fatma Gizem Karaoglan Yilmaz is an associate professor in the Department of Computer Technology & Information Systems at Bartin University in Turkey. She received his M.A. degree in Computer Education & Instructional Technology (CEIT) from Çukurova University in 2010. She received his Ph.D. degree in CEIT from Ankara University in 2014. She is interested in distance education, interactive learning environments, human-computer interaction, virtual reality, augmented reality and eye-tracking. Her articles have been published in various well-known journals such as Computers & Education, Computers in Human Behavior, Interactive Learning Environments, Journal of Educational Computing Research, Internet Research, etc. She has presented on a wide range of topics at national and international conferences.

Ramazan Yilmaz is an associate professor in the Department of Computer Technology & Information Systems at Bartin University in Turkey. He is the head of this department. In 2010, he received his M.A. degree in Computer Education & Instructional Technology (CEIT) from Gazi University. In 2014, he received his Ph.D. degree in CEIT from Ankara University. He is interested in virtual reality, smart learning environments, technology-enhanced learning, human-computer interaction, cyberpsychology, data mining, learning analytics, and eye-tracking. His articles have been published in various reputed journals such as Computers & Education, Computers in Human Behavior, Journal of Educational Computing Research, Internet Research, Interactive Learning Environments, etc. He has presented on a wide range of topics at national and international conferences.

Index

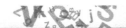

Recommended Reference Books

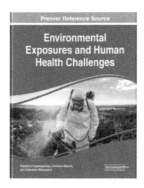

ISBN: 978-1-5225-7635-8
© 2019; 449 pp.
List Price: $255

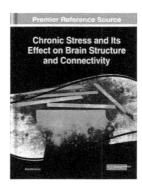

ISBN: 978-1-5225-7513-9
© 2019; 318 pp.
List Price: $225

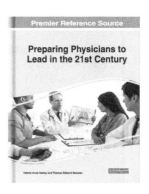

ISBN: 978-1-5225-7576-4
© 2019; 245 pp.
List Price: $245

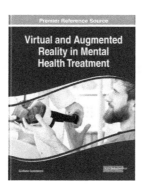

ISBN: 978-1-5225-7168-1
© 2019; 329 pp.
List Price: $265

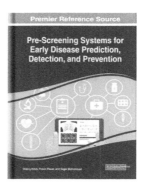

ISBN: 978-1-5225-7131-5
© 2019; 395 pp.
List Price: $245

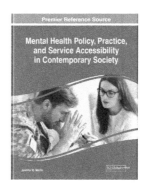

ISBN: 978-1-5225-7402-6
© 2019; 323 pp.
List Price: $245

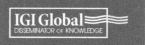

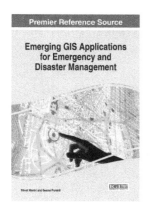
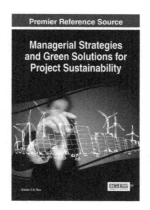
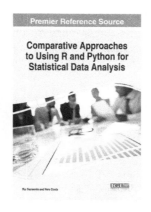
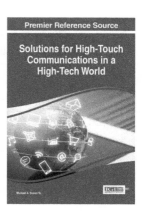

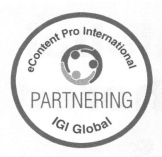

IGI Global Proudly Partners With eContent Pro International

Receive a 25% Discount on all Editorial Services

Editorial Services

IGI Global expects all final manuscripts submitted for publication to be in their final form. This means they must be reviewed, revised, and professionally copy edited prior to their final submission. Not only does this support with accelerating the publication process, but it also ensures that the highest quality scholarly work can be disseminated.

English Language Copy Editing

Let eContent Pro International's expert copy editors perform edits on your manuscript to resolve spelling, punctuaion, grammar, syntax, flow, formatting issues and more.

Scientific and Scholarly Editing

Allow colleagues in your research area to examine the content of your manuscript and provide you with valuable feedback and suggestions before submission.

Figure, Table, Chart & Equation Conversions

Do you have poor quality figures? Do you need visual elements in your manuscript created or converted? A design expert can help!

Translation

Need your documjent translated into English? eContent Pro International's expert translators are fluent in English and more than 40 different languages.

Email: customerservice@econtentpro.com   www.igi-global.com/editorial-service-partners

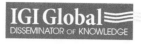

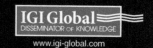

CPSIA information can be obtained
at www.ICGtesting.com
Printed in the USA
BVHW011213300320
575911BV00002BA/3